ADVERSE DRUG REACTIONS AND THE SKIN

To our families and colleagues

Adverse Drug Reactions and the Skin

STEPHEN M. BREATHNACH
MA MD PhD FRCP
Consultant Dermatologist,
St John's Dermatology Centre;
Senior Lecturer,
St John's Institute of Dermatology,
St Thomas's Hospital
London, UK

AND

HELMUT HINTNER
MD
Professor of Dermatology,
Department of Dermatology,
General Hospital,
Salzburg, Austria

OXFORD

BLACKWELL SCIENTIFIC PUBLICATIONS

LONDON EDINBURGH BOSTON

MELBOURNE PARIS BERLIN VIENNA

© 1992 by
Blackwell Scientific Publications
Editorial Offices:
Osney Mead, Oxford OX2 0EL
25 John Street, London WC1N 2BL
23 Ainslie Place, Edinburgh EH3 6AJ
3 Cambridge Center, Cambridge
  Massachusetts 02142, USA
54 University Street, Carlton
  Victoria 3053, Australia

Other Editorial Offices:
Librairie Arnette SA
2, rue Casimir-Delavigne
75006 Paris
France

Blackwell Wissenschafts-Verlag
Meinekestrasse 4
D-1000 Berlin 15
Germany

Blackwell MZV
Feldgasse 13
A-1238 Wien
Austria

First published 1992

Set by Setrite Typesetters,
Hong Kong
Printed and bound in Italy by
Vincenso Bona s.r.l., Turin

DISTRIBUTORS

Marston Book Services Ltd
PO Box 87
Oxford OX2 0DT
(*Orders*: Tel: 0865 791155
       Fax: 0865 791927
       Telex: 837515)

USA
Blackwell Scientific Publications, Inc.
3 Cambridge Center
Cambridge, MA 02142
(*Orders*: Tel: 800 759−6102
           617 225−0401)

Canada
Times Mirror
Professional Publishing, Ltd
5240 Finch Avenue East
Scarborough, Ontario M1S 5A2
(*Orders*: Tel: 800 268−4178
           416 298−1588)

Australia
Blackwell Scientific Publications
(Australia) Pty Ltd
54 University Street
Carlton, Victoria 3053
(*Orders*: Tel: 03 347−0300)

A catalogue record for this book is
available from the British Library

ISBN 0−632−03349−5

Contents

Preface

Medicine could not exist without drugs, and happily the overall incidence of adverse drug reactions is low considering the vast number of prescriptions dispensed. Nonetheless, complications resulting from therapy are familiar to everyone; drug eruptions are probably the most frequent of all manifestations of drug sensitivity. They are only too evident to the patient, may lead to loss of confidence in the doctor, and may frighten the doctor as well as the patient! We all know the classical situation where a patient on an acute ward or in the intensive care unit has been prescribed at least eight different drugs in the past fortnight and suddenly develops a widespread skin eruption. How does one tell the difference between a drug eruption and a viral exanthem or other relatively innocuous skin condition? How can the likely causative agent of a drug eruption be identified amongst an array of other innocent medications? Must all drugs be withdrawn, or is it possible to continue with an essential medication? What are the clinical pointers which indicate a risk of the rash developing into a potentially fatal condition such as exfoliative dermatitis or toxic epidermal necrolysis, and how should such patients be managed?

The aim of this book is to provide the reader with the background knowledge which will enable an informed approach to these difficult questions. In a field such as this, new information is constantly accumulating as further drugs are marketed. New reaction patterns, such as the eosinophilia–myalgia syndrome, neutrophilic eccrine hidradenitis, and drug eruptions in patients with AIDS are being recognized. Whilst we still remain woefully ignorant about the pathogenesis of many adverse drug reactions, recent advances in our knowledge of skin biology with regard to the skin immune system and cytokines are starting to provide insight into the mechanisms involved. We have attempted to provide a 'state of the art' text on adverse drug reactions and the skin. The skin has only a relatively limited number of ways in which it can react to injury, and thus certain patterns are recognized as characteristic of cutaneous drug reactions to particular medications. We have tried to make this book 'user-friendly' by providing full colour illustrations to accompany the discussion of these reactions patterns, combined with lists of the drugs most commonly implicated in their causation. In addition, we have provided in a separate section, and classified according to therapeutic groups, a systematic referenced discussion of the dermatological aspects of commonly prescribed individual medications, both systemic and topical (other than contact dermatitis). We trust that this book will prove useful as a reference text to a broad cross-section of the medical profession, including family practitioners, specialists in internal medicine, and dermatologists as well as to pharmacists in drug information units.

We gratefully acknowledge the assistance of our medical colleagues who provided clinical photographs. We especially thank Professor Peter Fritsch for granting us free access to the extensive slide collection at the Department of Dermatology, University of Innsbruck. Lastly, we wish to record our gratitude to the photography units at St John's Institute of Dermatology and at the University of Innsbruck, and to Mrs P.M. Tharratt, Librarian, St John's Institute of Dermatology, for helpful advice and expertise.

Stephen M. Breathnach
Helmut Hintner

Part 1
Epidemiology and Pathomechanisms

Chapter 1
Introduction and Incidence of Drug Reactions

1.1 Introduction

A drug may be defined as a chemical substance, or combination of substances, administered for the investigation, prevention or treatment of diseases or symptoms, real or imagined. The situation has become complicated with the advent of therapeutic agents which may be useful for improving the appearance, as with minoxidil for androgenetic alopecia and tretinoin for photo-aged skin; the distinction between drugs and cosmetics becomes blurred [1]. In addition, it is not always easy to differentiate between drugs and 'other chemicals', since chemicals of very diverse structure are increasingly added to foods and beverages as dyes, flavours or preservatives. Chemicals used in agriculture or in veterinary medicine may also contaminate human food and cause harmful side-effects.

An adverse drug reaction may be defined as an undesirable clinical manifestation resulting from administration of a particular drug; this includes reactions due to overdose, predictable side-effects, and unanticipated adverse manifestations. Adverse drug reactions may be said to be the inevitable price we pay for the benefits of modern drug therapy [2]. They are costly both in terms of the human illness caused and in economic terms, and can undermine the doctor−patient relationship [2,3]. Sometimes reactions could have been avoided, as in the recently reported cases of confusion between drugs with similar spelling of their brand names [4,5], or when adverse events result from human error [6]. Drug reactions, principally to corticosteroids and methotrexate, accounted for 32% of claims and 26% of dollar losses in dermatology malpractice suits in the US from 1963 to 1973 inclusive [7]. Medication side-effects, most frequently to corticosteroids, antibiotics and chemotherapeutic agents, represented 26% of lawsuits in a study of dermatology residency programmes in the US between 1964 and 1988 [8]. It is in everyone's interest to minimize the chances of the occurrence of adverse drug reactions, and to this end government regulatory bodies and the pharmaceutical industry collaborate to ensure adequate screening of new products. In addition to extensive *in vitro* and animal testing, prolonged and strictly controlled clinical trials are essential. Even so, hazards cannot be eliminated completely, for a serious reaction of low incidence may not be suspected until a very large number of patients have been treated with a new drug. Premarketing clinical trials conducted before a new drug is licensed will not identify adverse reactions occurring in less than 0.1–1% of patients; nor will they identify complications occurring only after prolonged administration, or with a long latency period, or those occurring only in susceptible patients, or when the drug is combined with some other factor, such as another drug [9,10]. Unnecessary adverse drug reactions have occurred because excessive doses may be used when a drug is first introduced on the market, since drug companies understandably wish to avoid the risk of inefficacy from too low a dosage in early clinical trials [11–13]. The US Food and Drug Administration now requires, before approval of a new drug, demonstration that a dose lower than that proposed is ineffective [14].

Another problem is that only a very small fraction of all adverse reactions are ever reported to monitoring agencies, and first warning is still often given by anecdotal reports published in medical journals [14,15]. Many of these reports are subsequently validated but a substantial proportion of poorly documented reports are not [15,16]. In an analysis of 5737 articles from 80 countries between 1972 and 1979, only half the reports contained enough information for the calculation of the frequency of a particular reaction [16]. The usefulness of anecdotal case reports is debatable [17]. Since incorrect reports may have serious legal and other consequences, a heavy responsibility rests with medical editors; a chance association or coincidental reaction should not be allowed to enter the literature. Criteria for assessment of potential drug reactions have been promulgated: these include recurrence on challenge, existence of a pharmacological basis for the reactions, the occurrence of immediate acute or local reactions at the time of administration, of previously known reactions with a new route of administration, or of repeated rare reactions, the presence of immunological abnormalities, and the exclusion of other drugs as alternative aetiologic candidates [15,18]. In the assessment of an unrecorded new reaction the existence of similar but unpublished reports to the manufacturers or, in the UK, the Committee on Safety of Medicines, is of particular importance.

1 Lavrijsen APM, Vermeer BJ. Cosmetics and drugs. Is there a need for a third group: cosmeceutics? *Br J Dermatol* 1991; **124**: 503–4.
2 Nolan L, O'Malley K. Adverse drug reactions in the elderly. *Br J Hosp Med* 1989; **41**: 446–57.
3 Kramer MS, Leventhal JM, Hutchinson TA, Feinstein AR. An algorithm for the operational assessment of adverse drug reactions. I. Background, description, and instructions for use. *JAMA* 1979; **242**: 623–32.
4 Fine SN, Eisdorfer RM, Miskovitz PF, Jacobson IM. Losec or Lasix? *N Engl J Med* 1990; **322**: 1674.
5 Faber J, Azzugnuni M, Di Romana S, Vanhaeverbeek M. Fatal confusion between 'Losec' and 'Lasix'. *Lancet* 1991; **337**: 1286–7.
6 Wright D, Mackenzie SJ, Buchan I, *et al*. Critical events in the intensive therapy unit. *Lancet* 1991; **338**: 676–8.

[4]

7 Altman J. Survey of malpractice claims in dermatology. *Arch Dermatol* 1975; **111**: 641−4.

8 Hollabaugh ES, Wagner RF Jr, Weedn VW, Smith EB. Patient personal injury litigation against dermatology residency programs in the United States, 1964− 1988. *Arch Dermatol* 1990; **126**: 618−22.

9 Bruinsma W. Drug monitoring in dermatology. *Int J Dermatol* 1986; **25**: 166−7.

10 Committee of Management, Prescribers' Journal. Adverse drug reactions. *Prescribers J* 1991; **31**: 1−3.

11 Venning GR. Rare and serious adverse reactions. *Med Toxicol* 1987; **2**: 235−41.

12 Herxheimer A. How much drug in the tablet? *Lancet* 1991; **337**: 346−8.

13 Venning GR. How much drug in the tablet? *Lancet* 1991; **337**: 670.

14 Leading Article. Crying wolf on drug safety. *Br Med J* 1982; **284**: 219−20.

15 Venning GR. Validity of anecdotal reports of suspected adverse drug reactions: the problem of false alarms. *Br Med J* 1982; **284**: 249−52.

16 Venulet J, Blattner R, von Bülow J, Berneker GC. How good are articles on adverse drug reactions? *Br Med J* 1982; **284**: 252−4.

17 Stern RS, Chan H-L. Usefulness of case report literature in determining drugs responsible for toxic epidermal necrolysis. *J Am Acad Dermatol* 1989; **21**: 317−22.

18 Stern RS, Wintroub BU. Adverse drug reactions: reporting and evaluating cutaneous reactions. *Adv Dermatol* 1987; **2**: 3−18

1.2 The incidence of drug reactions

Collection of data

It is difficult to obtain reliable information on the incidence of drug reactions, despite attempts at monitoring by government and the pharmaceutical industry. Moreover, the information which is available must be interpreted with considerable care, since data will be biased, depending on the method of collection [1]. Thus data on medical inpatients, especially from acute care facilities, may indicate a relatively high incidence, since these patients are generally sicker and receive more intensive drug treatment. By contrast, spontaneous reporting certainly underestimates the true incidence. National schemes for collating reported adverse drug reactions exist in many countries, and the World Health Organization's Adverse Reaction Collaborating Centre, in Uppsala, provides a very large database [1]. The UK's 'yellow card' reporting scheme solicits adverse drug reaction reports from doctors, dentists, Her Majesty's coroners, and drug manufacturers; the wide availability of reporting forms is important in encouraging reporting [1]. 'Pharmacovigilence' in France, which involves reporting to regional centres, and most other national schemes, also rely entirely on spontaneous reporting for the collection of adverse drug reaction information [2−4]. Institution of an adverse drug reaction reporting project in Rhode Island in the US substantially increased the rate of reporting of such reactions, since there was a more than 17-fold increase over a 2-year period [5].

Specialty-based systems for spontaneous reporting of adverse drug reactions have also been introduced, e.g. the Adverse Drug

Reaction Reporting System of the American Academy of Dermatology [6] and the Gruppo Italiano Studi Epidemiologici in Dermatologia [7]. However, in the UK, the specialty-based Cutaneous Reactions Database established at the Institute of Dermatology in 1988 was unfortunately closed in 1990 because of a meagre response [8]. The merits and disadvantages of spontaneous adverse drug reaction reporting have been widely discussed [9–11]; it has the advantage of being relatively inexpensive. Inherent difficulties with spontaneous reporting are that reactions associated with newly marketed drugs, those of unusual morphology, and reactions starting soon after initiation of therapy are more likely to be notified, and there may be strongly biased perceptions of what does and does not constitute an adverse drug reaction; at best only a crude estimate of true incidence is provided. All national spontaneous reporting systems are compromised by under-reporting [1]; in the UK surveys suggest that rarely more than 10% of serious reactions are notified to the Committee on Safety of Medicines [12,13]. A recent survey of 44 000 patients receiving one or other of seven new drugs undertaken by the Post Marketing Surveillance Unit of IMS International Ltd paints an even gloomier picture, and suggests that under-reporting by the spontaneous system may be as high as 98% when compared with information collected by the more objective 'event monitoring' system [2]. In a recent hospital study, the offer of a small fee increased the rate of reporting almost 50-fold [14]. The epidemiological assessment of adverse drug effects necessitates making use of information from all the disparate sources [15,16]. Thus pharmaco-epidemiology draws on clinical trials, spontaneous reporting systems, specialty-based reporting systems, case reports, prescription monitoring, case series, cohort studies, case-control studies, population-based registries using computerized material, and special surveillance programmes (e.g. the Boston Collaborative Drug Surveillance Program, in the US).

1 Rawlins MD, Breckenridge AM, Wood SM. National adverse drug reaction reporting — a silver jubilee. *Adverse Drug React Bull* 1989; **138**: 516–19.
2 Fletcher AP. Spontaneous adverse drug reaction reporting vs event monitoring: a comparison. *J R Soc Med* 1991; **84**: 341–4.
3 Moore N, Paux G, Begaud B, *et al.* Adverse drug reaction monitoring: doing it the French way. *Lancet* 1985; **ii**: 1056–9.
4 Guillaume JC, Roujeau JC, Chevrant-Breton J, *et al.* Comment imputer un accident cutané a un médicament. Application aux purpura vasculaires. *Ann Dermatol Vénéréol (Paris)* 1987; **114**: 721–4.
5 Scott HD, Thacher-Renshaw A, Rosenbaum SE, *et al.* Physician reporting of adverse drug reactions. Results of the Rhode Island Adverse Drug Reaction Reporting Project. *JAMA* 1990; **263**: 1785–8.
6 Stern RS, Bigby M. An expanded profile of cutaneous reactions to nonsteroid anti-inflammatory drugs. Reports to a specialty-based system for spontaneous reporting of adverse reactions to drugs. *JAMA* 1984; **252**: 1433–7.
7 Gruppo Italiano Studi Epidemiologici in Dermatologia. Spontaneous monitoring of adverse reactions to drugs by Italian dermatologists; a pilot study. *Dermatologica* 1991; **182**: 12–17.
8 Kobza Black A, Greaves MM. Cutaneous reactions database closure. *Br J Dermatol* 1990; **123**: 277.

9 Griffin JP, Weber JCP. Voluntary systems of adverse reaction reporting — Part I. *Adverse Drug React Acute Poisoning Rev* 1985; **4**: 213–30.

10 Griffin JP, Weber JCP. Voluntary systems of adverse reaction reporting — Part II. *Adverse Drug React Acute Poisoning Rev* 1986; **5**: 23–55.

11 Griffin JP, Weber JCP. Voluntary systems of adverse reaction reporting — Part III. *Adverse Drug React Acute Poisoning Rev* 1989; **8**: 203–15.

12 Rawlins MD. Spontaneous reporting of adverse drug reactions I: The data. *Br J Clin Pharmacol* 1988; **26**: 1–5.

13 Bem JL, Mann RD, Rawlins MD. Review of yellow cards 1986 and 1987. *Br Med J* 1988; **296**: 1319.

14 Feely J, Moriarty S, O'Connor P. Stimulating reporting of adverse drug reactions by using a fee. *Br Med J* 1990; **300**: 22–3.

15 Stern RS, Wintroub BU. Adverse drug reactions: reporting and evaluating cutaneous reactions. *Adv Dermatol* 1987; **2**: 3–18.

16 Stern RS. Epidemiologic assessment of adverse drug effects. *Semin Dermatol* 1989; **8**: 136–40.

General incidence of adverse drug reactions

The incidence of adverse drug reactions varies from 6 to 15% [1] to 30% [2], with at least 90 million courses of drug treatment given yearly in the US [3]. The reported percentage of patients who develop an adverse drug reaction during hospitalization varies markedly in different studies from 1.5 to 44% [4], although in most studies the incidence is about 10–20% [5–8]. About 3–8% of hospital admissions are a consequence of adverse drug reactions [9–11]. A recent survey of 30 195 randomly selected hospital records in 51 hospitals in the state of New York reported on the overall incidence of adverse events caused by medical treatment, of which 19% were the result of drug complications; the most frequently implicated classes of drug responsible were antibiotics, antitumour agents, and anticoagulants [12]. Of the adverse reactions related to drug treatment 18% were judged to have been caused by negligence [12]. Allergic–cutaneous complications constituted 14% of all drug-related complications in this study. Less information is available about the incidence among outpatients. In general practice it has been estimated that about 1 in 40 consultations are the result of adverse drug reactions [13], and eventually 41% of patients develop a reaction [14]. In one multicentre general practice study in the UK, the percentage of consultations involving an adverse drug reaction increased from 0.6% for patients aged 0–20 years to 2.7% for patients aged over 50 years [15]; in another study 2.5% of consultations were the result of iatrogenic illness [16]. Fatal reactions to drugs are more common than is generally realized. It was previously estimated that penicillin caused 300 deaths each year in the US alone [17]. Anaphylactic reactions to penicillin were reported in 1968 to occur in about 0.015%, and fatal reactions in up to 0.002% (i.e. 1 per 50 000), of treatment courses [18]. These figures may be somewhat less today, with use of newer β-lactam antibiotics. The risk of fatal aplastic anaemia with chloramphenicol therapy was reported as at least 1 in 60 000 [19], and the risk of a fatal outcome from treatment with monoamine oxidase inhibitors may be of the same order. It has been estimated that the incidence of fatality as a result of a drug reaction amongst inpatients ranges between 0.1 and 0.3% [8,20].

1 DeSwarte RD. Drug allergy — Problems and strategies. *J Allergy Clin Immunol* 1984; **74**: 209−21.
2 Jick H. Adverse drug reactions: The magnitude of the problem. *J Allergy Clin Immunol* 1984; **74**: 555−7.
3 Goldstein RA. Foreword. Symposium proceedings on drug allergy: prevention, diagnosis, treatment. *J Allergy Clin Immunol* 1984; **74**: 549−50.
4 Nolan L, O'Malley K. Adverse drug reactions in the elderly. *Br J Hosp Med* 1989; **41**: 446−57.
5 Simmons M, Parker JM, Gowdey CW, *et al*. Adverse drug reactions during hospitalization. *Can Med Assoc J* 1968; **98**: 175.
6 Gardner P, Watson LJ. Adverse drug reactions: A pharmacist-based monitoring system. *Clin Pharmacol Ther* 1970; **11**: 802−7.
7 Smidt WA, McQueen EG. Adverse reactions to drugs: A comprehensive hospital in-patient survey. *N Z Med J* 1972; **76**: 397−402.
8 Davies DM (ed.) *Textbook of Adverse Drug Reactions*, 3rd edn. Oxford University Press, Oxford, 1985, pp 1−11.
9 McKenney JM, Harrison WL. Drug-related hospital admissions. *Am J Hosp Pharm* 1976; **33**: 792−5.
10 Levy M, Kewitz H, Altwein W, *et al*. Hospital admissions due to adverse drug reactions: a comparative study from Jerusalem and Berlin. *Eur J Clin Pharmacol* 1980; **17**: 25−31.
11 Black AJ, Somers K. Drug-related illness resulting in hospital admission. *J R Coll Physicians* 1984; **18**: 40−1.
12 Leape LL, Brennan TA, Laird N, *et al*. The nature of adverse events in hospitalized patients. Results of the Harvard Medical Practice Study II. *N Engl J Med* 1991; **324**: 377−84.
13 Kellaway GSM, McCrae E. Intensive monitoring of adverse drug effects in patients discharged from acute medical wards. *N Z Med J* 1973; **78**: 525−8.
14 Martys CR. Adverse reactions to drugs in general practice. *Br Med J* 1979; **ii**: 1194−7.
15 Lumley LE, Walker SR, Hall CG, *et al*. The under-reporting of adverse drug reactions seen in general practice. *Pharmaceut Med* 1986; **1**: 205−12.
16 Mulroy R. Iatrogenic disease in general practice: its incidence and effects. *Br Med J* 1973; **ii**: 407−10.
17 Parker CW. Allergic reactions in man. *Pharmacol Rev* 1983; **34**: 85−104.
18 Idsøe O, Guthe T, Willcox RR, De Weck AL. Nature and extent of penicillin side reactions, with particular reference to fatalities from anaphylactic shock. *Bull WHO* 1968; **38**: 159−88.
19 Witts LJ. Adverse reactions to drugs. *Br Med J* 1965; **ii**: 1081−6.
20 Caranasos GJ, May FE, Stewart RB, Cluff LE. Drug-associated deaths of medical inpatients. *Arch Int Med* 1976; **136**: 872−5.

Differential risk of adverse drug reactions amongst patient groups

Certain patients groups are at increased risk of developing an adverse drug reaction. Women are more likely than men to develop adverse drug reactions [1]. The incidence of such reactions increases with the number of drugs taken both in hospital inpatients [2−4] and outpatients [5,6]. Although data are somewhat conflicting [7], the burden of evidence suggests that the incidence of adverse reactions increases with patient age [1,8]. While those over 65 years of age comprise only 11.7% of the population in the US, 31% of all drugs are prescribed for this age group [9]. Similarly, in the UK the elderly are dispensed twice as many prescriptions as the national average [10]. Adverse drug reactions contribute to the need for hospitalization in 10–17% of elderly inpatients [11–13]. In general, factors which may predispose the elderly to adverse drug reactions therefore include multiple drug therapy as well as changes in pharmacokinetics and pharmacodynamics associated with ageing.

Patients with the acquired immunodeficiency syndrome (AIDS) appear to be at increased risk for adverse drug reactions [14,15], especially from sulphonamides [16–19] including co-trimoxazole (trimethoprim-sulphamethoxazole) [20], amoxycillin and clavulanate [21] and thiacetazone [22,23]. This is probably the result both of increased use of drugs in this population, and of an absolute increase in risk. Human immunodeficiency virus (HIV)-positive individuals have a systemic glutathione deficiency, resulting in a decreased capacity to scavenge hydroxylamine derivatives of sulpha-methoxazole, which have been proposed as the reactive metabolites responsible for adverse reactions to this drug [20]. Not only is there an increased frequency of drug eruptions in HIV-positive indi-viduals, but there have been many reports of particularly severe reactions, ranging from erythema multiforme to toxic epidermal necrolysis (TEN) [15]. Patients with AIDS may be more likely to demonstrate multiple cutaneous drug reactions [15].

A high frequency of drug allergy among patients with Sjögren's syndrome (SS) has also been reported. In different series, drug allergy has been reported in 43% of SS patients compared with 9% of patients with systemic lupus erythematosus (SLE) without SS [24], 62% of SS patients [25], and 41% of rheumatoid arthritis patients with SS, compared with 17% of those without SS [26]. Sjögren's syndrome, like impaired lymphocyte response after mitogenic stimulation, which is associated with drug allergy, is linked to HLA-DR3 [27].

1 Davies DM (ed.) *Textbook of Adverse Drug Reactions*, 3rd edn. Oxford Uni-versity Press, Oxford, 1985, pp 1–11.
2 Vakil BJ, Kulkarni RD, Chabria NL, *et al*. Intense surveillance of adverse drug reactions. An analysis of 338 patients. *J Clin Pharmacol* 1975; **15**: 435–41.
3 May FE, Stewart RB, Cluff LE. Drug interactions and multiple drug admin-istration. *Clin Pharmacol Ther* 1977; **22**: 322–8.
4 Steel K, Gertman PM, Crescenzi C, Anderson J. Iatrogenic illness on a general medical service at a university hospital. *N Engl J Med* 1981; **304**: 638–42.
5 Kellaway GSM, McCrae E. Intensive monitoring of adverse drug effects in patients discharged from acute medical wards. *N Z Med J* 1973; **78**: 525–8.
6 Hutchinson TA, Flegel KM, Kramer MS, *et al*. Frequency, severity, and risk factors for adverse reactions in adult outpatients: a prospective study. *J Chronic Dis* 1986; **39**: 533–42.
7 Gurwitz JH, Avorn J. The ambiguous relation between aging and adverse drug reactions. *Ann Int Med* 1991; **114**: 956–66.
8 Nolan L, O'Malley K. Adverse drug reactions in the elderly. *Br J Hosp Med* 1989; **41**: 446–57.
9 Lamy PP. New dimensions and opportunities. *Drug Intell Clin Pharm* 1985; **19**: 399–402.
10 Black D, Denham MJ, Acheson RM, *et al*. Medication for the elderly. A report

of the Royal College of Physicians. *J R Coll Physicians Lond* 1984; **18**: 7−17.

11 Col N, Fanale JE, Kronholm P. The role of medication noncompliance and adverse drug reactions in hospitalizations of the elderly. *Arch Int Med* 1990; **150**: 841−5.

12 Levy M, Kewitz H, Altwein W, *et al*. Hospital admissions due to adverse drug reactions: a comparative study from Jerusalem and Berlin. *Eur J Clin Pharmacol* 1980; **17**: 25−31.

13 Williamson J, Chopin JM. Adverse reactions to prescribed drugs in the elderly: a multicentre investigation. *Age Ageing* 1980; **9**: 73−80.

14 Coopman SA, Stern RS. Cutaneous drug reactions in human immuno-deficiency virus infection. *Arch Dermatol* 1991; **127**: 714−17.

15 Porteous DM, Berger TG. Severe cutaneous drug reactions (Stevens−Johnson syndrome and toxic epidermal necrolysis) in human immunodeficiency virus infection. *Arch Dermatol* 1991; **127**: 740−1.

16 Jaffe HS, Amman A, Abrams DI, *et al*. Complication of cotrimoxazole in treatment of AIDS associated *Pneumocystis carinii* pneumonia in homosexual men. *Lancet* 1983; **ii**: 1109−11.

17 Gordin FM, Simon GL, Wofsy CB, Mills J. Adverse reactions to trimethoprim−sulfamethoxazole in patients with the acquired immunodeficiency syndrome. *Ann Intern Med* 1984; **100**: 495−9.

18 Mitsuyasu R, Groopman J, Volberding P. Cutaneous reaction to trimethoprim−sulfamethoxazole in patients with AIDS and Kaposi's sarcoma. *N Engl J Med* 1983; **308**: 1535−6.

19 De Raeve L, Song M, Van Maldergem L. Adverse cutaneous drug reactions in AIDS. *Br J Dermatol* 1988; **119**: 521−3.

20 van der Ven AJAM, Koopmans PP, Vree TB, van der Meer JWM. Adverse reactions to co-trimoxazole in HIV infection. *Lancet* 1991; **338**: 431−3.

21 Battegay M, Opravil M, Wütrich B, Lüthy R. Rash with amoxycillin−clavulanate therapy in HIV-infected patients. *Lancet* 1989; **ii**: 1100.

22 Nunn P, Kibuga D, Gathua S, *et al*. Cutaneous hypersensitivity reactions due to thiacetazone in HIV-1 seropositive patients treated for tuberculosis. Lancet 1991; **337**: 627−30.

23 Hira SK, Wadhawan D, Kamanga J, *et al*. Cutaneous manifestations of human immunodeficiency virus in Lusaka, Zambia. *J Am Acad Dermatol* 1988; **19**: 451−7.

24 Katz J, Marmary Y, Livneh A, Danon Y. Drug allergy in Sjögren's syndrome. *Lancet* 1991; **337**: 239.

25 Bloch KJ, Buchanan WW, Wohl MJ, Bunim JJ. Sjögrens's syndrome: a clinical, pathological and serological study of 62 cases. *Medicine* 1965; **44**: 187−231.

26 Williams BO, Onge RAST, Young A, *et al*. Penicillin allergy in rheumatoid arthritis with special reference to Sjögren's syndrome. *Ann Rheum Dis* 1969; **28**: 607−11.

27 Hashimoto S, Michalski JP, Berman MA, McCombs C. Mechanism of a lymphocyte abnormality associated with HLA-B8/DR3: role of interleukin-1. *Clin Exp Immunol* 1990; **79**: 227−32.

Frequency of all drug reactions in relation to types of medication

The incidence of reactions to a particular drug must obviously be related to the quantity prescribed [1]. Nearly one in every 10 prescriptions in the US in 1981 contained either hydrochlorothiazide or codeine [2]. One in every five prescriptions was for a diuretic or other cardiovascular drug, analgesics and antiarthritics constituted 13%, anti-infectives 13%, and sedatives and other psychotropics 11% of prescriptions. Of the 10 drugs most frequently reported by the yellow card system to the UK Committee on Safety of Medicines in the first 6 months of 1986, seven were non-steroidal anti-inflammatory agents (accounting for 74% of serious adverse reactions); the remaining drugs were the angiotensin converting enzyme (ACE) inhibitors enalapril and captopril (accounting for 19% of serious reactions) and co-trimoxazole (accounting for 7% of serious adverse reactions [3]. In another study, anti-inflammatory agents were the drugs responsible for almost 50% of the reactions necessitating admission to a general medical ward; most of the drug-related admissions to the hospital as a whole were caused by digoxin, phenytoin, tranquillizers, antihypertensives, cardiac depressants, and antineoplastic agents [4].

1 Committee on Safety of Medicines. CSM Update: Non-steroidal anti-inflammatory drugs and serious gastrointestinal reactions — 2. *Br Med J* 1986; **292**: 1190−1.
2 Baum C, Kennedy DL, Forbes MB, Jones JK. Drug use in the United States in 1981. *JAMA* 1984; **251**: 1293−7.
3 Mann RD. The yellow card data: the nature and scale of the adverse drug reactions problem. In Mann RD (ed.) *Adverse Drug Reactions.* Parthenon Publishing, Carnforth, Lancs, 1987, pp 5−66.
4 Black AJ, Somers K. Drug-related illness resulting in hospital admission. *J R Coll Physicians* 1984; **18**: 40−1.

Incidence of drug eruptions

Drug eruptions are probably the most frequent of all manifestations of drug sensitivity, although their incidence is difficult to determine. Most estimates are inaccurate because many mild and transitory eruptions are not recorded, and because skin disorders are sometimes falsely attributed to drugs. There have been several studies of the incidence of drug eruptions [1−6]. The reaction rate has been reported as about 2.2% [3,6]. A recent survey [5] of adverse cutaneous drug reactions in inpatients found one-third were fixed drug reactions, one-third exanthematous, and 20% were urticaria or angioedema. The relatively high frequency of fixed drug reactions in this series reflects the fact that the patients under study had been admitted to hospital. Antimicrobial agents were most frequently incriminated (42%), then antipyretic/anti-inflammatory analgesics (27%), with drugs acting on the central nervous system accounting for 10% of reactions. A few drugs gave specific reactions (e.g phenazone salicylate caused a fixed eruption, while penicillin and salicylates caused urticaria); however, most were capable of causing several types of eruption. Another large series [6] reported that exanthematous eruptions, urticaria and generalized pruritus were the commonest reactions. Of interest, and contributing to the difficulties in identifying the causative drugs, the average patient had received eight different medications. Antibiotics, blood products, and inhaled mucolytics together caused 75% of the eruptions; amoxycillin (51.4 cases/1000 exposed), trimethoprim−sulphamethoxazole (33.8 cases/1000 exposed), and ampicillin (33.2 cases/1000 exposed) caused the most reactions [6]. Desensitizing vaccines, muscle relaxants, intravenous anaesthetics, and radiological contrast media were the most frequent causes of anaphylaxis or anaphylactoid reactions reported to the UK Committee on Safety of Medicines in 1986–87 [7]; the chairman of the Committee accordingly advised in 1986 that desensitizing vaccines only be given where full cardiorespiratory resuscitation facilities are available. Quinidine, cimetidine, phenylbutazone, hydrochlorothiazide (especially in combination with amiloride), and frusemide have also been frequently implicated in drug eruptions [8,9]. In the US and in the UK, antibiotics, hypnotics and tranquillizers are the most frequent offenders; on a reaction per dose basis penicillin, warfarin and imipramine are the three drugs most frequently incriminated [10]. The prevalence of a history of penicillin allergy in the US population has been estimated to be between 5 and 10% [11]. A recent international study of 1790 patients from 11 countries documented the frequency of allergic reactions to long-term benzathine penicillin prophylaxis for rheumatic fever at 3.2%; anaphylaxis occurred in 0.2% (1.2/10 000 injections), and the fatality rate was 0.05% (0.31/10 000 injections) [12]. Reactions to sulphonamides may also affect up to 5% of those treated [13]. Cutaneous reactions to common drugs such as digoxin, antacids, phenacetin (acetominophen), nitroglycerine, spironolactone, meperidine, aminophylline, propranolol, prednisone, salbutamol and diazepam are very rare [8].

Even where the eruption is apparently the only manifestation, death can result from exfoliative dermatitis, erythema multiforme or epidermal necrolysis. The incidence of TEN has been estimated at 1.2 cases per million per year in France based on nationwide surveillance between 1981 and 1985 inclusive [14]. Another study, based on the data of the Group Health Cooperative of Puget Sound, Seattle, Washington (which covers about 260 000 individuals), investigated hospitalized patients from 1972 to 1986 inclusive. The incidence of erythema multiforme, Stevens–Johnson syndrome, and TEN was estimated at 1.8 cases per million person years for patients aged between 20 and 64 years; the incidence for patients aged less than 20, and 65 or greater, increased to 7 and 9 cases per million person years respectively [15]. The incidence of TEN was estimated at 0.5 per million per year. Reaction rates per 100 000 exposed individuals were as follows: phenobarbital 20; nitrofuranotin 7; sulphamethoxazole and trimethoprim, and ampicillin 3; and amoxycillin 2 [15]. An Italian study estimated the incidence of TEN at about 1.2 cases per million per year [16]. A study based on computerized Medicaid billing data for 1980–84 from the states of Michigan, Minnesota and Florida reported an incidence of Stevens–Johnson syndrome of 7.1, 2.6, and 6.8 per million per year respectively; penicillins, especially aminopenicillins, were most frequently implicated [17]. In West Germany, the overall annual risk of TEN and of Stevens–Johnson syndrome was estimated over the years 1981 through 1985 as 0.93 and 1.1 per million respectively; drugs most frequently implicated were antibiotics (sulphonamides and β-lactam agents), and analgesics and non-steroidal anti-inflammatory agents [18]. In this study, it was possible to attribute the cause of the TEN to a drug in 88% of cases.

1 Kaplan AP. Drug-induced skin disease. *J Allergy Clin Immunol* 1984; **74**: 573−9.
2 Kauppinen K. Cutaneous reactions to drugs. With special reference to severe mucocutaneous bullous eruptions and sulphonamides. *Acta Derm Venereol (Stockh)* 1972; **52** (Suppl 68): 1−89.
3 Arndt KA, Jick H. Rates of cutaneous reactions to drugs. A report from the Boston Collaborative Drug Surveillance Program. *JAMA* 1976; **235**: 918−22.
4 Kauppinen K, Stubb S. Drug eruptions: Causative agents and clinical types. A series of inpatients during a 10-year period. *Acta Derm Venereol (Stockh)* 1984; **64**: 320−4.
5 Alanko K, Stubb S, Kauppinen K. Cutaneous drug reactions: clinical types and causative agents. A five year survey of in-patients (1981−1985). *Acta Derm Venereol (Stockh)* 1989; **69**: 223−6.
6 Bigby M, Jick S, Jick H, Arndt K. Drug-induced cutaneous reactions. A report from the Boston Collaborative Drug Surveillance Program on 15 438 consecutive inpatients, 1975 to 1982. *JAMA* 1986; **256**: 3358−63.
7 Bem JL, Mann RD, Rawlins MD. Review of yellow cards 1986 and 1987. *Br Med J* 1988; **296**: 1319.
8 Kalish RS. Drug eruptions: a review of clinical and immunological features. *Adv Dermatol* 1991; **6**: 221−37.
9 Thestrup-Pedersen K. Adverse reactions in the skin from antihypertensive drugs. *Dan Med Bull* 1987; **34**: 3−5.
10 Davies DM (ed.) *Textbook of Adverse Drug Reactions*, 3rd edn. Oxford University Press, Oxford 1985, pp 1−11.
11 Green CR, Rosenblum A. Report of the Penicillin Study Group — American Academy of Allergy. *J Allergy Clin Immunol* 1971; **48**: 331−43.
12 International Rheumatic Fever Study Group. Allergic reactions to long-term benzathine penicillin prophylaxis for rheumatic fever. *Lancet* 1991; **337**: 1308−10.
13 Anonymous. Hypersensitivity to sulphonamides — A clue? (Editorial). *Lancet* 1986; **ii**: 958−9.
14 Roujeau J-C, Guillaume J-C, Fabre J-D, *et al.* Toxic epidermal necrolysis (Lyell syndrome). Incidence and drug etiology in France, 1981−1985. *Arch Dermatol* 1990; **126**: 37−42.
15 Chan H-L, Stern RS, Arndt KA, *et al.* The incidence of erythema multiforme, Stevens−Johnson syndrome, and toxic epidermal necrolysis. A population-based study with particular reference to reactions caused by drugs among outpatients. *Arch Dermatol* 1990; **126**: 43−7.
16 Naldi L, Locati F, Marchesi L, Cainelli T. Incidence of toxic epidermal necrolysis in Italy. *Arch Dermatol* 1990; **126**: 1103−4.
17 Strom BL, Carson JL, Halpern AC, *et al.* A population-based study of Stevens−Johnson syndrome. Incidence and antecedent drug exposures. *Arch Dermatol* 1991; **127**: 831−8.
18 Schöpf E, Stühmer A, Rzany B, *et al.* Toxic epidermal necrolysis and Stevens−Johnson syndrome. An epidemiologic study from West Germany. *Arch Dermatol* 1991; **127**: 839−42.

Chapter 2
Classification and Mechanisms of Drug Reactions

Drug reactions [1—12] may arise as a result of immunological drug allergy or, more commonly, by non-immunological mechanisms, and may be predictable (type A) or unpredictable (type B) (Table 2.1). About 80% of drug reactions are predictable, are usually dose-related, are a function of the known pharmacological actions of the drug, and occur in otherwise normal individuals. Side-effects are unavoidable at the regular prescribed dose. Unpredictable reactions are dose independent, not related to the pharmacological action of the drug, and may have a genetic basis. Intolerance refers to an

Table 2.1 Classification of adverse drug reactions

Non-immunological
Predictable
  Overdosage
  Side-effects
  Cumulation
  Delayed toxicity
  Facultative effects
  Drug interactions
  Metabolic alterations
  Teratogenicity
  Non-immunologic activation of effector pathways
  Exacerbation of disease
  Drug-induced chromosomal damage
Unpredictable
  Intolerance
  Idiosyncrasy

Miscellaneous
Jarisch—Herxheimer reactions
Infectious mononucleosis—ampicillin reaction

Immunological (unpredictable)
IgE-dependent (Type I) drug reactions
  Urticaria and anaphylaxis
Antibody-mediated (Type II) drug reactions
Immune complex-dependent (Type III) drug reactions
  Urticaria and anaphylaxis
  Serum sickness
  Vasculitis
  Arthus phenomenon
Cell-mediated (Type IV) drug reactions
  Jones—Mote hypersensitivity
  Classical delayed type hypersensitivity

---

expected drug reaction occurring at a lower dose, whilst idiosyncratic and hypersensitivity reactions are qualitatively abnormal unexpected responses. Type C reactions include those associated with prolonged therapy (e.g. analgesic nephropathy), and type D consists of delayed reactions (e.g. carcinogenesis and teratogenicity). The skin has a limited repertoire of morphological reaction patterns in response to a wide variety of stimuli, and it is therefore often impossible to identify an offending drug, or the pathological mechanism involved, on the basis of clinical appearances alone. We therefore remain relatively ignorant about the mechanisms underlying many clinical drug eruptions.

1 Van Arsdel PP. Allergy and adverse drug reactions. *J Am Acad Dermatol* 1982; **6**: 833−45.
2 Parker CW. Allergic reactions in man. *Pharmacol Rev* 1983; **34**: 85−104.
3 de Weck AL. Pathophysiologic mechanisms of allergic and pseudo-allergic reactions to foods, food additives and drugs. *Ann Allergy* 1984; **53**: 583−6.
4 Wintroub BU, Stern R. Cutaneous drug reactions: pathogenesis and clinical classification. *J Am Acad Dermatol* 1985; **13**: 833−45.
5 Rawlins MD, Thompson JW. Mechanisms of adverse drug reactions. In Davies DM (ed.) *Textbook of Adverse Drug Reactions*, 3rd edn. Oxford University Press, Oxford, 1985, pp 12−38.
6 De Swarte RD. Drug allergy: An overview. *Clin Rev Allergy* 1986; **4**: 143−69.
7 Stern RS, Wintroub BU, Arndt KA. Drug reactions. *J Am Acad Dermatol* 1986; **15**: 1282−8.
8 Blaiss MS, de Shazo RD. Drug allergy. *Pediatr Clin North Am* 1988; **35**: 1131−47.
9 Park BK, Coleman JW. The immunological basis of adverse drug reactions. A report on a Symposium held in Liverpool on 6th April 1988. *Br J Clin Pharmacol* 1988; **26**: 491−5.
10 Berg PA, Daniel PT, Holzschuh J, Brattig N. Medikamentöse Allergien. Diagnose und Immunpathogenese. *Dtsch Med Wochenschr* 1988; **113**: 65−73.
11 Ring J. Arzneimittelunverträglichkeit durch pseudo-allergische Reaktionen. *Wien Med Wochenschr* 1989; **6**: 130−4.
12 Kalish RS. Drug eruptions: a review of clinical and immunological features. *Adv Dermatol* 1991; **6**: 221−37.

2.1 Non-immunological drug reactions

Overdosage

The manifestations are a predictable exaggeration of the desired pharmacological actions of the drug, and are directly related to the total amount of drug in the body. Overdosage may be absolute, as a result of a prescribing or dispensing error, or of deliberate excess intake by the patient. It may also occur despite standard dosage due to varying individual rates of absorption, metabolism or excretion. An inappropriately large dose may be given to an infant or very old person or to one with renal impairment. Drug interactions may also cause drug overdosage.

Side-effects

These include unwanted or toxic effects which are not separable from the desired pharmacological action of the drug. Examples are the drowsiness induced by antihistamines, the atropine-like anticholinergic properties of some phenothiazines, many antihistamines, and tricyclic antidepressants, and the anagen alopecia caused by cytotoxic drugs.

Cumulative toxicity

Prolonged exposure may lead to cumulative toxicity. Accumulation of drugs in the skin may lead to colour disturbance, either as a result of deposition within phagocytic cells or mucous membranes (e.g. with prolonged administration of gold, silver, bismuth or mercury), or due to binding of the drug or a metabolite to a skin component (e.g. with high dose chlorpromazine therapy).

Delayed toxicity

Examples are the keratoses and skin tumours which appear many years after inorganic arsenic, and the delayed hepatotoxicity associated with methotrexate therapy.

Facultative effects

These include the consequences of drug-induced alterations in skin or mucous membrane flora. Antibiotics which destroy Gram-positive bacteria may allow the multiplication of resistant Gram-negative species. Broad spectrum antibiotics, corticosteroids, and immunosuppressive drugs may promote multiplication of *Candida albicans* and favour its transition from saphrophytism to pathogenicity. Corticosteroids promote the spread of tinea and erythrasma. Antibiotics such as clindamycin and tetracycline may be associated with pseudomembranous enterocolitis following bowel super-infection with *Clostridium difficile*.

Drug interactions

Interactions between two or more drugs administered simultaneously may occur before entry into the body in an intravenous drip, in the intestine, in the blood, and/or at tissue receptor sites, or indirectly by acceleration or slowing in the rate of drug metabolism or excretion. It should be remembered that adverse consequences of drug interactions may occur not only on introduction of a drug, but also on removal of a drug which causes acceleration of drug metabolism, since this may result in effective overdosage of the remaining drug. The subject of drug interactions has been extensively reviewed [1]. Combinations of drugs with potential adverse interactions continue to be prescribed [2].

Intestinal drug interactions

Examples are that phenobarbitone inhibits absorption of griseofulvin
[1], antacids inhibit absorption of tetracycline [3], and tetracycline
may decrease absorption of the oral contraceptive [4]. Whether the
latter is of real significance is a matter of debate [5].

Displacement from carrier or receptor sites

Most drugs are reversibly bound to carrier proteins in plasma or
extracellular fluid; bound drug acts as a reservoir, preventing
excessive fluctuation in the level of the active unbound fraction.
Displacement from a carrier protein augments drug activity, while
displacement from a receptor site diminishes it. Many acidic drugs
such as salicylates, coumarins, sulphonamides and phenylbutazone
are bound to plasma albumin and compete for binding sites. Thus
a sulphonamide may displace tolbutamide from albumin leading to
hypoglycaemia, or aspirin, sulphonamides, clofibrate or phenylbutazone may displace warfarin from albumin causing bleeding
and ecchymoses. Similarly, sulphonamides and aspirin may increase
methotrexate toxicity. Ciprofloxacin increases plasma levels of
theophylline.

Enzyme stimulation or inhibition

A drug may either stimulate or inhibit metabolic enzymes important
to its own degradation or that of another agent, with significant
clinical consequences. Thus some drugs induce synthesis of drug-
metabolizing enzymes in liver microsomes. The liver microsomal
hydroxylating system (which mediates metabolism of phenytoin
and debrisoquine) is based on cytochrome P450, and appears to be
a family of enzymes capable of acting on different substrates including barbiturates, fatty acids and endogenous steroids. The
cytochrome P450-dependent system also catalyses deamination (e.g.
amphetamine), dealkylation (e.g. morphine, azathioprine), sulphoxidation (e.g. chlorpromazine, phenylbutazone), desulphuration
(thiopentone), and dehalogenation (e.g. halogenated anaesthetics).
This lack of specificity accounts for the ability of an inducing agent
to stimulate metabolism of many other drugs, and of one drug to
inhibit metabolism of a structurally unrelated drug. Antibiotics, if
administered over a period (e.g. rifampicin for tuberculosis) can be
enzyme inducers. Barbiturates stimulate metabolism of griseofulvin,
phenytoin and coumarin anticoagulants, and griseofulvin induces
increased metabolism of coumarins. Similarly, rifampicin, phenytoin, and carbamazepine increase the metabolism of cyclosporin A
[6]. Drugs causing enzyme inhibition include chloramphenicol,
cimetidine, monoamine oxidase inhibitors, *p*-aminosalicylic acid,
pethidine and morphine. Dicoumarol, chloramphenicol and phenylbutazone inhibit metabolic inactivation of tolbutamide. Allopurinol

inhibits metabolism of azathioprine and mercaptopurine by xanthine oxidase. Cimetidine inhibits liver enzymes and decreases hepatic blood flow, therefore potentiating the action of some β-blockers (propranolol) and benzodiazepines, carbamazepine, warfarin, morphine, phenytoin and theophylline. Ketoconazole may potentiate oral anticoagulants [7] and erythromycin may potentiate carbamazepine [8]; both may potentiate cyclosporin. Nifedipine and cyclosporin are both metabolized by the same cytochrome P450 enzyme, P450cpn; cyclosporin potentiates the action of nifedipine, phenytoin and to a lesser extent valproate by decreasing P450cpn availability by competitive inhibition [9].

Altered drug excretion

Examples are the well-known probenecid-induced reduction in the renal excretion of penicillin, and aspirin-induced reduction in renal clearance of methotrexate.

1 Griffin JP, D'Arcy PF, Speirs CJ. *A Manual of Adverse Drug Interactions,* 4th edn. Wright (Butterworth & Co. Publishers Ltd), London, 1988.
2 Beers MH, Storrie MS, Lee G. Potential adverse drug interactions in the emergency room. An issue in the quality of care. *Ann Intern Med* 1990; **112**: 61−4.
3 Garty M, Hurwitz A. Effect of cimetidine and antacids on gastrointestinal absorption of tetracycline. *Clin Pharmacol Ther* 1980; **28**: 203−7.
4 Bacon JF, Shenfield GM. Pregnancy attributable to interaction between tetracycline and oral contraceptives. *Br Med J* 1980; **280**: 293.
5 Fleischer AB, Resnick SD. The effect of antibiotics on the efficacy of oral contraceptives. *Arch Dermatol* 1989; **125**: 1562−4.
6 Schofield OMV, Camp RDR, Levene GM. Cyclosporin A in psoriasis: interaction with carbamazepine. *Br J Dermatol* 1990; **122**: 425−6.
7 Smith AG. Potentiation of oral anticoagulants by ketoconazole. *Br Med J* 1984; **288**: 188−9.
8 Wroblewski BA, Singer WD, Whyte J. Carbamazepine-erythromycin interaction: Case studies and clinical significance. *JAMA* 1986; **255**: 1165−7.
9 McFadden JP, Pontin JE, Powles AV, *et al.* Cyclosporin decreases nifedipine metabolism. *Br Med J* 1989; **299**: 1224.

Metabolic changes

Drugs may induce cutaneous changes by their effects on nutritional or metabolic status. Thus drugs such as phenytoin which interfere with folate absorption or metabolism increase the risk of aphthous stomatitis, and isotretinoin may cause xanthomata by elevation of very low density lipoproteins [1].

1 Dicken CH. Eruptive xanthomas associated with isotretinoin (13-*cis*-retinoic acid). *Arch Dermatol* 1980; **116**: 951−2.

Teratogenicity and other effects on the fetus [1−5]

The advent of isotretinoin has focused the attention of dermatologists considerably on the problem of teratogenicity in general [5]. The

fetus is particularly at risk from drug-induced developmental malformations during the period of organogenesis, which lasts from
about the third to the tenth week of gestation. Thalidomide, retinoids
and cytotoxic drugs are proven teratogens. Heavy alcohol intake,
which produces the 'fetal alcohol syndrome', smoking, anticonvulsants (especially phenytoin and trimethadione), warfarin,
inhalational anaesthetics, lithium and quinine are probably teratogenic. High dose corticosteroids have been linked to cleft palate.
A major correlation has been found between the incidence of
glucocorticoid-induced cleft palate and the chromosome 8 segment
identified by *N*-acetyltransferase in mice [6]. 6-Aminonicotinamide-
induced cleft palate and phenytoin-induced cleft lip with or without
cleft palate are also influenced by this genetic region but not as
strongly. Sex hormones, psychotropic drugs, benzodiazepines, tetracycline, rifampicin, penicillamine, and the folate antagonists,
pyrimethamine and trimethoprim are possibly teratogenic and
should be avoided in the first trimester of pregnancy. The potential
adverse effects on the fetus and on the breast-fed infant of a number of
drugs frequently used by the dermatologist have been reviewed [4].

Drugs may also cause fetal damage later in pregnancy. Warfarin
may cause haemorrhage, and phenytoin near to term produces a
coagulation defect in the neonate, which is correctable by vitamin
K. Antithyroid drugs and iodides may cause neonatal goitre and
hypothyroidism. Fetal adrenal atrophy may follow high dose maternal corticosteroid therapy. The non-steroidal anti-inflammatory
drugs have various ill effects, although aspirin has been advocated
in pregnancy for the prevention of fetal growth retardation [7].
Tetracyclines are deposited in developing bones and cause discoloration and enamel hypoplasia of teeth [8]. Aminoglycoside
antibiotics are ototoxic, and chloroquine has caused a neonatal
chorioretinitis. Androgens and progestogens may virilize the fetus.
Stilboestrol administered from early pregnancy for several months
has been associated with female and male genital tract abnormalities,
and carcinoma of the vagina 20 years later in the offspring [9,10].

1 Ellis C, Fidler J. Drugs in pregnancy: adverse reactions. *Br J Hosp Med* 1982;
   28: 575−84.
2 Kalter H, Warkany J. Congenital malformations: Etiologic factors and their
   role in prevention. *N Engl J Med* 1983; **308**: 424−31, 491−7.
3 Ashton CH. Disorders of the fetus and infant. In Davies DM (ed.) *Textbook of
   Adverse Drug Reactions*, 3rd edn. Oxford University Press, Oxford, 1985,
   pp 77−127.
4 Stockton DL, Paller AS. Drug administration to the pregnant or lactating
   woman: A reference guide for dermatologists. *J Am Acad Dermatol* 1990; **23**:
   87−103.
5 Mitchell AA. Teratogens and the dermatologist. New knowledge, responsi-
   bilities, and opportunities. *Arch Dermatol* 1991; **127**: 399−401.
6 Karolyi J, Erickson RP, Liu S, Killewald L. Major effects on teratogen-induced
   facial clefting in mice determined by a single genetic region. *Genetics* 1990;
   126: 201−5.
7 Uzan S, Beaufils M, Breart G, *et al*. Prevention of fetal growth retardation

with low-dose aspirin: findings of the EPREDA trial. *Lancet* 1991; **337**: 1427−31.

8 Witkop CJ, Wolf RO. Hypoplasia and intrinsic staining of enamel following tetracycline therapy. *JAMA* 1963; **185**: 1008−11.

9 Wingfield M. The daughters of stilboestrol. Grown up now but still at risk. *Br Med J* 1991; **302**: 1414−15.

10 Anonymous. Diethylstilboestrol — effects of exposure *in utero*. *Drug Ther Bull* 1991; **29**: 49−50.

Anaphylactoid reactions
(non-immunologic activation of effector pathways)

Certain drugs, such as opiates, codeine, amphetamine, polymyxin B, *d*-tubocurarine, atropine, hydralazine, pentamidine, quinine and radiocontrast media, may release mast cell mediators directly to produce urticaria or angioedema [1−5]. Some drugs, such as radio-contrast media, may activate complement by an antibody-independent method [6]. Anaphylactic-like responses to cyclo-oxygenase inhibitors such as aspirin and other non-steroidal anti-inflammatory agents may in some way involve effects on pathways of arachidonic acid metabolism or on mast cell degranulation [7,8].

1 Schoenfeld MR. Acute allergic reactions to morphine, codeine, meperidine hydrochloride and opium alkaloids. *N Y State J Med* 1960; **60**: 2591−3.

2 Comroe JH, Dripps RD. Histamine-like action of curare and tubocurarine injected intracutaneously and intra-arterially in man. *Anesthesiology* 1946; **7**: 260−2.

3 Greenberger PA. Contrast media reactions. *J Allergy Clin Immunol* 1984; **74**: 600−5.

4 Assem ESK, Bray K, Dawson P. The release of histamine from human basophils by radiological contrast agents. *Br J Radiol* 1983; **56**: 647−52.

5 Rice MC, Lieberman P, Siegle RL, Mason J. *In vitro* histamine release induced by radiocontrast media and various chemical analogs in reactor and control subjects. *J Allergy Clin Immunol* 1983; **72**: 180−6.

6 Arroyave CM, Bhatt KN, Crown NR. Activation of the alternative pathway of the complement system by radiographic contrast media. *J Immunol* 1976; **117**: 1866−9.

7 Morassut P, Yang W, Karsh J. Aspirin intolerance. *Semin Arthritis Rheum* 1989; **19**: 22−30.

8 Ring J. Arzneimittelunverträglichkeit durch pseudo-allergische Reaktionen. *Wien Med Wochenschr* 1989; **6**: 130−4.

Exacerbation of disease

Examples of adverse drug effects on pre-existing skin conditions include: lithium exacerbation of acne and psoriasis, β-blocker induction of a psoriasiform dermatitis [1] and corticosteroid withdrawal resulting in exacerbation of psoriasis; cimetidine, penicillin or sulphonamide exacerbation of lupus erythematosus (LE); and vasodilator exacerbation of rosacea. Sometimes a drug may unmask a latent condition, as when barbiturates precipitate symptoms of porphyria.

1 Abel EA, Dicicco LM, Orenberg EK, *et al.* Drugs in exacerbation of psoriasis. *J Am Acad Dermatol* 1986; **15**: 1007–22.

Intolerance

The characteristic effects of the drug are produced to an exaggerated extent by an abnormally small dose. This may simply represent an extreme within normal biological variation. Alternatively, the intolerance may be contributed to by delayed metabolism or excretion due to impaired hepatic or renal function, or by genetic variation in the rate of drug metabolism.

Idiosyncrasy

This term describes an uncharacteristic response, not predictable from animal experiments, and not mediated by an immunological mechanism. The cause is often unknown, but genetic variation in metabolic pathways may be involved. Such genetic abnormalities include: glucose-6-phosphate dehydrogenase (G-6-PD) deficiency [1,2], hereditary methaemoglobinaemia, porphyria, glucocorticoid glaucoma, and malignant hyperthermia of anaesthesia, all of which are characterized by unusual pharmacological responses to various drugs.

1 Beutler E. Glucose-6-phosphate dehydrogenase deficiency. *Lancet* 1991; **324**: 169–74.
2 Magon AM, Leipzig RM, Zannoni VG, Brewer GJ. Interactions of glucose-6-phosphate dehydrogenase deficiency with drug acetylation and hydroxylation reactions. *J Lab Clin Med* 1981; **97**: 764–70.

Pharmacogenetic mechanisms and genetic influences underlying intolerance and idiosyncratic reactions [1–3]

The pharmacokinetics of drugs, including their absorption, plasma protein binding, distribution, metabolism and elimination, may be influenced by genetic factors. Oxidation, hydrolysis, and acetylation are the three metabolic pathways most subject to genetic influence. Genetic factors also influence pharmacodynamics, i.e. tissue or organ responsiveness. Thus genetic variations in all these areas may underlie both intolerance and idiosyncrasy.

Examples of genetically mediated intolerance include pupil size responses to phenylephrine and parasympatholytics [4] and the very rare dominantly inherited familial resistance to coumarin anticoagulants, the result of mutation in the receptor for vitamin K and anticoagulants [5]. Low red cell G-6-PD levels, inherited as a sex-linked dominant [6], are common in Negroes, certain Levantine peoples, and Philippinos, and result in a chronic deficit of reduced glutathione sulphydryl (SH) groups. G-6-PD reduces NADP while oxidizing glucose-6-phosphate, thus providing a source of reducing power that maintains sulphydryl groups and aids in the detoxification of free radicals and peroxides; in its absence red blood cells are vulnerable to oxidative damage [6]. Affected individuals are at risk of acute haemolysis on exposure to the drugs listed in Table 2.2, all of which may oxidize the few reduced SH groups in older red cells. Phenacetin (acetominophen) and aspirin appear safe to use [6].

Oxidation

Anticonvulsants, many hypnotics, tricyclic antidepressants, anticoagulants, various anti-inflammatory and anxiolytic agents are eliminated by oxidation. For many drugs, oxidation rates vary as a continuous spectrum within the population. Genetic differences in metabolism of sulphonamides may underlie idiosyncratic toxicity [7−12]. Oxidative metabolism of sulphonamides by cytochrome P450 enzymes and N-acetylation yields a reactive hydroxylamine intermediate which is inactivated by glutathione conjugation. The hydroxylamine metabolite is toxic to lymphocytes, and the lymphocyte toxicity is markedly increased in patients with a history of hypersensitivity or with glutathione synthetase deficiency. Phenytoin is also metabolized by the cytochrome P450 enzyme system into a reactive arene-oxide intermediate [13]. Phenytoin hypersensitivity syndrome appears to be associated with an inherited deficiency of epoxide hydrolase, which is primarily responsible for detoxifying the toxic arene-oxide intermediate [13−15]. Activated phenytoin has been shown to be toxic to lymphocytes from patients with phenytoin reactions, and to a lesser degree, to lymphocytes from their parents [15]. Impaired metabolism of phenacetin and phenformin, inherited as a result of genetic polymorphism in liver microsomal oxidation, may result in adverse reactions [16,17]. The induction of liver enzymes responsible for drug oxidation may itself be under genetic control [18]. There is a fourfold increase in toxicity with penicillamine in patients with rheumatoid arthritis

Table 2.2 Drugs and chemicals causing haemolytic anaemia in patients with G-6-PD deficiency (after [6]).

Acetanilid
Doxorubicin
Furazolidone
Methylene blue
Nalidixic acid
Niridazole
Nitrofurantoin
Phenazopyridine
Primaquine (antimalarial)
Sulphonamides
   Sulphamethoxazole
   Dapsone

with a genetically determined poor capacity to sulphoxidate the structurally related mucolytic agent, carbocisteine [19].

Hydrolysis

Genetic influence on drug hydrolysis is well illustrated in the case of suxamethonium, which normally results in only very brief neuromuscular blockade due to rapid hydrolysis by plasma pseudocholinesterase. Genetically determined atypical cholin-esterases cannot hydrolyse the drug, leading to prolonged apnoea in affected individuals [20]; conversely, dominantly inherited resistance to suxamethonium, mediated by a highly active cholin-esterase, has been reported [21].

Acetylation

Isoniazid, many sulphonamides, hydralazine, dapsone, pro-cainamide, etc. are inactivated by conversion to acetyl conjugates. Acetylation rates vary greatly, with a bimodal frequency distribution, and there is marked ethnic variation. Rapid inactivation is domi-nantly inherited, and is commonest amongst Eskimos and Japanese and least common amongst certain Mediterranean Jews. The LE-like syndrome due to procainamide may occur more in fast acety-lators, implying that a conjugate and not the parent compound is responsible [22]. Slow acetylators, in whom higher and more per-sistent drug levels occur, are more liable to develop adverse re-actions to isoniazid (pellagra-like syndrome and peripheral neuritis), dapsone (haemolysis) [23], and hydralazine (LE-like syndrome) [24,25].

Influence of HLA types

An association between HLA types and susceptibility to drug erup-tions has been reported on several occasions, particularly in relation to gold (HLA-DRw3 and HLA-B8) and penicillamine toxicity [19,26−29]. Penicillamine toxicity is associated with HLA pheno-types as follows [19]: HLA-DR3 and B8 are associated with renal toxicity, DR3, B7 and DR2 with haematological toxicity, A1 and DR4 with thrombocytopenia, and cutaneous adverse reactions are linked to HLA-DRw6. A positive association with Aw33 and B17/Bw58 haplotypes, and a negative association with the A2 haplotype, has been reported in southern Chinese patients with drug eruptions after exposure to allopurinol [30]. Aspirin-sensitive asthma is associated with HLA-DQw2 [31]. HLA-linkage associations with certain bullous disorders have been reported [32]. The above findings suggest that there may be genetic predisposition to develop certain drug eruptions.

1 Rawlins MD, Thompson JW. Mechanisms of adverse drug reactions. In Davies

DM (ed.) *Textbook of Adverse Drug Reactions*, 3rd edn. Oxford University Press, Oxford, 1985, pp 12–38.

2 Shear NH, Bhimji S. Pharmacogenetics and cutaneous drug reactions. *Semin Dermatol* 1989; **8**: 219–26.

3 Lennard MS, Tucker GT, Woods HF. Inborn 'errors' of drug metabolism. Pharmacokinetic and clinical implications. *Clin Pharmacokinet* 1990; **19**: 257–63.

4 Bertler Å, Smith SE. Genetic influences in drug responses of the eye and the heart. *Clin Sci* 1971; **40**: 403–10.

5 O'Reilly RA. The second reported kindred with hereditary resistance to oral anticoagulant drugs. *N Engl J Med* 1970; **282**: 1448–51.

6 Beutler E. Glucose-6-phosphate dehydrogenase deficiency. *Lancet* 1991; **324**: 169–74.

7 Shear NH, Spielberg SP. *In vitro* evaluation of a toxic metabolite of sulfadiazide. *Can J Physiol Pharmacol* 1985; **63**: 1370–2.

8 Shear NH, Spielberg SP. An *in vitro* lymphocytotoxicity assay for studying adverse reactions to sulphonamides. *Br J Dermatol* 1985; **113**: 112–13.

9 Shear N, Spielberg S, Grant D, *et al.* Differences in metabolism of sulfonamides predisposing to idiosyncratic toxicity. *Ann Intern Med* 1986; **105**: 179–84.

10 Anonymous. Hypersensitivity to sulphonamides — A clue? (Editorial). *Lancet* 1986; **ii**: 958–9.

11 Rieder MJ, Uetrecht J, Shear NH, *et al.* Synthesis and *in vitro* toxicity of hydroxylamine metabolites of sulphonamides. *J Pharmacol Exp Ther* 1988; **244**: 724–8.

12 Rieder MJ, Uetrecht J, Shear NH, *et al.* Diagnosis of sulfonamide hypersensitivity reactions by *in-vitro* 'rechallenge' with hydroxylamine metabolites. *Ann Intern Med* 1989; **110**: 286–9.

13 Shear NH, Spielberg SP. Anticonvulsant hypersensitivity syndrome. *In vitro* assessment of risk. *J Clin Invest* 1988; **82**: 1826–32.

14 Spielberg SP, Gordon GB, Blake DA, *et al.* Predisposition to phenytoin hepatotoxicity assessed *in vitro*. *N Engl J Med* 1981; **305**: 722–7.

15 Spielberg SP. *In vitro* assessment of pharmacogenetic susceptibility to toxic drug metabolites in humans. *Fed Proc* 1984; **43**: 2308–13.

16 Shahidi NT. Acetophenetidin sensitivity. *Am J Dis Child* 1967; **113**: 81–2.

17 Eichelbaum M. Defective oxidation of drugs: Pharmacokinetic and therapeutic implications. *Clin Pharmacokinet* 1982; **7**: 1–22.

18 Vessell ES, Passananti T, Greene FE, Page JG. Genetic control of drug levels and of the induction of drug-metabolizing enzymes in man: individual variability in the extent of allopurinol and nortryptiline inhibition of drug metabolism. *Ann N Y Acad Sci* 1971; **179**: 752–3.

19 Dasgupta B. Adverse reactions profile: 2. Penicillamine. *Prescribers J* 1991; **31**: 72–7.

20 Harris H. Enzymes and drug sensitivity. The genetics of serum cholinesterase 'deficiency' in relation to suxamethonium apnoea. *Proc R Soc Med* 1964; **57**: 503–6.

21 Neitlich HW. Increased plasma cholinesterase activity and succinylcholine resistance: A genetic variant. *J Clin Invest* 1966; **45**: 380–7.

22 Davies DM, Beedie MA, Rawlins MD. Antinuclear antibodies during procainamide treatment and drug acetylation. *Br Med J* 1975; **iii**: 682–4.

23 Ellard GA, Gammon PT, Savin LA, Tan RSH. Dapsone acetylation in dermatitis herpetiformis. *Br J Dermatol* 1974; **90**: 441–4.

24 Perry HM Jr, Sakamoto A, Tan EM. Relationship of acetylating enzyme to hydralazine toxicity. *J Lab Clin Med* 1967; **70**: 1020–1.

25 Russell GI, Bing RF, Jones JA, *et al.* Hydralazine sensitivity: clinical features, autoantibody changes and HLA-DR phenotype. *Q J Med* 1987; **65**: 845–52.

26 Wooley PH, Griffin J, Payani GS, *et al.* HLA-DR antigens and toxic reaction to sodium aurothiomalate and D-penicillamine in patients with rheumatoid arthritis. *N Engl J Med* 1980; **303**: 300–2.

27 Latts JR, Antel JP, Levinson DJ, *et al.* Histocompatibility antigens and gold toxicity: a preliminary report. *J Clin Pharmacol* 1980; **20**: 206–9.

28 Bardin T, Dryll A, Debeyre N, *et al.* HLA system and side effects of gold salts

and D-penicillamine treatment of rheumatoid arthritis. *Ann Rheum Dis* 1982; **41**: 599–601.

29 Emery P, Panayi GS, Huston G, *et al*. D-penicillamine induced toxicity in rheumatoid arthritis: the role of sulphoxidation status and HLA-DR3. *J Rheumatol* 1984; **11**: 626–32.

30 Chan SH, Tan T. HLA and allopurinol drug eruption. *Dermatologica* 1989; **179**: 32–3.

31 Mullarkey MF, Thomas PS, Hansen JA, *et al*. Association of aspirin-sensitive asthma with HLA-DQw2. *Am Rev Respir Dis* 1986; **133**: 261–3.

32 Roujeau J-C, Bracq C, Huyn NT, *et al*. HLA phenotypes and bullous cutaneous reactions to drugs. *Tissue Antigens* 1986; **28**: 251–4.

Drug-induced chromosomal damage [1–3]

This may be studied by examining the chromosomes of patients or animals exposed to drugs, or *in vitro* by the addition of drugs to cell cultures; substances capable of inducing chromosomal damage are termed clastogens. Effects may be dose related, but *in vitro* results may not be representative of the *in vivo* situation. Antimitotic and antibiotic agents have been the most studied, but psychotropics, anticonvulsants, hallucinogens, immunosuppressants, and oral contraceptives have also been investigated and shown to cause in varying degree chromosomal damage. Damage ranges from staining variations through 'gaps' in staining, chromosome breaks, gross aberrations such as deletions, fragments, translocations, inversions, etc. to polyploidy. Such damage may be stable and retained over a succession of cell divisions, or transient.

1 Shaw MW. Human chromosome damage by chemical agents. *Ann Rev Med* 1970; **21**: 409–32.

2 Bender MA, Griggs HG, Bedford JS. Mechanisms of chromosomal aberration production. III. Chemicals and ionizing radiation. *Mutat Res* 1974; **23**: 197–212.

3 Rawlins MD, Thompson JW. Mechanisms of adverse drug reactions. In Davies DM (ed.) *Textbook of Adverse Drug Reactions*, 3rd edn. Oxford University Press, Oxford: 1985, pp 12–38.

2.2 Miscellaneous reactions

Jarisch–Herxheimer reaction

This is the focal exacerbation of lesions of infective origin when potent antimicrobial therapy is initiated, and is classically observed in the treatment of early syphilis with penicillin; it may also occur 3 days after starting griseofulvin therapy, during therapy with diethyl-carbamazine for onchocerciasis and thiabendazole for strongyloidiasis, and with penicillin or minocycline for erythema chronicum migrans due to *Borrelia burgdorferi* infection [1]. The reaction has been attributed to sudden release of pharmacologically and/or immunologically active substances from killed microorganisms or damaged tissues. There is, however, little evidence that it is an

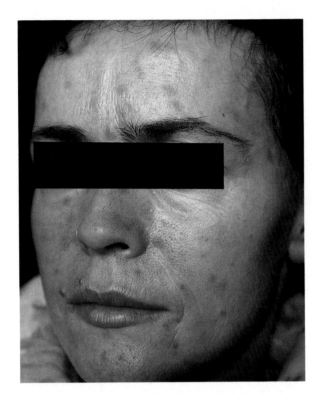

Figure 2.1 Jarisch–Herxheimer reaction with prominent facial lesions, following penicillin therapy for secondary syphilis.

allergic reaction [2]. Clinically there may be fever, rigors, lymphadenopathy, arthralgia, and transient macular or urticarial eruptions (Fig 2.1); a vesicular eruption has also been described [3].

1 Weber K. Jarisch–Herxheimer-Reaktion bei Erythema-migrans-Krankheit. *Hautarzt* 1984; **35**: 588–90.
2 Skog E, Gudjónsson H. On the allergic origin of the Jarisch–Herxheimer reaction. *Acta Derm Venereol (Stockh)* 1966; **46**: 136–43.
3 Rosen T, Rubin H, Ellner K, *et al*. Vesicular Jarisch–Herxheimer reaction. *Arch Dermatol* 1989; **125**: 77–81.

Infectious mononucleosis–ampicillin reaction

Ampicillin almost always causes a severe morbilliform eruption when given to a patient with infectious mononucleosis or lymphatic leukaemia (Fig. 2.2). The reaction occurs much less frequently with amoxycillin. The exact mechanism responsible is not known.

2.3 Immunological drug reactions

Allergic hypersensitivity reactions result from immunological sensitization to a drug, by previous exposure to that drug or to a chemically related cross-reacting substance [1–7]. Although drugs frequently elicit an immune response, clinically evident hypersensitivity reactions are manifest only in a small proportion of exposed individuals. Thus, using highly sensitive passive haem-

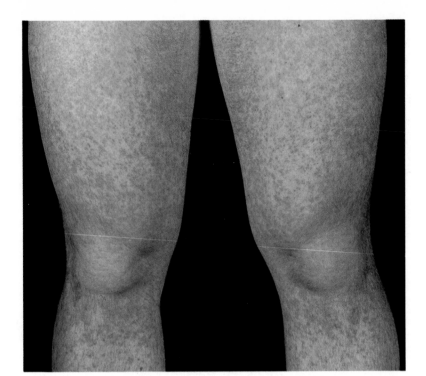

Figure 2.2 Maculopapular erythema in a patient with glandular fever treated with ampicillin.

agglutination assays, IgM class antibodies to the penicilloyl group (the major hapten determinant derived from penicillin) are detectable in almost 100% of normal individuals, even in the absence of a history of penicillin therapy; 40% of patients receiving more than 2 g of penicillin for more than 10 days develop IgG class antibodies [8]. Macromolecular drugs such as protein or peptide hormones, insulin or dextran are antigenic in their own right. By contrast, most drugs are small organic molecules with a molecular mass of less than 1 kDa; conjugation of free drug as a hapten with a macromolecular carrier is then required to initiate an immune response. Fortunately, many drugs have only a limited capacity to form covalent bonds with tissue proteins. Clinical sensitization may also result from allergy to reactive drug metabolites as haptens, or to minor contaminants.

Clinical features distinguishing allergic from non-allergic drug reactions

Prior exposure before sensitization should have been without adverse effect. If there has been no previous exposure, there should be a latent period of several days of uneventful therapy before the reaction supervenes, during which primary sensitization occurs. Thereafter, reactions may develop within minutes (or even seconds) and certainly within 24 hours. Allergic reactions do not resemble the pharmacological action of the drug, may follow exposure to

[27]

doses far below the therapeutic level, and are reproducible on re-administration (if judged safe).

Factors concerned in the development of hypersensitivity

The route of administration of a drug may affect its immunogenicity and the nature of any allergy. Topical drug exposure is more likely to result in sensitization than oral administration, and favours development of contact dermatitis; thus poison ivy is a potent contact sensitizer, but oral ingestion may promote tolerance. Anaphylaxis is more likely to be associated with intravenous drug administration. However, anaphylaxis may sometimes occur as fast after oral penicillin administration [9]. Whether allergy develops or not may also depend on the antigenic load in terms of degree of drug exposure, and individual genetic variation in drug absorption and metabolism. Thus, as stated above, a lupus-like syndrome with antinuclear antibody formation following hydralazine therapy occurs more frequently in slow acetylators of the drug [10]. Hydralazine-related systemic lupus erythematosus (SLE) is 10 times more frequent in HLA-DR4 positive patients than in the population at large, and is commoner in females. Allergic drug reactions are less common in childhood and possibly in the aged; in the latter, this may be related to impaired immunological responsiveness. Immuno-suppression may increase the risk by inhibiting the regulatory function of suppressor T cells [11]. Environmental factors may also affect susceptibility to drug hypersensitivity, as for example the well-recognized increase in ampicillin-induced morbilliform eruptions associated with infectious mononucleosis, and photo-allergic reactions to drugs such as thiazide diuretics or phenothiazines.

The duration of hypersensitivity

The duration of allergic sensitivity is unpredictable. Although there is a general tendency for immunological responses to a drug to fall off with time, provided the patient is not re-exposed to the drug or a related substance, this can never be relied on; where necessary, safe confirmatory procedures (if available) should be carried out.

1 de Weck AL. Pathophysiologic mechanisms of allergic and pseudo-allergic reactions to foods, food additives and drugs. *Ann Allergy* 1984; **53**: 583–6.
2 Wintroub BU, Stern R. Cutaneous drug reactions: pathogenesis and clinical classification. *J Am Acad Dermatol* 1985; **13**: 833–45.
3 Rawlins MD, Thompson JW. Mechanisms of adverse drug reactions. In Davies DM (ed.) *Textbook of Adverse Drug Reactions*, 3rd edn. Oxford University Press, Oxford, 1985, pp 12–38.
4 De Swarte RD. Drug allergy: An overview. *Clin Rev Allergy* 1986; **4**: 143–69.
5 Stern RS, Wintroub BU, Arndt KA. Drug reactions. *J Am Acad Dermatol* 1986; **15**: 1282–8.
6 Blaiss MS, de Shazo RD. Drug allergy. *Pediatr Clin North Am* 1988; **35**: 1131–47.
7 Kalish RS. Drug eruptions: a review of clinical and immunological features. *Adv Dermatol* 1991; **6**: 221–37.

8 Weiss ME, Adkinson NF. Immediate hypersensitivity reactions to penicillin and related antibiotics. *Clin Allergy* 1988; **18**: 515–40.
9 Simmonds J, Hodges S, Nicol F, Barnett D. Anaphylaxis after oral penicillin. *Br Med J* 1978; **ii**: 1404.
10 Perry HM Jr, Sakamoto A, Tan EM. Relationship of acetylating enzyme to hydralazine toxicity. *J Lab Clin Med* 1967; **70**: 1020–1.
11 Lakin JD, Grace WR, Sell KW. IgE antipolymyxin B antibody formation in a T-cell depleted bone marrow transplant patient. *J Allergy Clin Immunol* 1975; **56**: 94–103.

2.4 Types of immunological reaction

IgE-dependent (Type I) drug reactions: urticaria and anaphylaxis [1]

In vivo cross-linkage by polyvalent drug–protein conjugates of two or more specific IgE molecules, fixed to sensitized tissue mast cells or circulating basophil leucocytes, triggers the cell to release a variety of chemical mediators including histamine, peptides such as eosinophil chemotactic factor of anaphylaxis, lipids such as leukotriene C_4 or prostaglandin D_2, and a variety of pro-inflammatory cytokines [2]. These in turn have effects on a variety of target tissues including skin, respiratory, gastrointestinal and/or cardiovascular systems. Eosinophil degranulation may also result in release of pro-inflammatory mediators [3]. Dilation and increased permeability of small blood vessels with resultant oedema and hypotension, contraction of bronchiolar smooth muscle and excessive mucus secretion, and chemotaxis of inflammatory cells including polymorphs and eosinophils occurs. Clinically this may produce pruritus, urticaria, bronchospasm, laryngeal oedema, and in severe cases, anaphylactic shock with hypotension and possible death. Immediate reactions occur within minutes of drug administration; accelerated reactions may occur within hours or days, and are generally urticarial but may involve laryngeal oedema. Penicillins are the commonest cause of IgE-dependent drug eruptions; the frequency of Type I reactions to β-lactam antibiotics is about 2% [4].

1 Champion RH, Greaves MW, Kobza Black A (eds.) *The Urticarias.* Churchill Livingstone, Edinburgh, 1985.
2 Schwartz LB. Mast cells and their role in urticaria. *J Am Acad Dermatol* 1991; **25**: 190–204.
3 Leiferman KM. A current perspective on the role of eosinophils in dermatologic diseases. *J Am Acad Dermatol* 1991; **24**: 1101–12.
4 Sullivan TJ, Wedner HJ, Shatz GS, *et al.* Skin testing to detect penicillin allergy. *J Allergy Clin Immunol* 1981; **68**: 171–80.

Antibody-mediated (Type II) drug reactions

Binding of antibody to cells may lead to cell damage following complement-mediated cytolysis. The classical example of immune complex formation between a drug (as hapten) bound to the surface of a cell (in this case, platelets) and IgG class antibody, with subsequent complement fixation, was the purpura caused by apronalide (Sedormid). A further example is the thrombocytopenic purpura which may result from antibodies to quinidine–platelet conjugates [1,2]. A number of drugs including penicillin, quinine and sulphonamides may rarely produce a haemolytic anaemia by this method. Methyldopa very occasionally induces a haemolytic anaemia mediated by autoantibodies directed against red cell antigens.

1 Christie DJ, Weber RW, Mullen PC, *et al*. Structural features of the quinidine and quinine molecules necessary for binding of drug-induced antibodies to human platelets. *J Lab Clin Med* 1984; **104**: 730–40.
2 Gary M, Ilfeld D, Kelton JG. Correlation of a quinidine-induced platelet-specific antibody with development of thrombocytopenia. *Am J Med* 1985; **79**: 253–5.

Immune complex-dependent (Type III) drug reactions

Urticaria and anaphylaxis

Immune complexes may activate the complement cascade, with resultant formation of anaphylatoxins such as the complement protein fragments C3a and C5a, which trigger release of mediators from mast cells and basophils directly, resulting in urticaria or anaphylaxis.

Serum sickness [1–4]

Serum sickness-like reactions and other immune complex-mediated conditions necessitate a drug antigen to persist in the circulation for long enough for antibody, largely of IgG or IgM class, to be synthesized and to combine with it to form circulating antibody–antigen immune complexes. They therefore develop about 6 days or more after drug administration. Serum sickness occurs when antibody combines with antigen in antigen excess, leading to slow removal of persistent complexes by the mononuclear phagocyte system. It was usually seen in the context of serum therapy with large doses of heterologous antibody, as with horse antiserum for the treatment of diphtheria. It has been reported more recently with antilymphocyte globulin therapy. Clinical manifestations of serum sickness include fever, arthritis, nephritis, neuritis, oedema, and an urticarial or papular rash.

Vasculitis [5–14]

Drug-induced immune complexes play a part in the pathogenesis of cutaneous necrotizing vasculitis (Fig. 2.3) Deposition of immune complexes on vascular endothelium results in activation of the complement cascade, with generation of the anaphylatoxins C3a and C5a which have chemotactic properties. Vasoactive amines and

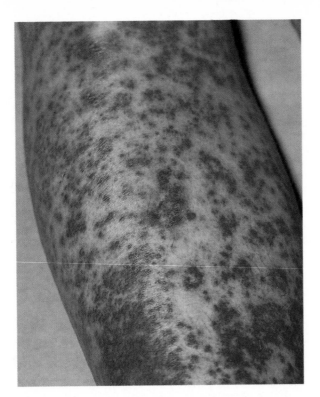

Figure 2.3 Palpable purpura related to necrotizing vasculitis.

pro-inflammatory cytokines are released from basophils and mast cells, with resultant increased vascular permeability and attraction of neutrophil polymorphonuclear cells. Immune complex interaction with platelets via their Fc receptors causes platelet aggregation and microthrombus formation. Release by neutrophils of lysosomal enzymes contributes further to local inflammation. These events lead to the histological appearance of leucocytoclastic vasculitis. Deposition of immunoglobulins and complement in and around blood vessel walls is detectable by direct immuno-fluorescence staining of skin biopsies. Hydralazine and the hydroxylamine metabolite of procainamide bind to complement component C4 and inhibit its function; this may impair clearance of immune complexes, and predispose to development of a LE syndrome [13].

The Arthus reaction [14]

The Arthus reaction is a localized form of immune complex vasculitis. Intradermal or subcutaneous injection of antigen into a sensitized individual with circulating precipitating antibodies, usually of IgG_1 class, leads to local immune complex formation and the cascade of events described above. Clinically, there is erythema and oedema (see Fig. 15.7, p. 316), haemorrhage, and occasionally necrosis at the injection site, which reaches a peak at 4–10 hours, and then gradually wanes. The initial polymorph infiltrate may be replaced by a mononuclear cell infiltrate.

[31]

1 Yancey KB, Lawley TJ. Circulating immune complexes: Their immuno-chemistry, biology, and detection in selected dermatologic and systemic diseases. *J Am Acad Dermatol* 1984; **10**: 711−31.

2 Lawley TJ, Bielory L, Gascon P, *et al.* A prospective clinical and immunologic analysis of patients with serum sickness. *N Engl J Med* 1984; **311**: 1407−13.

3 Erffmeyer JE. Serum sickness. *Ann Allergy* 1986; **56**: 105−9.

4 Lin RY. Serum sickness syndrome. *Am Fam Physician* 1986; **33**: 157−62.

5 Fauci AS, Haynes EF, Katz P. The spectrum of vasculitis; clinical, pathologic, immunologic and therapeutic considerations. *Ann Intern Med* 1978; **89**: 660−76.

6 Herrmann WA, Kauffmann RH, van Es LA *et al.* Allergic vasculitis. A histo-logical and immunofluorescent study of lesional and non-lesional skin in relation to circulating immune complexes. *Arch Dermatol Res* 1980; **269**: 179−87.

7 Mackel SE, Jordon RE. Leukocytoclastic vasculitis. A cutaneous expression of immune complex disease. *Arch Dermatol* 1983; **118**: 296−301.

8 Wenner NP, Safai B. Circulating immune complexes in Henoch−Schönlein purpura. *Int J Dermatol* 1983; **22**: 383−5.

9 Price N, Sams WM Jr. Vasculitis. *Dermatol Clin* 1983; **1**: 475−91.

10 Sanchez NP, Van Hale HM, Su WPD. Clinical and histopathologic spectrum of necrotizing vasculitis. Report of findings in 101 cases. *Arch Dermatol* 1985; **121**: 220−4.

11 Sams WM. Hypersensitivity angiitis. *J Invest Dermatol* 1989; **93**: 78S−81S.

12 Smoller BR, McNutt NS, Contreras F. The natural history of vasculitis. What the histology tells us about pathogenesis. *Arch Dermatol* 1990; **126**: 84−9.

13 Sim E. Drug-induced immune complex disease. *Complement Inflamm* 1989; **6**: 119−26.

14 Hay F. Hypersensitivity − Type III. In Roitt I, Brostoff J, Male D (eds) *Immunology*, 2nd edn. Gower Medical Publishing, London, 1989, pp 21.1−21.10.

Cell-mediated (Type IV) reactions

The role of delayed type cell-mediated immune reactions in contact drug hypersensitivity, as with penicillin [1], is well established, but the importance of such mechanisms involving specific effector lymphocytes in other varieties of cutaneous drug allergy is uncertain. It is nevertheless thought that a number of drug reactions, including erythema multiforme, toxic epidermal necrolysis, lichenoid reactions, lupus-like reactions, and some morbilliform reactions, involve T lymphocyte responses to altered self. The potential mechanisms involved are reviewed below.

1 Stejskal VDM, Forsbeck M, Olin R. Side chain-specific lymphocyte responses in workers with occupational allergy induced by penicillins. *Int Arch Allergy Appl Immunol* 1987; **82**: 461−4.

The skin immune system and cutaneous inflammation

Cell-mediated immune reactions involve interactions between bone marrow-derived cells, including T and B lymphocytes and cells of monocyte−macrophage lineage, which express amongst other sur-face markers, class II major histocompatibility complex (MHC) antigens (i.e. HLA-DR). These interactions are under the control of the immune response or MHC genes, which in the human are located on chromosome 6 [1]. It has only comparatively recently been appreciated that the skin contains all the elements of an intrinsic immune system [2,3], comprising lymphocytes [4], resident antigen-presenting cells in the epidermis (CD1⁺HLA-DR⁺ Langerhans cells) [5,6] and dermis (perivascular macrophage-like cells, including factor XIIIa⁺ dermal dendritic cells) [7,8], and keratinocytes which secrete a wide range of pro-inflammatory cytokines with chemotactic and/or immunoregulatory properties; the latter include the interleukins IL-1, IL-3, IL-6 and IL-8, as well as tumour necrosis factor-α (TNF-α), transforming growth factors α and β, and granulocyte macrophage colony stimulating factor [9,10]. Langerhans cells pick up and process antigen, and migrate to the regional lymph nodes; they may interact with sensitized T lymphocytes in the epidermis, dermis, or the regional nodes [2,3,5,6]. Interactions between Langerhans cells, keratinocytes and T lymphocytes are critical to the development of contact sensitization and to cell-mediated immune reactions as a whole [3,5,6,11]. Keratinocytes, other than those associated with the acrosyringium, do not normally express class II MHC/HLA-DR antigen, but may acquire HLA-DR expression in a wide variety of lymphocyte-mediated skin disorders as a result of T lymphocyte secretion of γ-interferon [12,13].

Recruitment of inflammatory cells into the extravascular spaces of the dermis is dependent upon attachment of adhesion molecules on the inflammatory cells, such as lymphocyte function associated antigen 1 (LFA-1), to ligands on endothelial cells, such as intercellular adhesion molecule 1 (ICAM-1), endothelial leucocyte adhesion molecule-1 (ELAM-1) and vascular cell adhesion molecule 1 (VCAM-1) [14−18]. While ICAM-1 and VCAM-1 show no tissue-specific restriction, the selectin ELAM-1 has been reported to act as a vascular addressin for memory T cell homing to the skin, since the ligand for ELAM-1 on T cells is highly restricted to a specific subset of memory T cells, and ELAM-1 shows biased expression on inflamed endothelium of skin [18]. ICAM-1 is not constitutively expressed by either endothelial cells or keratinocytes, but may be induced on these cells by the action of the T lymphocyte cytokine γ-interferon; lymphocytes adhere to endothelium in skin biopsy material incubated with γ-interferon *in vitro* [19,20]. Since expression of these adhesion molecules is modulated by the action of cytokines, it has been proposed that keratinocyte production of cytokines such as IL-1 and TNF-α following various noxious stimuli is sufficient to initiate cutaneous inflammation in an antigen-independent fashion [16]. The dermal dendrocyte may be involved in dermal recruitment of inflammatory cells [21]. Amplification and persistence of inflammation would then be dependent on antigen-dependent mechanisms involving T cell−Langerhans cell or T cell−dermal macrophage interactions [16,21]. Epidermal keratinocytes express ICAM-1 in a whole range of skin disorders characterized by cutaneous lymphocyte infiltration, presumably as a result of T lymphocyte production of γ-interferon. Keratinocyte expression of

ICAM-1 may be important in determining the exocytosis of leucocytes into the epidermis [15,20].

Lymphocytes activated by incubation with IL-2 are able to destroy keratinocytes *in vitro* by a non-specific mechanism, and pretreatment of the keratinocytes with γ-interferon, with consequent keratinocyte ICAM-1 expression, increases keratinocyte destruction [22]. Thus keratinocytes may be non-specifically damaged as 'innocent bystanders' during the course of a lymphocyte-mediated reaction. Keratinocyte HLA-DR expression is thought to represent an immunoregulatory phenomenon, which tends to down-regulate cutaneous cell-mediated immune reactions. In addition, HLA-DR expression by keratinocytes may lead to their increased destruction by cytotoxic T cells.

Apart from immunohistochemical investigations characterizing the phenotype of mononuclear cells in the cutaneous infiltrate, studies on the role of the skin immune system in drug eruptions are exceedingly few, reflecting the fact that much of the information reviewed above has been discovered only very recently. Keratinocytes have been shown to express HLA-DR and ICAM-1 in lesions of fixed drug eruption [23,24]. Nevertheless, it is clear that interactions between the various elements of the skin immune system must be fundamental to many varieties of adverse drug reaction occurring in the skin. Further insight into the immunological mechanism involved in drug eruptions may be obtained by extrapolating from studies on cutaneous graft-versus-host disease.

1 Roitt I, Brostoff J, Male D (eds) *Immunology* 2nd edn. Gower Medical Publishing, London, 1989.
2 Streilein JW. Skin-associated lymphoid tissues (SALT): origins and functions. *J Invest Dermatol* 1983; **80**: 12S–16S.
3 Bos JD (ed.) *Skin Immune System (SIS).* CRC Press, Boca Raton, Florida, 1990.
4 Bos JD, Zonneveld I, Das PK, *et al.* The skin immune system: Distribution and immunophenotype of lymphocyte populations in normal human skin. *J Invest Dermatol* 1987; **88**: 569–73.
5 Breathnach SM. The Langerhans cell. *Br J Dermatol* 1988; **119**: 463–9.
6 Schuler G (ed.) *Epidermal Langerhans Cells.* CRC Press, Boca Raton, Florida, 1991.
7 Sontheimer RD. Perivascular dendritic macrophages as immunobiological constituents of the human dermal microvascular unit. *J Invest Dermatol* 1989; **93**: 96S–101S.
8 Cerio R, Griffiths CEM, Cooper KD, *et al.* Characterization of factor XIIIa positive dermal dendritic cells in normal and inflamed skin. *Br J Dermatol* 1989; **121**: 421–31.
9 Luger TA, Schwarz T. Evidence for an epidermal cytokine network. *J Invest Dermatol* 1990; **95**: 100S–104S.
10 McKenzie RC, Sauder DN. The role of keratinocyte cytokines in inflammation and immunity. *J Invest Dermatol* 1990; **95**: 105S–107S.
11 Breathnach SM, Katz SI. Cell mediated immunity in cutaneous disease. *Hum Pathol* 1986; **17**: 161–7.
12 Auböck J, Romani N, Grubauer G, Fritsch P. HLA-DR expression on keratinocytes is a common feature of diseased skin. *Br J Dermatol* 1986; **114**: 465–72.
13 Basham TY, Nickoloff BJ, Merigan TC, Morhenn VB. Recombinant gamma

interferon induces HLA-DR expression on cultured human keratinocytes. *J Invest Dermatol* 1984; **83**: 88−90.

14 Rothlein R, Dustin ML, Marlin SD, *et al*. A human intercellular adhesion molecule (ICAM-1) distinct from LFA-1. *J Immunol* 1986; **137**: 1270−4.

15 Nickoloff BJ. Role of interferon-γ in cutaneous trafficking of lymphocytes with emphasis on molecular and cellular adhesion events. *Arch Dermatol* 1988; **124**: 1835−43.

16 Barker JNWN, Mitra RS, Griffiths CEM, *et al*. Keratinocytes as initiators of inflammation. *Lancet* 1991; **337**: 211−14.

17 Norris P, Poston RN, Thomas DS, *et al*. The expression of endothelial leucocyte adhesion molecule-1 (ELAM-1), intercellular adhesion molecule-1 (ICAM-1), and vascular cell adhesion molecule-1 (VCAM-1) in experimental cutaneous inflammation: a comparison of ultraviolet B erythema and delayed hypersensitivity. *J Invest Dermatol* 1991; **96**: 763−70.

18 Mackay CR. Skin-seeking memory T cells. *Nature* 1991; **349**: 737−8.

19 Dustin ML, Singer KH, Tuck DT, *et al*. Adhesion of T lymphoblasts to epidermal keratinocytes is regulated by interferon gamma and is mediated by intercellular adhesion molecule 1 (ICAM-1). *J Exp Med* 1988; **157**: 1323−40.

20 Nickoloff BJ, Griffiths CEM. T lymphocytes and monocytes bind to keratinocytes in frozen sections of biopsy specimens of normal skin treated with gamma interferon. *J Am Acad Dermatol* 1989; **20**: 736−43.

21 Nickoloff BJ, Griffiths CEM. Lymphocyte trafficking in psoriasis: a new perspective emphasizing the dermal dendrocyte with active dermal recruitment mediated via endothelial cells followed by intra-epidermal T-cell activation. *J Invest Dermatol* 1990; **95**: 35S−37S.

22 Kalish RS. Non-specifically activated human peripheral blood mononuclear cells are cytotoxic for human keratinocytes *in vitro*. *J Immunol* 1989; **142**: 74−80.

23 Murphy GF, Guillén FJ, Flynn TC. Cytotoxic T lymphocytes and phenotypically abnormal epidermal dendritic cells in fixed cutaneous eruption. *Hum Pathol* 1985; **16**: 1264−71.

24 Shiohara T, Nickoloff BJ, Sagawa Y, *et al*. Fixed drug eruption. Expression of epidermal keratinocyte intercellular adhesion molecule-1 (ICAM-1). *Arch Dermatol* 1989; **125**: 1371−6.

Graft-versus-host disease as a model for drug eruptions

Graft-versus-host disease (GVHD) classically occurs as a result of donor T lymphocyte responses to 'foreign' transplantation antigens on recipient tissues, following the injection of lymphoid cells from an immunocompetent donor animal into a histo-incompatible recipient animal incapable of rejecting them [1−3]. Our concept of the requirements for the development of GVHD has undergone slight modification with the reported occurrence of GVHD following sygeneic (identical twin) or autologous marrow transplantation [4−5], especially following cessation of cyclosporin A therapy [6].

GVHD in its acute and chronic forms shares clinical, histological and immunological features with several important lymphocyte-mediated skin diseases, and may therefore provide us with valuable insights into their pathogenesis [1,2,7−11]. The similarity between the spectrum of clinical and histological skin changes resulting from adverse reactions to the sulphydryl group of drugs (tiopronin, D-penicillamine, captopril, and gold sodium thiomalate, which either have a thiol group or release sulphydryl compounds) and GVHD has been noted [12]. In acute graft-versus-host disease, cutaneous findings include a pruritic maculopapular rash, often on the palms, soles and ears; this may progress to erythroderma, with bulla formation, or necrolysis. Histologically, there is an upper dermal perivascular infiltrate, with scattered vacuolated dyskeratotic keratinocytes in the basal and spinous layers, lymphoid exocytosis into the epidermis, and satellite cell necrosis, in which lymphocytes are seen adjacent to dyskeratotic keratinocytes [13]. In certain cases, full thickness epidermal necrosis occurs. In chronic GVHD, skin changes may produce a widespread lichen planus-like eruption or a papulosquamous dermatitis; abnormalities of pigmentation, alopecia, and onychodysplasia may result. In severe forms, chronic GVHD may resemble scleroderma, with induration, joint contractures, atrophy and chronic ulceration; a sicca syndrome may develop. Histologically, there may be epidermal atrophy, a lichenoid upper dermal infiltrate, and later changes of sclerosis of the dermis and subcutaneous fat [14].

The fact that acute GVHD resembles changes seen in erythema multiforme or toxic epidermal necrolysis, that early chronic cutaneous GVHD mimics lichen planus, and that late chronic cutaneous GVHD resembles LE or scleroderma, might suggest that epidermal damage in idiopathic or drug-induced variants of these skin diseases is also mediated by cytotoxic T cells. Immunohistochemical studies have shown that the majority of intra-epidermal T cells in human GVHD are of suppressor/cytotoxic phenotype [15−17]. Langerhans cells, which express class II MHC antigen, may be a particular target for destruction in GVHD; by extrapolation, drug-haptenated Langerhans cells may be foci of destruction in drug eruptions [1,2,10,18]. Epidermal cells can certainly act as targets for cytotoxic T cells, since primed hapten-specific cytotoxic T cells will lyse haptenated murine epidermal cells *in vitro* [19]. Further evidence for the ability of cytotoxic T cells to mediate epidermal damage is the finding that cloned cytotoxic T cells produce immunologically specific destruction of allogeneic epidermis following intradermal injection into histo-incompatible mice [20].

It is of interest that the syngeneic GVHD which follows withdrawal of cyclosporin A appears to be mediated by autoreactive cytotoxic T cells with specificity for class II MHC antigen [21]. Class II MHC-autoreactive T lymphocyte clones also develop in a murine model of chronic GVHD [22]. Thus one could envisage that some drug eruptions may develop as a result of autoreactive cytotoxic T cell clones directed against a drug−class II MHC antigen complex, either as a result of failure of deletion of these clones, or due to a failure of autoregulatory T lymphocytes. Soluble mediators or cytokines, in particular TNFα, may have a central role as a mediator of GVHD [23]. Alternatively, cells with the phenotypic characteristics of natural killer cells rather than of cytotoxic T lymphocytes may cause the cutaneous damage in GVHD [24], and perhaps also in certain drug eruptions. A GVHD-like illness which may follow infusion of autologous peripheral blood cells treated with IL-2 (as part of an anticancer protocol) appears to be mediated by lymphokine-activated killer cells differing from both cytotoxic T cells and natural killer cells [25,26].

1 Breathnach SM. Current understanding of the aetiology and clinical implications of cutaneous graft-vs-host disease. *Br J Dermatol* 1986; **114**: 139−43.

2 Breathnach SM, Katz SI. Immunopathology of cutaneous graft-versus-host disease. *Am J Dermatopathol* 1987; **9**: 343−8.

3 Ferrara JLM, Deeg HJ. Graft-versus-host disease. *N Engl J Med* 1991; **324**: 667−74.

4 Hood AF, Vogelsang GB, Black LP, *et al*. Acute graft-vs-host disease. Development following autologous and syngeneic bone marrow transplantation. *Arch Dermatol* 1987; **123**: 745−50.

5 Ferrara JLM. Syngeneic graft-vs-host disease. *Arch Dermatol* 1987; **123**: 741−2.

6 Hess AD, Fischer AC. Immune mechanisms in cyclosporine-induced syngeneic graft-versus-host disease. *Transplantation* 1989; **48**: 895−900.

7 Saurat H. Cutaneous manifestations of graft-versus-host disease. *Int J Dermatol* 1981; **20**: 249−56.

8 James WD, Odom RB. Graft-vs-host disease. *Arch Dermatol* 1983; **119**: 683−9.

9 Gleichman E, Pals ST, Rolinck AG, *et al*. Graft-versus-host reactions: clues to the etiopathogenesis of a spectrum of immunological diseases. *Immunol Today* 1984; **5**: 324−32.

10 Breathnach SM, Katz SI. Cell mediated immunity in cutaneous disease. *Hum Pathol* 1986; **17**: 161−7.

11 Tanaka K, Sullivan KM, Shulman HM, *et al*. A clinical review: cutaneous manifestations of acute and chronic graft-versus-host disease following bone marrow transplantation. *J Dermatol (Tokyo)* 1991; **18**: 11−17.

12 Kitamura K, Aihara M, Osawa J, *et al*. Sulfhydryl drug-induced eruption: a clinical and histological study. *J Dermatol (Tokyo)* 1990; **17**: 44−51.

13 Sale GE, Lerner KG, Barker EA, *et al*. The skin biopsy in the diagnosis of acute graft-versus-host disease in man. *Am J Pathol* 1977; **89**: 621−36.

14 Shulman HM, Sale GE, Lerner KG, *et al*. Chronic cutaneous graft-versus-host disease in man. *Am J Pathol* 1978; **91**: 545−70.

15 Lampert IA, Janossy G, Suitters AJ, *et al*. Immunological analysis of the skin in graft-versus-host disease. *Clin Exp Immunol* 1982; **50**: 123−31.

16 Gomes MA, Schmitt DS, Souteyrand P, *et al*. Lichen planus and chronic graft-versus-host reaction. *In situ* identification of immunocompetent cell phenotypes. *J Cutan Pathol* 1982; **9**: 249−57.

17 Sloane JP, Thomas JA, Imrie SF, *et al*. Morphological and immunohistological changes in the skin in allogeneic bone marrow recipients. *J Clin Pathol* 1984; **37**: 919−30.

18 Breathnach SM, Shimada S, Kovac Z, Katz SI. Immunologic aspects of acute cutaneous graft-vs-host disease: decreased density and antigen-presenting capacity of Ia$^+$ Langerhans cells and absent antigen-presenting capacity of Ia$^+$ keratinocytes. *J Invest Dermatol* 1986; **86**: 226−34.

19 Tamaki K, Fujiwara H, Levy RB, *et al*. Hapten-specific TNP-reactive cytotoxic effector cells using epidermal cells as targets. *J Invest Dermatol* 1981; **77**: 225−9.

20 Tyler JD, Galli SJ, Snider ME, *et al*. Cloned cytolytic T lymphocytes destroy allogeneic tissue *in vivo*. *J Exp Med* 1984; **159**: 234−43.

21 Hess AD, Horwitz L, Beschorner WE, Santos GW. Development of graft-vs.-host disease-like syndrome in cyclosporine-treated rats after syngeneic bone marrow transplantation. I. Development of cytotoxic T lymphocytes with apparent polyclonal anti-Ia specificity, including autoreactivity. *J Exp Med* 1985; **161**: 718−30.

22 Parkman R. Clonal analysis of murine graft-versus-host disease: I. Phenotypic and functional analysis of T lymphocyte clones. *J Immunol* 1986; **136**: 3543−8.

23 Piguet PF. Tumor necrosis factor and graft-vs-host disease. In Burakoff SJ, Deeg HJ, Ferrara J, Atkinson K (eds) *Graft-vs.-Host Disease: Immunology,*

Pathophysiology, and Treatment. Marcel Dekker, New York, 1990, pp 225–76.
24 Guillen FJ, Ferrara J, Hancock WW, *et al.* Acute cutaneous graft-versus-host disease to minor histocompatibility antigens in a murine model. Evidence that large granular lymphocytes are effector cells in the immune response. *Lab Invest* 1986; **55**: 35–42.
25 Lotze MT, Matory YL, Ettinghausen SE, *et al. In vivo* administration of purified human interleukin 2: II. Halflife, immunologic effects, and expansion of peripheral lymphoid cells *in vivo* with recombinant IL-2. *J Immunol* 1985; **135**: 2865–75.
26 Sondel PM, Hank JA, Kohler PC, *et al.* Destruction of autologous human lymphocytes by interleukin 2-activated cytotoxic cells. *J Immunol* 1986; **137**: 502–11.

Jones–Mote (cutaneous basophil) hypersensitivity

Suboptimal immunization, as with soluble protein antigens in incomplete Freund's adjuvant, leads on challenge in the guinea-pig model to basophil infiltration, thought to be mediated by T lymphocyte cytokine production [1]. The equivalent human reaction may be mediated by mast cells. The reaction is optimal some 7–10 days after induction. Cutaneous swelling is maximal 24 hours after antigen challenge. Challenge by intravenous injection of antigen causes a generalized macular erythema with eosinophilia [2]. It has been proposed that Jones–Mote hypersensitivity may provide a model to explain the pathomechanisms operative in some morbilliform drug eruptions [3].

1 Katz SI. Recruitment of basophils in delayed hypersensitivity reactions. *J Invest Dermatol* 1978: **71**: 70–5.
2 Dvorak HF, Hammond ME, Colvin RB, *et al.* Systemic expression of cutaneous basophil hypersensitivity. *J Immunol* 1977; **118**: 1549–57.
3 Kalish RS. Drug eruptions: a review of clinical and immunological features. *Adv Dermatol* 1991; **62**: 221–37.

Part 2
Patterns of Clinical Disease

Chapter 3
Types of Clinical Reaction

The mucocutaneous reactions which may result from adverse drug reactions have been the subject of extensive reviews [1–14]. The skin usually reacts to noxious stimuli by one of a fairly limited range of morphological responses. This chapter outlines the common drug-induced reaction patterns; the reader is further referred to later sections relating to discussion of adverse effects of individual drugs. It is unfortunate that, while certain drugs are commonly associated with a specific reaction, most drugs are in fact capable of causing several different types of eruption. In most patterns of reaction to drugs, the histological changes are no more distinctive than are the clinical features [15]. For example, urticaria, erythema multiforme, toxic epidermal necrolysis (TEN), and exfoliative dermatitis provoked by drugs cannot be differentiated from the same reactions resulting from other causes.

1 Kauppinen K. Cutaneous reactions to drugs. With special reference to severe mucocutaneous bullous eruptions and sulphonamides. *Acta Derm Venereol (Stockh)* 1972; **52** (Suppl 68): 1–89.
2 Kauppinen K, Stubb S. Drug eruptions: Causative agents and clinical types. A series of in-patients during a 10-year period. *Acta Derm Venereol (Stockh)* 1984; **64**: 320–4.
3 Davies DM (ed.) *Textbook of Adverse Drug Reactions*, 3rd edn. Oxford University Press, Oxford, 1985.
4 Bork K. *Kutane Arzneimittelnebenwirkungen. Unerwünschte Wirkungen systemisch verabreichter Medikamente an Haut und hautnahen Schleimhäuten bei Erwachsenen und Kindern.* Schattauer, Stuttgart, 1985.
5 Fellner MJ, Zeide DA (eds) Unexpected drug reactions. *Clin Dermatol* 1986; **4** (1).
6 Stern RS, Wintroub BU. Adverse drug reactions: reporting and evaluating cutaneous reactions. *Adv Dermatol* 1987; **2**: 3–18.
7 Seymour RA, Walton JG. *Adverse Drug Reactions in Dentistry*. Oxford University Press, Oxford, 1988.
8 Bork K. *Cutaneous Side Effects of Drugs*. WB Saunders, Philadelphia, 1988.
9 Dukes MNG (ed.) *Meylers Side Effects of Drugs*, 11th edn. Elsevier Science Publishers, Amsterdam, 1988.
10 Alanko K, Stubbs S, Kauppinen K. Cutaneous drug reactions: clinical types and causative agents. A five year survey of in-patients (1981–1985). *Acta Derm Venereol* 1989; **69**: 223–6.
11 Shear NH (ed.) Adverse reactions to drugs. *Semin Dermatol* 1989; **8**: 135–226.
12 Bruinsma WA. *A Guide to Drug Eruptions: The European File of Side Effects in Dermatology*, 5th edn. The File of Medicines, Oosthuizen, The Netherlands, 1990.
13 Kalish RS. Drug eruptions: a review of clinical and immunological features. *Adv Dermatol* 1991; **6**: 221–37.

14 Pavan-Langston D, Dunkel EC. *Handbook of Ocular Drug Therapy and Ocular Side Effects of Systemic Drugs*. Little, Brown, Boston, 1991.
15 Lever WF, Schaumburg-Lever G. *Histopathology of the Skin*, 7th edn. JB Lippincott, Philadelphia, 1990.

3.1 Exanthematic (maculopapular) reactions

Drug aetiology

These are the most frequent of all cutaneous reactions to drugs, and can occur after almost any drug at any time up to 2 weeks after administration. Ampicillin, amoxycillin, and sulphonamides are amongst the most frequent causes of a morbilliform eruption [1]. The commoner causes of an exanthematic drug eruption are listed in Table 3.1. In the case of some drugs such as penicillin and its derivatives, the eruption may first develop more than 2 weeks after initiation of therapy, or as much as 2 weeks after cessation of therapy. It is not possible to identify the offending drug by the nature of the eruption.

Clinical features

The clinical features are variable; the reaction may be accompanied by mild fever, pruritus and eosinophilia. Lesions may be scarlatiniform, rubelliform, or morbilliform (Fig. 3.1), or may consist of a profuse eruption of small papules showing no close resemblance to any infective exanthem. Less common are eruptions with large macules, polycylic and gyrate erythema, reticular eruptions (Fig. 3.2), and sheet-like erythema. The distribution is also variable, but it is generally symmetrical. Drug eruptions often start on the trunk, and may initially be pronounced at sites of therapeutic manipulation or trauma (Fig. 3.3). The trunk and extremities are usually involved, and not uncommonly intertriginous areas may be favoured, but the face may be spared. Palmar (Fig. 3.4) and plantar lesions may occur, and sometimes the eruption is generalized. Purpuric lesions, especially on the legs (Figs 3.5 & 3.6), and erosive stomatitis may develop. There may be relative sparing of pressure areas. Localized alterations in vascular supply may result in unusual variations. Thus, a predominantly unilateral erythematous maculopapular eruption occurred on the hemiplegic side of a patient with a head injury following phenytoin therapy, presumably as a result of altered vasomotor control [2]. A generalized drug reaction sparing a nevus depigmentosus has also been described [3].

If the administration of the drug is continued, an exfoliative dermatitis may develop. However, occasionally the eruption subsides despite continuation of the medication. Maculopapular drug eruptions usually fade with desquamation (Fig. 3.7), sometimes with postinflammatory hyperpigmentation, after 2 weeks. Morbilliform drug eruptions usually, but not always, recur on rechallenge.

Table 3.1 Drugs causing exanthematic reactions

Most common
Ampicillin and penicillin
Phenylbutazone and other
   pyrazolones
Sulphonamides
Phenytoin
Carbamazepine
Gold
Gentamicin

Less common
Cephalosporins
Barbiturates
Thiazides
Naproxen
Isoniazid
Phenothiazines
Quinidine
Meprobamate
Atropine

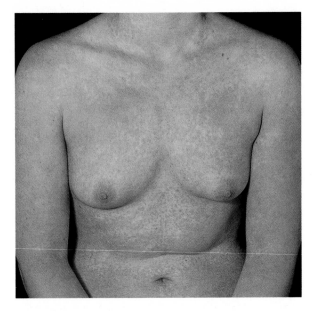

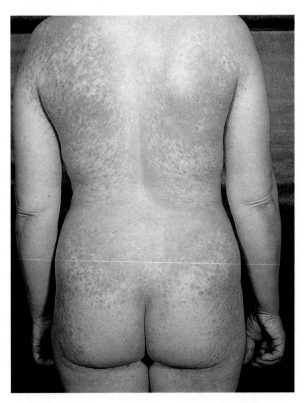

Figure 3.1 Generalized morbilliform erythematous drug eruption.

Figure 3.2 Widespread reticular erythematous drug eruption.

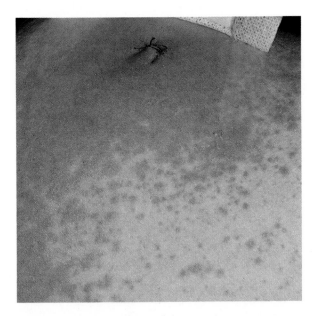

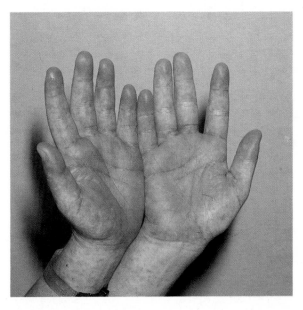

Figure 3.3 Maculopapular erythema due to trimethoprim-sulphamethoxazole(co-trimoxazole), centred around an incision site

Figure 3.4 Palmar erythema as a manifestation of a drug eruption to trimethoprim−suphamethoxazole (co-trimoxazole).

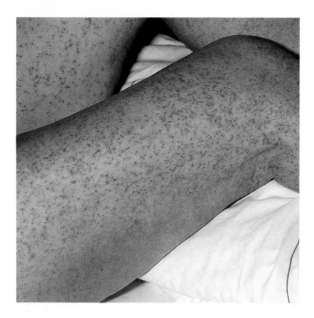

Figure 3.5 Mild purpuric changes in a drug eruption due to aztreonam.

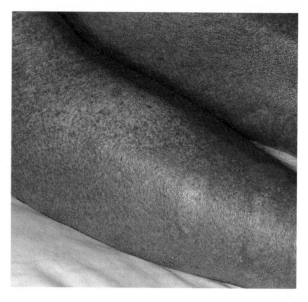

Figure 3.6 Marked purpura complicating a maculopapular eruption due to carbamazepine.

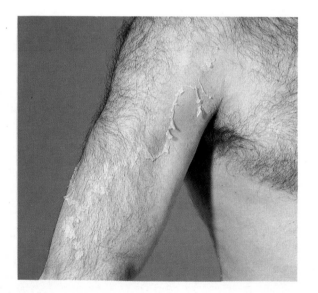

Figure 3.7 Desquamation subsequent to a generalized drug eruption caused by epicillin.

It is useful, in differentiating exanthematic drug eruptions from viral exanthemata, to remember that viral rashes may start on the face and progress to involve the trunk, and are more often accompanied by conjunctivitis, lymphadenopathy and fever.

Histology

Histological appearances are usually unremarkable, with mild perivascular lymphohistiocytic and eosinophil infiltration, with occasional red blood cell extravasation (Fig. 3.8).

[44]

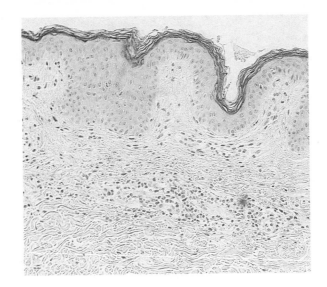

Figure 3.8 Lymphohistiocytic perivascular dermal infiltrate in a maculopapular drug eruption.

1 Porter J, Jick H. Amoxicillin and ampicillin rashes equally likely. *Lancet* 1980; **i**: 1037.
2 Basak P, Kanwar AJ, Mistri G. Drug rash in a hemiplegic. *Arch Dermatol* 1990; **126**: 688−9.
3 Naik RPC, Srinivas CR, Das PC. Generalized drug reaction sparing nevus depigmentosus. *Arch Dermatol* 1986; **122**: 509−10.

3.2 Purpura

Clinical features

Purpura occurs as a result of haemorrhage into the skin. A purpuric element to a drug eruption is not uncommon, but primarily purpuric drug-induced rashes also occur (Fig. 3.9). Accentuation of purpura may be seen in relation to application of a sphygmomanometer cuff, or at the site of application of suction cups for electrocardiography (Fig. 3.10).

Drug aetiology

Many drugs may interfere with platelet aggregation [1], but with the exception of aspirin this does not usually result in bleeding. A number of drugs have been implicated in the development of drug-induced purpura [2−4]. Several mechanisms may be involved. These include altered coagulation after anticoagulants or some cephalosporins, allergic and non-allergic thrombocytopenia, altered platelet function (as after valproic acid), or vascular causes, including steroid-induced fragility and loss of support. Cytotoxic drug therapy may result in non-allergic purpura due to bone marrow depression, with a platelet count of less than 30 000/mm^3. Bleomycin may induce thrombocytopenia by causing endothelial damage and consequent platelet aggregation [5]. A large number of drugs has been reported

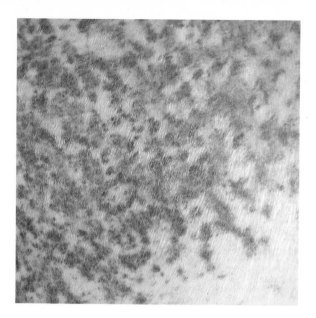

Figure 3.9 Purpuric drug eruption.

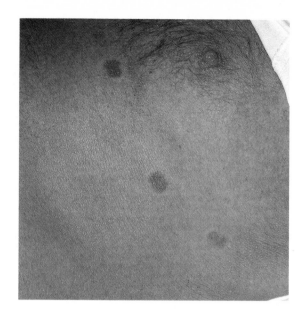

Figure 3.10 Accentuation of purpuric eruption at sites of electrocardiogram suction cups.

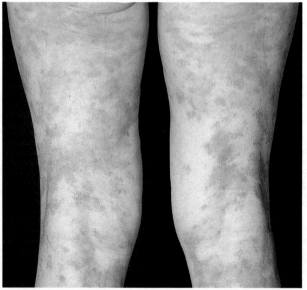

Figure 3.11 Pigmented purpuric eruption of capillaritis.

to cause allergic thrombocytopenia [2−4]. Heparin may cause purpura with overdosage or due to an allergic thrombocytopenia [6]. The classical example of complement-mediated destruction of platelets, following immune complex formation between a drug (as hapten) bound to the platelet surface and IgG class antibody, was the purpura caused by apronalide (Sedormid). Quinine, quinidine [7,8] and chlorothiazide may also cause allergic purpura. Tissue plasminogen activator (alteplase) has been associated with painful purpura [9]. A purpuric vasculitis-like rash followed secondary spread of a contact dermatitis to balsam of Peru [10].

[46]

Capillaritis (pigmented purpuric eruption) (Fig. 3.11) may be due to carbromal or more rarely to meprobamate [11,12], carbamazepine, and phenacetin; it may be due to formation of antibody to a drug–capillary endothelial cell complex [12]. Chronic pigmented purpura is recorded with thiamine propyldisulphide and chlordiazepoxide [13].

1 George JN, Shattil SJ. The clinical importance of acquired abnormalities of platelet function. *N Engl J Med* 1991; **324**: 27–39.
2 Miescher PA, Graf J. Drug-induced thrombocytopenia. *Clin Haematol* 1980; **9**: 505–19.
3 Moss RA. Drug-induced immune thrombocytopenia. *Am J Haematol* 1980; **9**: 439–46.
4 Bork K. *Cutaneous Side Effects of Drugs.* WB Saunders, Philadelphia, 1988.
5 Hilgard P, Hossfeld DK. Transient bleomycin-induced thrombocytopenia. A clinical study. *Eur J Cancer* 1978; **14**: 1261–4.
6 Babcock RB, Dumper CW, Scharfman WB. Heparin-induced thrombocytopenia. *N Engl J Med* 1976; **295**: 237–41.
7 Christie DJ, Weber RW, Mullen PC, *et al.* Structural features of the quinidine and quinine molecules necessary for binding of drug-induced antibodies to human platelets. *J Lab Clin Med* 1984; **104**: 730–40.
8 Gary M, Ilfeld D, Kelton JG. Correlation of a quinidine-induced platelet-specific antibody with development of thrombocytopenia. *Am J Med* 1985; **79**: 253–5.
9 DeTrana C, Hurwitz RM. Painful purpura: an adverse effect to a thrombolysin. *Arch Dermatol* 1990; **126**: 690–1.
10 Bruynzeel DP, van den Hoogenband HM, Koedijk F. Purpuric vasculitis-like eruption in a patient sensitive to balsam of Peru. *Contact Dermatitis* 1984; **11**: 207–9.
11 Peterson WC, Manick KP. Purpuric eruptions associated with use of carbromal and meprobamate. *Arch Dermatol* 1967; **95**: 40–2.
12 Carmel WJ, Dannenberg T. Nonthrombocytopenic purpura due to Miltown (2-methyl-2-n-propyl-1,3-propanediol dicarbamate). *N Engl J Med* 1956; **255**: 770–1.
13 Nishioka K, Katayama I, Masuzawa M, *et al.* Drug-induced chronic pigmented purpura. *J Dermatol (Tokyo)* 1989; **16**: 220–2.

3.3 Annular erythema

Annular or gyrate erythema represents a distinctive reaction pattern [1]. Erythema annulare centrifugum, in which the areas of annular erythema migrate slowly with time over the body surface, has been reported in association with chloroquine and hydroxychloroquine [2], oestrogens, cimetidine (Fig. 3.12) [3], penicillin, salicylates, and piroxicam, as well as with hydrochlorothiazide [4], spironolactone [5], thiacetazone [6], and the phenothiazine levomepromazin [7]. Annular erythema has occurred with vitamin K [8].

1 Hurley HJ, Hurley JP. The gyrate erythemas. *Semin Dermatol* 1984; **3**: 327–36.
2 Ashurst PJ. Erythema annulare centrifugum. Due to hydroxychloroquine sulfate and chloroquine sulfate. *Arch Dermatol* 1967; **95**: 37–9.
3 Merrett AC, Marks R, Dudley FJ. Cimetidine-induced erythema annulare centrifugum: no cross-sensitivity with ranitidine. *Br Med J* 1981; **283**: 698.
4 Goette DK, Beatrice E. Erythema annulare centrifugum caused by hydrochlorothiazide-induced interstitial nephritis. *Int J Dermatol* 1988; **27**: 129–30.

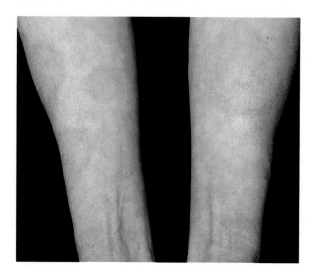

Figure 3.12 Annular erythematous eruption caused by cimetidine.

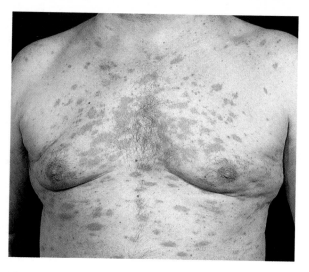

Figure 3.13 Pityriasiform eruption related to gold therapy.

5 Carsuzaa F, Pierre C, Dubegny M. Érytheme annulaire centrifuge a l'aldactone. *Ann Dermatol Vénéréol (Paris)* 1987; **114**: 375–6.
6 Ramesh V. Eruption resembling erythema annulare centrifugum. *Australas J Dermatol* 1987; **28**: 44.
7 Blazejak T, Hölzle E. Phenothiazin-induziertes Pseudolymphom. *Hautarzt* 1990; **41**: 161–3.
8 Kay MH, Duvic M. Reactive annular erythema after intramuscular vitamin K. *Cutis* 1986; **37**: 445–8.

3.4 Pityriasis rosea-like eruptions

Pityriasiform rashes consist of oval erythematous lesions with scaling adherent peripherally as a collarette, arranged with their long axes running down and out from the spine along the lines of the ribs. The best known drug cause of these eruptions is gold therapy (Fig. 3.13), but several other drugs have been implicated, including metronidazole [1], captopril [2] and isotretinoin [3], and are listed in Table 3.2.

Table 3.2 Drugs causing pityriasis rosea-like drug reactions

Arsenicals
Bismuth
Gold
Barbiturates
β-Blockers
Clonidine
Captopril
Griseofulvin
Isotretinoin
Metronidazole
Pyribenzamine
Methoxypromazine

1 Maize JC, Tomecki J. Pityriasis rosea-like drug eruption secondary to metronidazole. *Arch Dermatol* 1977; **113**: 1457–8.
2 Wilkin JK, Kirkendall WM. Pityriasis rosea-like rash from captopril. *Arch Dermatol* 1982; **118**: 186–7.
3 Helfman RJ, Brickman M, Fahey J. Isotretinoin dermatitis simulating acute pityriasis rosea. *Cutis* 1984; **33**: 297–300.

3.5 Psoriasiform eruptions

Psoriasiform eruptions typically consist of erythematous plaques surmounted by large dry silvery scales (Fig. 3.14). A number of drugs [1,2], principally β-blockers [1–4], antimalarials [5–8], lithium salts [9–11], and non-steroidal anti-inflammatory agents, have been reported to exacerbate psoriasis (Table 3.3). The effects of

[48]

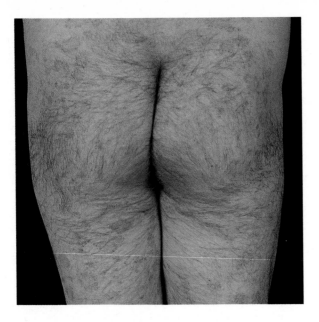

Figure 3.14 Psoriasiform drug eruption.

Table 3.3 Drugs reported to exacerbate psoriasis

Antimalarials
β-Blockers
Lithium salts
Non-steroidal anti-inflammatory agents
   Ibuprofen
   Indomethacin (but see text)
   Meclofenamate sodium
   Pyrazolone derivatives (phenylbutazone, oxyphenbutazone)
Miscellaneous
   Captopril
   Chlorthalidone
   Cimetidine
   Clonidine
   Gemfibrozil
   Interferon
   Methlydopa
   Penicillamine
   Penicillin
   Terfenadine
   Trazodone

chloroquine on psoriasis are variable. In a recent report, 88% of 50 psoriatics who were treated with standard doses of chloroquine noted no change in their psoriasis [7]; however, erythroderma has been provoked [8]. Generalized pustular psoriasis may develop following cessation of oral steroid therapy, or withdrawal of potent topical steroid therapy for plaque lesions [12]. Other drugs implicated in the worsening of established psoriasis in isolated reports include: tetracycline [13,14], gold therapy [15], potassium iodide [16], captopril and chlorthalidone [17,18], clonidine [19], the hypolipidaemic agent gemfibrozil [20], penicillin [21], ampicillin [22], terfenadine

[23], trazodone [24], and α-interferon [25–27]. Psoriatic patients frequently receive non-steroidal anti-inflammatory agents for management of the associated arthritis. Whilst in general it seems that such drugs do not appear to have an obvious direct adverse effect on psoriasis, indomethacin [28–30], diclofenac [30], phenylbutazone and oxyphenbutazone [31], ibuprofen [32], and meclofenamate [33] have been associated with worsening of psoriasis. However, indomethacin in a standard dose of 75 mg daily had no significant harmful effect on psoriasis in a series of patients treated with the Ingram regime (coal tar bath, followed by a sub-erythemal dose of ultraviolet B phototherapy, and dithranol in Lassar's paste) [34].

1 Bruinsma W. The file of side effects to the skin: A guide to drug eruptions. *Semin Dermatol* 1989; **8**: 141–3.

2 Abel EA, Dicicco LM, Orenberg EK, *et al*. Drugs in exacerbation of psoriasis. *J Am Acad Dermatol* 1986; **15**: 1007–22.

3 Heng MCY, Heng MK. Beta-adrenoceptor antagonist-induced psoriasiform eruption. Clinical and pathogenetic aspects. *Int J Dermatol* 1988; **27**: 619–27.

4 Gold MH, Holy AK, Roenigk HH Jr. Beta-blocking drugs and psoriasis. A review of cutaneous side effects and retrospective analysis of their effects on psoriasis. *J Am Acad Dermatol* 1988; **19**: 837–41.

5 Kuflik EG. Effect of antimalarial drugs on psoriasis. *Cutis* 1980; **26**: 153–8.

6 Nicolas J-F, Mauduit G, Haond J, *et al*. Psoriasis grave induit par la chloroquine (nivaquine). *Ann Dermatol Vénéréol (Paris)* 1988; **115**: 289–93.

7 Katugampola G, Katugampola S. Chloroquine and psoriasis. *Int J Dermatol* 1990; **29**: 153–4.

8 Slagel GA, James WD. Plaquenil-induced erythroderma. *J Am Acad Dermatol* 1985; **12**: 857–62.

9 Skott A, Mobacken H, Starmark JE. Exacerbation of psoriasis during lithium treatment. *Br J Dermatol* 1977; **96**: 445–8.

10 Lowe NJ, Ridgway HB. Generalized pustular psoriasis precipitated by lithium. *Arch Dermatol* 1978; **114**: 1788–9.

11 Sasaki T, Saito S, Aihara M, *et al*. Exacerbation of psoriasis during lithium treatment. *J Dermatol (Tokyo)* 1989; **16**: 59–63.

12 Boxley JD, Dawber RPR, Summerly R. Generalised pustular psoriasis on withdrawal of clobetasol propionate ointment. *Br Med J* 1975; **2**: 225–6.

13 Tsankov N, Botev-Zlatkov N, Lazarova AZ, *et al*. Psoriasis and drugs: influence of tetracyclines on the course of psoriasis. *J Am Acad Dermatol* 1988; **19**: 629–32.

14 Bergner T, Przybilla B. Psoriasis and tetracyclines. *J Am Acad Dermatol* 1990; **23**: 770.

15 Smith DL, Wernick R. Exacerbation of psoriasis by chrysotherapy. *Arch Dermatol* 1991; **127**: 268–270.

16 Shelley WB. Generalized pustular psoriasis induced by potassium iodide. *JAMA* 1967; **201**: 1009–14.

17 Wolf R, Dorfman B, Krakowski A. Psoriasiform eruption induced by captopril and chlorthalidone. *Cutis* 1987; **40**: 162–4.

18 Hauschild TT, Bauer R, Kreysel HW. Erstmanifestation einer eruptiv-exanthematischen Psoriasis vulgaris unter Captoprilmedikation. *Hautarzt* 1986; **37**: 274–7.

19 Wilkin J. Exacerbation of psoriasis during clonidine therapy. *Arch Dermatol* 1981; **117**: 4.

20 Fisher DA, Elias PM, LeBoit PL. Exacerbation of psoriasis by the hypolipidemic agent, gemfibrozil. *Arch Dermatol* 1988; **124**: 854–5.

21 Katz M, Seidenbaum M, Weinrauch L. Penicillin-induced generalised pustular psoriasis. *J Am Acad Dermatol* 1987; **17**: 918–20.

22 Saito S, Ikezawa Z. Psoriasiform intradermal test reaction to ABPC in a patient with psoriasis and ABPC allergy. *J Dermatol (Tokyo)* 1990; **17**: 677–83.

23 Harrison PV, Stones RN. Severe exacerbation of psoriasis due to terfenadine. *Clin Exp Dermatol* 1988; **13**: 271.

24 Barth JH, Baker H. Generalised pustular psoriasis precipitated by trazodone in the treatment of depression. *Br J Dermatol* 1986; **115**: 629–30.

25 Quesada JR, Gutterman JU. Psoriasis and alpha-inteferon. *Lancet* 1986; **i**: 1466–8.

26 Hartmann F, von Wussow P, Deicher H. Psoriasis — exacerbation bei therapie mit alpha-Interferon. *Dtsch Med Wochenschr* 1989; **114**: 96–8.

27 Jucgla A, Marcoval J, Curco N, Servitje O. Psoriasis with articular involvement induced by interferon alfa. *Arch Dermatol* 1991; **127**: 910–11.

28 Katayama H, Kawada A. Exacerbation of psoriasis induced by indomethacin. *J Dermatol (Tokyo)* 1981; **8**: 323–7.

29 Powles AV, Griffiths CEM, Seifert MH, Fry L. Exacerbation of psoriasis by indomethacin. *Br J Dermatol* 1987; **117**: 799–800.

30 Sendagorta E, Allegue F, Rocamora A, Ledo A. Generalized pustular psoriasis precipitated by diclofenac and indomethacin. *Dermatologica* 1987; **175**: 300–1.

31 Reshad H, Hargreaves GK, Vickers CFH. Generalized pustular psoriasis precipitated by phenylbutazone and oxyphenbutazone. *Br J Dermatol* 1983; **109**: 111–13.

32 Ben-Chetrit E, Rubinow O. Exacerbation of psoriasis by ibuprofen. *Cutis* 1986; **38**: 45.

33 Meyerhoff JO. Exacerbation of psoriasis with meclofenamate. *N Engl J Med* 1983; **309**: 496.

34 Sheehan-Dare RA, Goodfield MJD, Rowell NR. The effect of oral indomethacin on psoriasis treated with the Ingram regime. *Br J Dermatol* 1991; **125**: 253–5.

3.6 Erythroderma and exfoliative dermatitis

Clinical features

A widespread confluent erythema (erythroderma), often associated with desquamation (exfoliative dermatitis) is one of the most danger-ous patterns of cutaneous reaction to drugs [1–5]. It may follow exanthematic eruptions (Fig. 3.15) or may develop, as in some reactions to arsenicals and the heavy metals, as erythema and exu-dation in the flexures, rapidly generalizing. The eruption may start several weeks after initiation of the therapy. An eczematous derma-titis in patients previously sensitized by contact may also become universal.

Complications

Complications of this widespread erythematous and exfoliating dis-order (Fig. 3.16) include hypothermia, fluid and electrolyte loss, infection, cardiac failure, stress-induced gastrointestinal ulceration and haemorrhage, malabsorption, and venous thrombosis due to imposed bed rest and impaired circulation [5].

Drug aetiology

The main drugs implicated are listed in Table 3.4. In one large series, sulphonamides, antimalarials and penicillin were most fre-

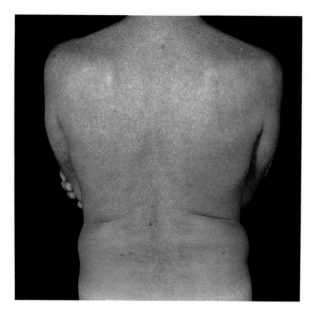 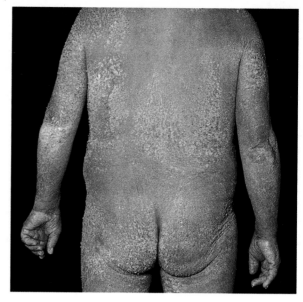

Figure 3.15 Erythrodermic drug eruption in a patient treated with penicillin and oxyphenbutazone.

Figure 3.16 Severe exfoliative dermatitis caused by a drug eruption.

Table 3.4 Drugs causing erythroderma and exfoliative dermatitis

Allopurinol
p-Aminosalicylic acid
Ampicillin
Barbiturates
Captopril
Carbamazepine
Cefoxitin
Chloroquine
Chlorpromazine
Cimetidine
Diltiazem
Gold
Griseofulvin
Hydantoins
Isoniazid
Lithium
Nitrofurantoin
D-Penicillamine
Penicillin
Phenylbutazone
Quinidine
Streptomycin
Sulphonamides
Sulphonylureas
Thiacetazone

quently implicated [1]. In another series from India [3], the commonest associated drugs were isoniazid (20%), thiacetazone (15%), topical tar (15%), and a variety of homoeopathic medicines (20%), with phenylbutazone, streptomycin, and sulphadiazine each accounting for 5% of cases. Phenytoin is a well-recognized cause [6]. Recently incriminated drugs have included captopril, cefoxitin, cimetidine, and ampicillin [7].

1 Nicolis GD, Helwig EB. Exfoliative dermatitis. A clinicopathologic study of 135 cases. *Arch Dermatol* 1973; **108**: 788–97.
2 Hasan T, Jansén DT. Erythroderma: A follow-up of fifty cases. *J Am Acad Dermatol* 1983; **8**: 836–4.
3 Sehgal VN, Srivastava G. Exfoliative dermatitis. A prospective study of 80 patients. *Dermatologica* 1986; **173**: 278–84.
4 Sage T, Faure M. Conduite a tenir devant les érythrodermies de l'adulte. *Ann Dermatol Vénéréol (Paris)* 1989; **116**: 747–52.
5 Irvine C. 'Skin failure' — a real entity: discussion paper. *J R Soc Med* 1991; **84**: 412–13.
6 Danno K, Kume M, Ohta M, *et al.* Erythroderma with generalized lymphadenopathy induced by phenytoin. *J Dermatol (Tokyo)* 1989; **16**: 392–6.
7 Saito S, Ikezawa Z. Psoriasiform intradermal test reaction to ABPC in a patient with psoriasis and ABPC allergy. *J Dermatol (Tokyo)* 1990; **17**: 677–83.

3.7 Anaphylaxis and anaphylactoid reactions

Clinical features

This systemic reaction, which usually develops within minutes to hours (the vast majority within the first hour), is often severe and may be fatal [1,2]. Biphasic reactions, in which symptoms are delayed or recurrent and appear many hours after an initial reaction, occur occasionally [3]. In less severe cases, there may be premonitory dizziness or faintness, skin tingling and reddening of the bulbar conjunctiva, followed by urticaria, angioneurotic oedema, bronchospasm, abdominal pain, and vasomotor collapse. Swelling of the lips and tongue may impair swallowing and ventilation; upper airway obstruction may develop as a result of oedema of the larynx, epiglottis or surrounding tissue. It usually develops on second exposure to a drug, but may develop during the first treatment if this lasts sufficiently long for sensitization to occur. However, anaphylaxis is unlikely to occur with a drug taken continuously for several months; by contrast, intermittent administration may predispose to anaphylaxis [1]. It is commoner after parenteral than oral drug administration. β-Blockers enhance anaphylactic reactions caused by other allergens, and may make resuscitation more difficult [4,5].

Drug aetiology

The principal drug causes are shown in Table 3.5. Antibiotics (especially penicillin) and radiocontrast media are the most common known causes of anaphylactic events [2]; the incidence of such reactions for each is about 1 in 5000 exposures [6,7], of which less than 10% are fatal [2]. The risk for recurrent anaphylactic reactions is 10–20% for penicillins [6] and 20–40% for radiocontrast media [8]. Anaphylaxis may be caused by massive release of histamine and other mediators, following cross-linkage of IgE on mast cells and basophils, as with allergy to penicillin, and to some muscle relaxants [9]. Histamine is probably the main mediator responsible for the clinical manifestations [10].

Anaphylactoid reactions are those which clinically resemble an immediate immune response but in which the mechanism is undetermined. Potential causes include complement activation by immune complexes, with generation of anaphylatoxins such as C3a or C5a which can trigger release of mediators from mast cells or basophils directly. Some drugs and agents, such as mannitol and radiographic contrast media, can stimulate mediator release by an as yet unknown direct mechanism independent of IgE or complement. Anaphylactoid reactions may be produced by non-steroidal analgesics and anti-inflammatory reagents [11,12], including aspirin and other salicylates, indomethacin, phenylbutazone, propyphenazone, metimazol and tolmetin [13], as well as by radiographic contrast media, *d*-tubocurarine, benzoic acid preservatives [14], tartrazine dyes, and sulphite preservatives [15]. Patients with anaphylactic reactions to the pyrazolone group of anti-inflammatory agents may demonstrate contact urticaria at 30–60 minutes on patch testing [16].

1 Sussman GL, Dolovich J. Prevention of anaphylaxis. *Semin Dermatol* 1989; **8**: 158–65.

Table 3.5 Drugs causing urticaria or anaphylaxis

Animal sera
Vaccines containing egg protein
Desensitizing agents including
   pollen vaccines
Antibiotics
   Penicillins
   Cephalosporins
   Aminoglycosides
   Tetracyclines
   Sulphonamides
Antifungal agents
   Fluconazole
   Ketoconazole
Blood products
Angiotensin converting enzyme
   inhibitors
Radiographic contrast media
Non-steroidal anti-inflammatory
   agents (NSAIDs)
   Salicylates
   Other NSAIDs
      (e.g. phenylbutazone,
      aminopyrine, propyphenazone,
      metamizol, tolmetin)
Narcotic analgesics
Anaesthetic agents (local and general)
Muscle relaxants
   Suxamethonium
   Curare
Dextrans
Mannitol
Sorbitol complexes
Enzymes
   Trypsin
   Streptokinase
   Chymopapain
Steroids
   Progesterone
   Hydrocortisone
Polypeptide hormones
   Insulin
   Corticotrophin
   Vasopressin
Food and drug additives
   Benzoates
   Sulphites
   Tartrazine dyes
Hydantoins
Hydralazine
Quinidine
Anticancer drugs
Vitamins
Protamine

2 Bochner BS, Lichtenstein LM. Anaphylaxis. *N Engl J Med* 1991; **324**: 1785−90.

3 Stark BJ, Sullivan RJ. Biphasic and protracted anaphylaxis. *J Allergy Clin Immunol* 1986; **78**: 76−83.

4 Hannaway PJ, Hopper GDK. Severe anaphylaxis and drug-induced beta-blockade. *N Engl J Med* 1983; **308**: 1536.

5 Toogood JH. Risk of anaphylaxis in patients receiving beta-blocker drugs. *J Allergy Clin Immunol;* 1988; **81**: 1−5.

6 Weiss ME, Adkinson NF. Immediate hypersensitivity reactions to penicillin and related antibiotics. *Clin Allergy* 1988; **18**: 515−40.

7 Ansell G, Tweedie MCK, West DR, *et al.* The current status of reactions to intravenous contrast media. *Invest Radiol* 1980; **15** (Suppl 6): S32−S39.

8 Greenberger P, Patterson R, Kelly J, *et al.* Administration of radiographic contrast media in high-risk patients. *Invest Radiol* 1980; **15** (Suppl 6): S40−S43.

9 Vervloet D, Nizankowska E, Arnaud A, *et al.* Adverse reactions to suxamethonium and other muscle relaxants under general anesthesia. *J Allergy Clin Immunol* 1983; **71**: 552−9.

10 Kaliner M, Shelhamer JH, Ottesen EA. Effects of infused histamine: correlation of plasma histamine levels and symptoms. *J Allergy Clin Immunol* 1982; **69**: 283−9.

11 Antépara I, Martín-Gil D, Dominguez MA, Oehling A. Adverse drug reactions produced by analgesic drugs. *Allergol Immunopathol* 1981; **9**: 545−54.

12 Stevenson DD. Diagnosis, prevention and treatment of adverse reactions to aspirin (ASA) and nonsteroidal anti-inflammatory drugs (NSAID). *J Allergy Clin Immunol* 1984; **74**: 617−22.

13 Rossi AC, Knapp DE. Tolmetin-induced anaphylactoid reactions. *N Engl J Med* 1982; **307**: 499−500.

14 Michils A, Vandermoten G, Duchateau J, Yernault J-C. Anaphylaxis with sodium benzoate. *Lancet* 1991; **337**: 1424−5.

15 Twarog FJ, Leung DYM. Anaphylaxis to a component of isoetharine (sodium bisulfite). *JAMA* 1982; **248**: 2030−1.

16 Maucher OM, Fuchs A. Kontakturtikaria im Epikutantest bei Pyrazolonallergie. *Hautarzt* 1983: **34**; 383−6.

3.8 Urticaria

Clinical features

Urticaria is, after an exanthematous eruption, the second most common type of drug reaction. Urticaria involves circumscribed, raised, oedematous, erythematous wheals widely scattered on the body (Fig. 3.17); it may accompany systemic anaphylaxis or 'serum sickness' reactions [1−3]. Individual lesions rarely persist for more than 24 hours. Urticaria usually occurs within 36 hours of drug administration; on rechallenge, lesions may develop within minutes. Angioedema [4], involving oedema of the deep dermis or subcutaneous and submucosal areas (Fig. 3.18), is more rarely seen than urticaria as an adverse drug reaction, and occurs in less than 1% of patients receiving the particular drug.

Drug aetiology

The commoner drug causes of urticaria/angioedema are listed in Table 3.5. The frequency of urticaria/angioedema or anaphylactic responses to aspirin and other non-steroidal anti-inflammatory drugs is about 1% in an outpatient population [5] and is familial [6].

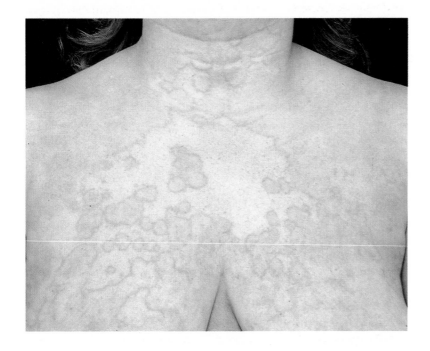

Figure 3.17 Urticarial eruption with characteristic wheals.

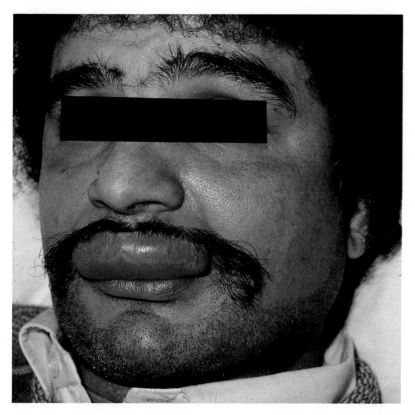

Figure 3.18 Angioedema of the upper lip in a patient treated with penicillin and aspirin.

Aspirin (salicylates) may also aggravate chronic urticaria [1,2,7−9]. In addition, an unsuspected agent, e.g. the yellow dye tartrazine, may really be responsible for an urticaria attributed to aspirin or another drug [6,8]. The analgesic codeine is also a cause of urticaria [10]. While penicillin is a very well documented cause of acute urticaria, the role of this drug in the aetiology of chronic urticaria is controversial [11]. Urticaria develops in about 1% of patients receiving blood transfusions [12]. There have been numerous papers on the potential role of food and drug additives [13−18], including preservatives such as benzoic acid, butylated hydroxyanisole (BHA), butylated hydroxytoluene (BHT) [19], sulphites [20] and rarely aspartame [21], as well as tartrazine dyes [22,23], in the development of chronic urticaria. However, a recent study suggested that common food additives are seldom if ever of significance in urticaria [24]. Urticaria may follow alcohol consumption [25]. Urticarial and papular plaques have been reported as a presentation of contact allergy to proflavine and to permanent waving lotion [26].

Some drugs, for example aspirin, are capable of inducing urticaria by either an allergic or a pharmacological mechanism. Allergic urticaria is the cutaneous manifestation of a Type I reaction mediated by IgE antibodies, or of a Type III reaction in which the antigen forms a complement-fixing complex with antibody, resulting in histamine release following generation of anaphylatoxins; penicillin allergy may cause urticaria by either mechanism. Certain drugs, such as opiates, codeine, amphetamine, polymyxin B, *d*-tubocurarine, atropine, hydralazine, pentamidine, quinine and radiocontrast media, may release mast cell mediators directly (see Chapter 2: anaphylactoid reactions). Cyclooxygenase inhibitors, such as aspirin and indomethacin, and angiotensin converting enzyme inhibitors, such as captopril and enalapril, may cause urticaria or angioedema by pharmacological mechanisms. Cyclooxygenase inhibition may lead to amplified mast cell degranulation and enhanced biosynthesis of lipoxygenase products of arachidonic acid, which cause vasodilation and oedema [27]. Angiotensin converting enzyme inhibitors may potentiate bradykinin activity; they have been reported to enhance bradykinin-induced cutaneous wheals in normal individuals [28,29].

1 Champion RH, Greaves MW, Kobza Black A (eds) *The Urticarias*. Churchill Livingstone, Edinburgh, 1985.
2 Soter NA. Acute and chronic urticaria and angioedema. *J Am Acad Dermatol* 1991; **25**: 146−54.
3 Soter NA. Treatment of urticaria and angioedema: low-sedating H_1-type antihistamines. *J Am Acad Dermatol* 1991; **24**: 1084−7.
4 Greaves M, Lawlor F. Angioedema: manifestations and management. *J Am Acad Dermatol* 1991; **25**: 155−65.
5 Chaffee FH, Settipane GA. Aspirin intolerance. I. Frequency in an allergic population. *J Allergy Clin Immunol* 1974; **53**: 193−9.
6 Settipane GA, Pudupakkam RK. Aspirin intolerance. III. Subtypes, familial occurrence and cross reactivity with tartrazine. *J Allergy Clin Immunol* 1975; **56**: 215−21.

7 Juhlin L, Michäelsson G, Zetterström O. Urticaria and asthma induced by food-and-drug additives in patients with aspirin hypersensitivity. *J Allergy Clin Immunol* 1972; **50**: 92−8.

8 Doeglas HMG. Reactions to aspirin and food additives in patients with chronic urticaria, including the physical urticarias. *Br J Dermatol* 1975; **93**: 135−44.

9 Settipane RA, Constantine HP, Settipane GA. Aspirin intolerance and recurrent urticaria in normal adults and children. Epidemiology and review. *Allergy* 1980; **35**: 149−54.

10 De Groot AC, Conemans J. Allergic urticarial rash from oral codeine. *Contact Dermatitis* 1986; **14**: 209−14.

11 Boonk WJ, Van Ketel WG. The role of penicillin in the pathogenesis of chronic urticaria. *Br J Dermatol* 1982; **106**: 183−90.

12 Shulman IA. Adverse reactions to blood transfusion. *Texas Med* 1990; **85**: 35−42.

13 Juhlin LG, Michäelsson G, Zetterström O. Urticaria and asthma induced by food-and-drug additives in patients with aspirin hypersensitivity. *J Allergy* 1972; **50**: 92−8.

14 Levantine AJ, Almeyda J. Cutaneous reactions to food and drug additives. *Br J Dermatol* 1977; **91**: 359−62.

15 Simon RA. Adverse reactions to drug additives. *J Allergy Clin Immunol* 1984; **74**: 623−30.

16 Hannuksela M, Lahti A. Peroral challenge tests with food additives in urticaria and atopic dermatitis. *Int J Dermatol* 1986; **25**: 178−80.

17 Supramaniam G, Warner JO. Artificial food additives intolerance in patients with angioedema and urticaria. *Lancet* 1986; **ii**: 907−9.

18 Juhlin L. Additives and chronic urticaria. *Ann Allergy* 1987; **59**: 119−23.

19 Goodman DL, McDonnell JT, Nelson HS, *et al*. Chronic urticaria exacerbated by the antioxidant food preservatives, butylated hydroxyanisole (BHA) and butylated hydroxytoluene (BHT). *J Allergy Clin Immunol* 1990; **86**: 570−5.

20 Settipane GA. Adverse reactions to sulfites in drugs and foods. *J Am Acad Dermatol* 1984; **10**: 1077−80.

21 Kulczycki A Jr. Aspartame-induced urticaria. *Ann Intern Med* 1986; **104**: 207−8.

22 Neuman I, Elian R, Nahum H, *et al*. The danger of 'yellow dyes' (tartrazine) to allergic subjects. *J Allergy* 1972; **50**: 92−8.

23 Miller K. Sensitivity to tartrazine. *Br Med J* 1982; **285**: 1597−8.

24 Hannuksela M, Lahti A. Peroral challenge tests with food additives in urticaria and atopic dermatitis. *Int J Dermatol* 1986; **25**: 178−80.

25 Ormerod AD, Holt PJA. Acute urticaria due to alcohol. *Br J Dermatol* 1983; **108**: 723−4.

26 Goh CL. Urticarial papular and plaque eruptions. A noneczematous manifestation of allergic contact dermatitis. *Int J Dermatol* 1989; **28**: 172−6.

27 Stevenson DD, Lewis RA. Proposed mechanisms of aspirin sensitivity reactions. *J Allergy Clin Immunol* 1987; **80**: 788−90.

28 Wood SM. Angio-oedema and urticaria associated with angiotensin converting enzyme inhibitors. *Br Med J* 1987; **294**: 91−2.

29 Ferner RE. Effects of intradermal bradykinin after inhibition of angiotensin converting enzyme. *Br Med J* 1987; **294**: 1119−20.

3.9 Serum sickness

Clinical features

Serum sickness may occur from between 5 days and up to 3 weeks after initial exposure, and is a manifestation of a Type III immune complex-mediated reaction [1−4]. Serum sickness in its complete form combines fever, urticaria (often figurate or polycyclic), angioedema, joint pain and swelling (especially of the hands and feet), lymphadenopathy, and occasionally nephritis or endocarditis, with eosinophilia. Rarely, neuritis develops and is not always fully reversible, with pain in the neck, shoulder or arm. In minor forms of serum sickness, fever, urticaria and transitory joint tenderness may be the only manifestations.

Drug aetiology

This reaction may be produced by amongst other drugs heterologous serum [1,2], aspirin, penicillin [3], streptomycin, sulphonamides, thiouracils and globulin preparations. Serum sickness developed in a series of patients treated with intravenous infusions of horse antithymocyte globulin for bone marrow failure [1,2]. A characteristic serpiginous, erythematous and purpuric eruption developed on the hands and feet at the borders of palmar and plantar skin. Circulating immune complexes, low serum C4 and C3 levels, and elevated plasma C3a anaphylatoxin levels, were found. Direct immunofluorescence revealed the presence of immunoreactants including IgM, C3, IgE, and IgA in the walls of dermal blood vessels [1,2].

1 Lawley TJ, Bielory L, Gascon P, *et al*. A prospective clinical and immunologic analysis of patients with serum sickness. *N Engl J Med* 1984; **311**: 1407–13.
2 Bielory L, Yancey KB, Young NS, *et al*. Cutaneous manifestations of serum sickness in patients receiving antithymocyte globulin. *J Am Acad Dermatol* 1985; **13**: 411–17.
3 Erffmeyer JE. Serum sickness. *Ann Allergy* 1986; **56**: 105–9.
4 Lin RY. Serum sickness syndrome. *Am Fam Physician* 1986; **33**: 157–62.

3.10 Erythema multiforme and the Stevens–Johnson syndrome

Clinical features of erythema multiforme

Erythema multiforme is a very well recognized pattern of adverse cutaneous drug reaction [1–8], although as it is more commonly precipitated by various infections, many instances may have been wrongly blamed on drugs. Clinically, macular, papular, or urticarial lesions, as well as the classical iris or 'target lesions' (Figs 3.19 & 3.20), sometimes with central vesicles, bullae or purpura, are distributed preferentially on the distal extremities, especially the dorsa of the hands and the extensor forearms. Lesions may involve the palms or trunk, as well as the oral (Figs 3.21 & 3.22) and genital mucous membranes. Occasionally, mucous membrane involvement is all that is seen.

Drug aetiology of erythema multiforme

In a prospective study of cases of erythema multiforme, only 10% were drug related [4]. However, re-exposure has confirmed a drug

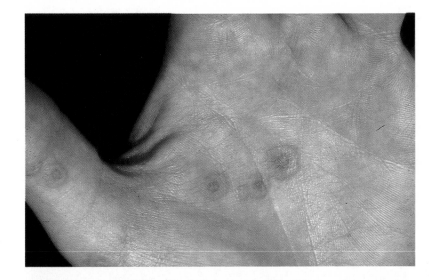

Figure 3.19 Typical target lesions of erythema multiforme.

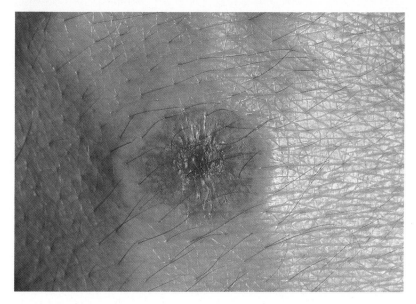

Figure 3.20 Close-up view of a target lesion in erythema multiforme.

cause in many instances, so that sulphonamides and co-trimoxazole, barbiturates, pyrazolone derivatives (phenylbutazone), phenolphthalein, rifampicin, penicillins, hydantoin derivatives, carbamazepine, phenothiazines, chlorpropamide, thiazide diuretics, and sulphones have all been implicated (Table 3.6). Recent reports have incriminated phenazone, minoxidil, fenbrufen, mianserin, sulindac, methaqualone, ceftazidime [9], and trazodone [10]. Progesterone has also been implicated [11]. Erythema multiforme may follow vaccination. A large number of topical medications may induce erythema multiforme-like eruptions [12], including: balsam of Peru, chloramphenicol, econazole, ethylenediamine, furazolidone, mafenide acetate cream used to treat burns, the muscle relaxant mephensin, neomycin, nifuroxime, promethazine, scopolamine, sulphonamides

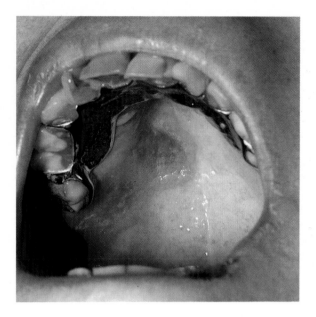 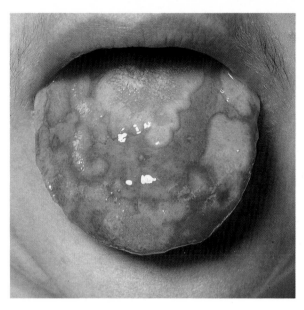

Figure 3.21 Erosions on the hard palate in a patient with drug-related erythema multiforme.

Figure 3.22 Extensive erosions of the tongue in drug-related erythema multiforme.

[13,14], ophthalmic anticholinergic preparations (scopolamine hydrobromide and tropicamide drops) [15], vitamin E, and the antimycotic agent pyrrolnitrin, as well as proflavine [16]. In addition, contact with a number of environmental substances may induce erythema multiforme-like reactions [17], including: nickel, formaldehyde, trichloroethylene, phenyl sulphone derivative, the insecticide methyl parathion, nitrogen mustard, epoxy compounds [18], and also trinitrotoluene [19].

Clinical features of the Stevens—Johnson syndrome

The Stevens—Johnson syndrome [1—3,7,8,20] comprises fever, malaise, myalgia, arthralgia, and extensive erythema multiforme of the trunk (Fig. 3.23), with occasional skin blisters and erosions covering less than 10% of the body's surface area. Abnormalities of liver function may be present [8]. Stevens—Johnson syndrome (Figs 3.24 & 3.25) should be differentiated from TEN, in which sheet-like erosions involve more than 10% of the body surface, and in which there is severe involvement of conjunctival, corneal, irideal, buccal, labial and genital mucous membranes.

Drug aetiology of Stevens—Johnson syndrome

Drugs potentially causing Stevens—Johnson syndrome are listed in Table 3.6. A retrospective study from Malaysia reported that the most common causes of Stevens—Johnson syndrome were sulphonamides, tetracycline, and the penicillin derivatives [5]. In the US, non-steroidal anti-inflammatory drugs were reported to be an important cause [21]. Severe Stevens−Johnson-like reactions have been described resulting from sulphonamides with or without trimethoprim [22−24] and following malaria prophylaxis with Fansidar (pyrimethamine and sulphadoxine) [25,26]. Patients with acquired immunodeficiency syndrome (AIDS) seem to be at an increased risk of developing severe Stevens−Johnson reactions to co-trimoxazole, possibly because of a systemic glutathione deficiency and a resultant decreased capacity to scavenge hydroxylamine derivatives of sulphamethoxazole, and thiacetazone [27−29]. Re-exposure to drugs suspected of causing a reaction has resulted in fatality and should not be carried out for diagnostic purposes [1].

Histology of erythema multiforme/Stevens−Johnson syndrome

Histological analysis distinguishes three types of lesion in the erythema multiforme/Stevens−Johnson syndrome spectrum [30−33]. The dermal type, seen in macular and most papular lesions, shows perivascular infiltration with lymphocytes, with variable eosinophil infiltration and papillary oedema; bullae may be due to subepidermal or intra-epidermal separation. The mixed dermal and epidermal type, seen in papular, plaque and target lesions, is characterized by dermal changes of a mononuclear cell infiltrate in a perivascular distribution and at the dermo-epidermal junction, upper dermal red cell extravasation, and subepidermal bulla formation, in conjunction with epidermal basal cell hydropic change, scattered individually necrotic keratinocytes, spongiosis, mononuclear cell exocytosis, and areas of epidermal necrosis. The histology of the epidermal type, seen in some target lesions of erythema multiforme, and in Stevens−Johnson syndrome, resembles that of TEN, with a sparse dermal perivascular infiltrate, mononuclear cell exocytosis, and extensive necrosis of the epidermis leading to sub-epidermal or intra-epidermal blistering.

Immunopathogenesis of erythema multiforme/Stevens−Johnson syndrome

Deposits of IgM and C3 may be found in the walls of superficial blood vessels in erythema multiforme [4,6,34−37], especially in lesions less than 24 hours old [34]. Circulating immune complexes have been reported [35,36], and it has been proposed that immune complex deposition may be important in the pathogenesis. However, the clinical features are quite unlike those of an immune complex vasculitis, and the vascular changes may occur as a result of a secondary phenomenon. Herpes simplex genome has been identified in the lesions of herpes-induced erythema multiforme [38], which suggests that virus-specific T lymphocytes might mediate the skin changes in this situation. By extrapolation, it is possible that drug hapten-specific T cells could be involved in the pathogenesis of

Table 3.6 Drugs causing erythema multiforme or Stevens−Johnson syndrome

Antibiotics
Sulphonamides
  Trimethoprim−sulphamethoxazole
  Sulphadoxine−pyrimethamine
Sulphones
Penicillins
Ceftazidime
Griseofulvin
Rifampicin
Tetracyclines

Non-steroidal anti-inflammatory agents
Salicylates
Fenbrufen
Ibuprofen
Sulindac
Pyrazolone derivatives
  Antipyrine
  Phenylbutazone
  Phenazone

Metals
Arsenic
Bromides
Mercury
Gold
Iodides

Anticonvulsants
Barbiturates
Carbamazepine
Hydantoin derivatives
Trimethadione

Antihypertensives
Frusemide
Hydralazine
Minoxidil
Thiazide diuretics

Drugs acting on the CNS
Mianserin
Phenothiazines
Trazodone

Miscellaneous
Chlorpropamide
Codeine
Cyclophosphamide
Methaqualone
Nitrogen mustard
Pentazocine
Phenolphthalein
Progesterone
Vaccination

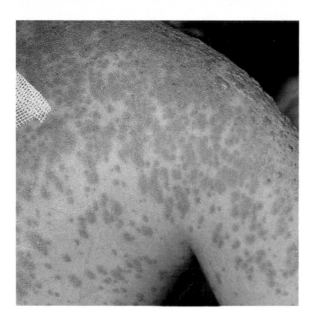

Figure 3.23 Extensive erythema multiforme lesions in Stevens—Johnson syndrome caused by salazosulphapyridine.

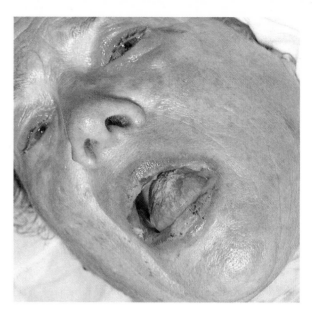

Figure 3.24 Severe ocular and oral mucous membrane involvement in Stevens—Johnson syndrome following vaccination with tetanus toxoid.

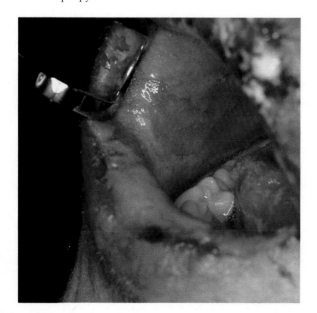

Figure 3.25 Extensive involvement of the lip and buccal mucous membrane in Stevens—Johnson syndrome; patient receiving multiple drug therapy.

drug-induced erythema multiforme and Stevens—Johnson syndrome. An alternative theory, in view of the multiplicity of potential triggering factors for the conditions, would be that these diverse stimuli trigger induction of an autoimmune reaction resulting in the common clinical presentation.

1 Bianchine JR, Macaraeg PVJ, Lasagna L, *et al*. Drugs as etiologic factors in the Stevens—Johnson syndrome. *Am J Med* 1968; **44**: 390−405.
2 Kauppinen K. Cutaneous reactions to drugs. With special reference to severe

mucocutaneous bullous eruptions and sulphonamides. *Acta Derm Venereol (Stockh)* 1972; **52** (Suppl 68): 1–89.

3 Böttiger LE, Strandberg I, Westerholm B. Drug-induced febrile mucocutaneous syndrome. With a survey of the literature *Acta Med Scand* 1975; **198**: 229–33.

4 Huff JC, Weston WL, Tonnesen MG. Erythema multiforme: A critical review of characteristics, diagnostic criteria, and causes. *J Am Acad Dermatol* 1983; **8**: 763–75.

5 Gebel K, Hornstein OP. Drug-induced oral erythema multiforme. Results of a long-term retrospective study. *Dermatologica* 1984; **168**: 35–40.

6 Howland WW, Golitz LE, Weston WL, Huff JC. Erythema multiforme: Clinical, histopathologic, and immunologic study. *J Am Acad Dermatol* 1984; **10**: 438–46.

7 Ruiz-Maldonado R. Acute disseminated epidermal necrosis types 1, 2, and 3: Study of sixty cases. *J Am Acad Dermatol* 1985; **13**: 623–35.

8 Nethercott JR, Choi BC. Erythema multiforme (Stevens–Johnson syndrome) — chart review of 123 hospitalized patients. *Dermatologica* 1985; **171**: 383–96.

9 Pierce TH, Vig SJ, Ingram PM. Ceftazidime in the treatment of lower respiratory tract infection. *J Antimicrob Chemother* 1983; **12** (Suppl A): 21–5.

10 Ford HE, Jenike MA. Erythema multiforme associated with trazadone therapy. *J Clin Psychiatry* 1985; **46**: 294–5.

11 Wojnarowska F, Greaves MW, Peachey RDG, *et al.* Progesterone-induced erythema multiforme. *J R Soc Med* 1985; **78**: 407–8.

12 Fisher AA. Erythema multiforme-like eruptions due to topical medications: Part II. *Cutis* 1986; **37**: 158–61.

13 Gottschalk HR, Stone OJ. Stevens–Johnson syndrome from ophthalmic sulfonamide. *Arch Dermatol* 1976; **112**: 513–14.

14 Genvert GI, Cohen EJ, Donnenfeld ED, Blecher MH. Erythema multiforme after use of topical sulfacetamide. *Am J Ophthalmol* 1985; **99**: 465–8.

15 Guill MA, Goette DK, Knight CG, *et al.* Erythema multiforme and urticaria. Eruptions induced by chemically related ophthalmic anticholinergic reagents. *Arch Dermatol* 1979; **115**: 742–3.

16 Goh CL. Erythema multiforme-like and purpuric eruption due to contact allergy to proflavine. *Contact Dermatitis* 1987; **17**: 53–4.

17 Fisher AA. Erythema multiforme-like eruptions due to topical miscellaneous compounds: Part III. *Cutis* 1986; **37**: 262–4.

18 Whitfield MJ, Rivers JK. Erythema multiforme after contact dermatitis in response to an epoxy sealant. *J Am Acad Dermatol* 1991; **25**: 386–8.

19 Goh CL. Erythema multiforme-like eruption from trinitrotoluene allergy. *Int J Dermatol* 1988; **27**: 650–1.

20 Ting HC, Adam BA. Stevens–Johnson syndrome, a review of 34 cases. *Int J Dermatol* 1985; **24**: 587–91.

21 Stern R, Bigby M. An expanded profile of cutaneous reactions to nonsteroidal anti-inflammatory drugs. *JAMA* 1984; **252**: 1433–7.

22 Carrol OM, Bryan PA, Robinson RJ. Stevens–Johnson syndrome associated with long-acting sulfonamides. *JAMA* 1966; **195**: 691–3.

23 Azinge NO, Garrick GA. Stevens–Johnson syndrome (erythema multiforme) following ingestion of trimethoprim–sulfamethoxazole on two separate occasions in the same person. A case report. *J Allergy Clin Immunol* 1978; **62**: 125–6.

24 Aberer W, Stingl G, Wolff K. Stevens–Johnson-Syndrom und toxische epidermale Nekrolyse nach Sulfonamideinnahme. *Hautarzt* 1982; **33**: 484–90.

25 Hornstein OP, Ruprecht KW. Fansidar-induced Stevens–Johnson syndrome. *N Engl J Med* 1982; **307**: 1529–30.

26 Miller KD, Lobel HO, Satriale RF, *et al.* Severe cutaneous reactions among American travelers using pyrimethamine–sulfadoxine (Fansidar) for malaria prophylaxis. *Am J Trop Med Hyg* 1986; **35**: 451–8.

27 Porteous DM, Berger TG. Severe cutaneous drug reactions (Stevens–Johnson syndrome and toxic epidermal necrolysis) in human immunodeficiency virus infection. *Arch Dermatol* 1991; **127**: 740–1.

28 De Raeve L, Song M, Van Maldergem L. Adverse cutaneous drug reactions in AIDS. *Br J Dermatol* 1988; **119**: 521–3.

29 van der Ven AJAM, Koopmans PP, Vree TB, van der Meer JWM. Adverse reactions to co-trimoxazole in HIV infection. *Lancet* 1991; **338**: 431−3.

30 Lever WF, Schaumburg-Lever G. *Histopathology of the Skin*, 7th edn. JB Lippincott, Philadelphia, 1990.

31 Ackermann AB, Ragaz A. Erythema multiforme. *Am J Dermatopathol* 1985; **8**: 133−9.

32 Lever WF. My concept of erythema multiforme. *Am J Dermatopathol* 1985; **8**: 141−2.

33 Reed RJ. Erythema multiforme. A clinical syndrome and a histologic complex. *Am J Dermatopathol* 1985; **8**: 143−52.

34 Kazmierowski JA, Wuepper KD. Erythema multiforme: Immune complex vasculitis of the superficial cutaneous microvasculature. *J Invest Dermatol* 1978; **71**: 366−9.

35 Imamura S, Yanase K, Taniguchi S, *et al*. Erythema multiforme: Demonstration of immune complexes in the sera and skin lesions. *Br J Dermatol* 1980; **102**: 161−6.

36 Bushkell LL, Mackel SE, Jordon RE. Erythema multiforme: Direct immunofluorescence studies and detection of circulating immune complexes. *J Invest Dermatol* 1980; **74**: 372−4.

37 Finan MC, Schroeter AL. Cutaneous immunofluorescence studies of erythema multiforme: Correlation with light microscopic patterns and etiologic agents. *J Am Acad Dermatol* 1984; **10**: 497−506.

38 Brice SL, Krzemien D, Weston WL, *et al*. Detection of herpes simplex virus DNA in cutaneous lesions of erythema multiforme. *J Invest Dermatol* 1989; **93**: 183−7.

3.11 Toxic epidermal necrolysis (TEN)

Clinical features

There is a degree of overlap between Stevens−Johnson syndrome and TEN; Stevens−Johnson syndrome may evolve into TEN, and several drugs can produce both entities [1−11]. Clinically, TEN presents with a prodromal period with flu-like symptoms (malaise, fever, rhinitis, and conjunctivitis), sometimes accompanied by difficulty in urination, which usually lasts 2−3 days; however, it may last from 1 day to 3 weeks before signs of skin involvement develop. The acute phase of TEN is characterized by persistent fever, mucous membrane involvement and generalized epidermal sloughing, and lasts from 8 to 12 days. There may be an initial 'burning' maculopapular, urticarial or erythema multiforme-like eruption. There is rapid progression to areas of confluent erythema, often starting in the axillae and groins, followed by blistering and sloughing of large areas of skin (Figs 3.26−3.28). Nikolsky's sign, the ability to extend the area of superficial sloughing by gentle lateral pressure on the surface of the skin at an apparently unaffected site, may be positive. Blisters on the palms and soles may remain intact, although the whole of the skin of these regions may be denuded. The process tends to occur in waves, over a 3-day period, but involvement of the whole of the body surface occurs within 24 hours in about 10% of cases.

Mucous membranes (particularly the buccal, and less commonly the genital, perianal, nasal, conjunctival, tracheal, bronchial, pharyngeal and oesophageal ones) are often involved (Fig. 3.29). Mucous

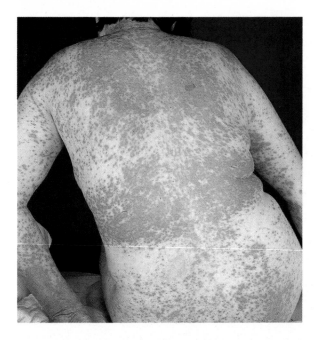

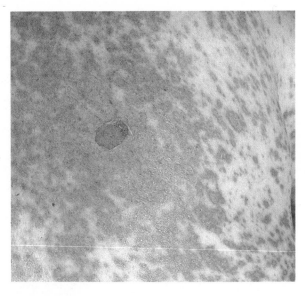

Figure 3.27 Close-up view of eroded area in toxic epidermal necrolysis (site of positive Nikolsky's test).

Figure 3.26 Widespread erythema and incipient blistering, with focal erosion, in early toxic epidermal necrolysis caused by co-trimoxazole (trimethoprim–sulphamethoxazole).

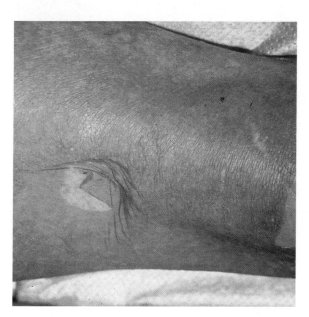

Figure 3.28 Generalized epidermal sloughing in toxic epidermal necrolysis due to co-trimoxazole (trimethoprim–sulphamethoxazole).

membrane lesions may precede the skin lesions by up to 3 days in one-third of cases [10]. Urethritis develops in up to two-thirds of patients, and may lead to urinary retention. Stomatitis and mucositis lead to impaired oral intake with consequent malnutrition and dehydration. Intestinal involvement has been documented [12]. Healing occurs by re-epithelialization; this may occur within a few days on the anterior thorax, but is slower on the back and at intertriginous areas. Most patients completely heal their skin lesions in about 3–4 weeks, but mucosal lesions take longer, and the glans penis may take up to 2 months to heal over.

[65]

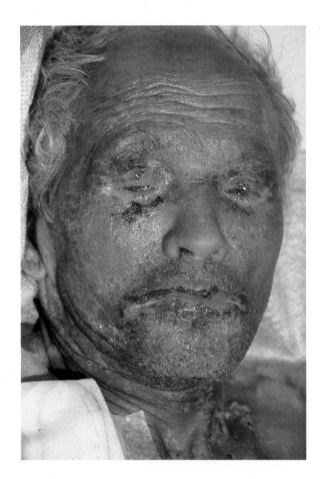

Figure 3.29 Severe involvement of ocular and labial mucous membranes in toxic epidermal necrolysis due to co-trimoxazole (trimethoprim-sulphamethoxazole).

Complications

Mucocutaneous complications of TEN [11] include wound infections, pigmentary changes (either hyperpigmentation or hypopigmentation), nail shedding or dystrophy, hypohidrosis, scarring alopecia, and hypertrophic scarring which may lead to contractures. Development of melanocytic naevi has been reported [13]. Mucosal involvement may lead to chronic xerostomia, oesophageal strictures, phimosis, and chronic orogenital erosions. Ocular complications occur in 40–50% of survivors [10] and include [14]: conjunctivitis, pseudomembrane formation, photophobia, ectropion, entropion with trichiasis, symblepharon, and corneal vascularization, corneal opacities, and corneal ulceration and scarring [4,15,16]. Blindness may result. Lacrimal duct destruction may result in xerophthalmia. A Sjögren-like sicca syndrome may be seen [17]. Ankylosymblepharon (fusion of eyelids to each other and to the globe) may follow secondary infection.

Pneumonia or pneumonitis occurs in up to 30% of patients, contributed to by sloughing of the tracheobronchial tree. Anaemia or leucopenia, due to selective depletion of $CD4^+$ helper T cells, is moderately common [10]. Disseminated intravascular coagulation is documented. Septicaemia, primarily the result of *Staphylococcus aureus* or *Pseudomonas*, but on occasion due to Gram-negative organisms or *Candida*, may result from infection of the skin, lungs, urinary tract catheters, and intravenous (especially central) lines. There is an appreciable mortality as a result of TEN, of the order of 20–30%, which is due to infection in more than half the cases [10]. Elderly patients and those with extensive TEN have a worse prognosis. Hypovolaemia, gastrointestinal haemorrhage, and pulmonary emboli are also causes of death. It has been claimed that severe granulocytopenia is a poor prognostic indicator [18], although this has been disputed on the basis that lymphopenia is more usually found in severe TEN [19].

Drug aetiology

A large number of different drugs have been implicated [11], but the commonest triggers (Table 3.7) include anti-epileptic drugs (phenytoin, barbiturates and carbamazepine), sulphonamides, ampicillin, allopurinol, and non-steroidal anti-inflammatory drugs (especially pyrazolone derivatives, e.g phenylbutazone, and oxicam derivatives), and pentamidine [1–11,20]. The absolute incidence of phenytoin-induced TEN is very low, with nine cases reported in the US over the past decade, compared with 2 million Americans who take phenytoin [11]. In France, a recent survey showed two main classes of drug were most often responsible: antibacterial agents (especially sulphonamides); non-steroidal anti-inflammatory agents including isoxicam, oxyphenbutazone, and fenbufen; and phenytoin [21]. Isoxicam and oxyphenbutazone were withdrawn from the French market accordingly. The incidence of erythema multiforme, Stevens–Johnson syndrome, and TEN in a US series with the following drugs was reported as follows: phenobarbital 20, nitrofurantoin 7, co-trimoxazole and ampicillin each 3, and amoxycillin 2 per 100 000 exposed patients [22]. In India by contrast, one-third of cases are the result of drugs used for the treatment of tuberculosis, especially thiacetazone and isoniazid [23]. Review of the English language literature from 1966 to 1987 suggested that allopurinol, non-steroidal anti-inflammatory agents, phenytoin and the sulphonamide antibiotics were most frequently responsible [24]. A recent study from the US reported that penicillins, especially aminopenicillins, were most frequently implicated [25]. In West Germany, drugs most frequently implicated were antibiotics (sulphonamides and β-lactam agents) and analgesics and non-steroidal anti-inflammatory agents [26]. Griseofulvin [27,28], and immunization with diphtheria–pertussis–tetanus (DPT), measles, poliomyelitis, smallpox and influenza vaccines [11], are less frequently implicated. A single case of fatal TEN following the second exposure to diatrizoate solution for excretory pyelography has been documented [29].

Identification of the responsible drug is often difficult, because patients frequently take more than one medication (an average of

Table 3.7 Drugs causing toxic epidermal necrolysis

Antibiotics
Sulphonamides
Penicillins
   Amoxycillin
   Ampicillin
Ethambutol
Isoniazid
Streptomycin
Tetracycline
Thiacetazone

Non-steroidal anti-inflammatory agents
Pyrazolone derivatives
   Phenylbutazone
   Oxyphenbutazone
Oxicam derivatives
   Isoxicam
Fenbufen
Salicylates

Anticonvulsants
Barbiturates
Carbamazepine
Phenytoin

Miscellaneous
Allopurinol
Chlorpromazine
Dapsone
Gold
Griseofulvin
Nitrofurantoin
Pentamidine
Tolbutamide
Vaccination

4.4 in one series) [7,30]. A helpful guide-line is that most drugs which cause TEN have been first given between 1 and 3 weeks previously [10,11]; another very suggestive guide is that of recurrence within 48 hours on administration of a drug previously recorded as having caused a similar reaction. A given drug is unlikely to be responsible for TEN if it was first given 24 hours previously, or if the duration of treatment exceeds 3 weeks [7,11]. However, phenytoin-induced TEN may occur any time between 2 and 8 weeks after initiation of therapy, and may progress despite discontinuation of phenytoin days or weeks earlier [31]. Unfortunately, there is no reliable test to confirm the aetiological role of a given drug in an individual case [10], and the *in vitro* lymphocyte transformation test [32] is of no value.

Histology

The histology [33] of early lesions is characterized by moderate perivascular mononuclear cell infiltration in the papillary dermis, with epidermal spongiosis and exocytosis. Satellite cell necrosis, with close apposition of mononuclear cells to necrotic keratinocytes, may be seen. In established TEN, there is full thickness necrosis of the epidermis (Fig. 3.30), with little in the way of any dermal abnormality.

Immunopathogenesis

The general consensus is that TEN has an immunological basis [34]. It has been suggested that there may be a genetic susceptibility to TEN; HLA-A29, HLA-B12, and HLA-DR7 were linked with sulphonamide-induced TEN in a study from France [35]. Patients with systemic lupus erythematosus may be at an increased risk of developing TEN [36]. Moreover, TEN bears clinical and histological similarities to graft-versus-host disease, a T cell-mediated disease [5,34,37−41]. Lymphocytopenia with depletion in the circulating helper/inducer subset of T lymphocytes has been reported in patients with TEN [39].

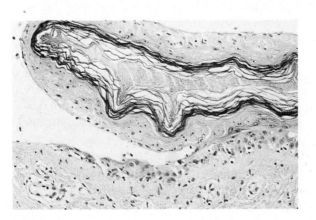

Figure 3.30 Full thickness necrosis of folded, stripped-off epidermis in toxic epidermal necrolysis.

[68]

There have been few reports on the immunophenotyping of cells in the cutaneous inflammatory infiltrate in TEN. CD8$^+$ suppressor/cytotoxic T lymphocytes were prominent along the dermo-epidermal junction and within the involved epidermis, while CD4$^+$ helper/inducer T cells predominated within the dermis, in a patient with bromisovalum-induced TEN [42]. In another case report of TEN, the majority of inflammatory cells were of helper/inducer T cell phenotype [40]. There have been several cases in which skin tests (intradermal and/or patch tests) have demonstrated delayed hypersensitivity to the offending drug [42–44]. Immunohistochemical localization of immunoglobulins and complement to the intercellular region of the basal layer of the epidermis was reported in two cases [45]; however, this has not been a consistent finding in other studies [10].

Differential diagnosis from staphylococcal scalded skin syndrome

Drug-induced TEN is rare in children, in whom it must be distinguished from the staphylococcal scalded skin syndrome (SSSS), in which blister formation results from intra-epidermal, subcorneal splitting caused by a toxin produced by *Staphylococcus aureus* group II, phage type 71 [46]. However, SSSS may occur in adults (Fig. 3.31) and therefore forms an important differential diagnosis of TEN. Examination of frozen sections of the roof of a blister will enable rapid distinction between the two, since the level of splitting is subcorneal in SSSS (Fig. 3.32), and much lower in drug-induced TEN, where the full thickness of the necrotic epidermis forms the roof of the blister (Fig. 3.30) [47,48].

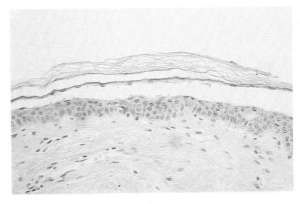

Figure 3.32 Subcorneal splitting of the epidermis in staphylococcal scalded skin syndrome.

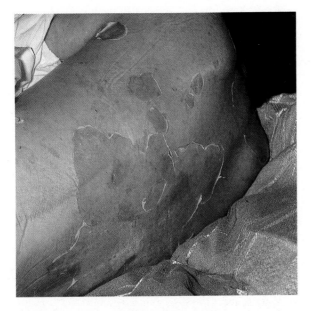

Figure 3.31 Widespread superficial sloughing of the skin in staphylococcal scalded skin syndrome.

1 Kauppinen K. Cutaneous reactions to drugs. With special reference to severe mucocutaneous bullous eruptions and sulphonamides. *Acta Derm Venereol (Stockh)* 1972; **52** (Suppl 68): 1–89.

2 Lyell A. Toxic epidermal necrolysis (the scalded skin syndrome): A reappraisal. *Br J Dermatol* 1979; **100**: 69–86.

3 Rasmussen JE. Toxic epidermal necrolysis. *Med Clin North Am* 1980; **64**: 901–20.

4 Chan HL. Observations on drug-induced toxic epidermal necrolysis in Singapore. *J Am Acad Dermatol* 1984; **10**: 973–8.

5 Heng MCY. Drug-induced toxic epidermal necrolysis. *Br J Dermatol* 1985; **113**: 597–600.

6 Fabrizio PJ, McCloshey WW, Jeffrey LP. Drugs causing toxic epidermal necrolysis. *Drug Intell Clin Pharm* 1985; **19**: 733–5.

7 Guillaume J-C, Roujeau J-C, Penso D, *et al*. The culprit drugs in 87 cases of toxic epidermal necrolysis (Lyell's syndrome). *Arch Dermatol* 1987; **123**: 1166–70.

8 Revuz J, Penso D, Roujeau J-C, *et al*. Toxic epidermal necrolysis. Clinical findings and prognosis factors in 87 patients. *Arch Dermatol* 1987; **123**: 1160–5.

9 Editorial. Toxic epidermal necrolysis. Unmuddying the waters. *Arch Dermatol* 1987; **123**: 1153–6.

10 Roujeau J-C, Chosidow O, Saiag P, Guillaume J-C. Toxic epidermal necrolysis (Lyell syndrome). *J Am Acad Dermatol* 1990; **23**: 1039–58.

11 Avakian R, Flowers FP, Araujo OE, Ramos-Caro FA. Toxic epidermal necrolysis: a review. *J Am Acad Dermatol* 1991; **25**: 69–79.

12 Chosidow O, Delchier J-C, Chaumette M-T, *et al*. Intestinal involvement in drug-induced toxic epidermal necrolysis. *Lancet* 1991; **337**: 928.

13 Burns DA, Sarkany I. Junctional naevi following toxic epidermal necrolysis. *Clin Exp Dermatol* 1978; **3**: 323–6.

14 De Felice GP, Caroli R, Autelitano A. Long-term complications of toxic epidermal necrolysis (Lyell's disease): clinical and histopathologic study. *Ophthalmologica* 1987; **195**: 1–6.

15 Ruiz-Maldonado R. Acute disseminated epidermal necrosis types 1, 2 and 3: study of 60 cases. *J Am Acad Dermatol* 1985; **13**: 623–35.

16 Tham TCK, Allen G, Hayes D, *et al*. Possible association between toxic epidermal necrolysis and ciprofloxacin. *Lancet* 1991; **338**: 522.

17 Roujeau J-C, Phlippoteau C, Koso M, *et al*. Sjögren-like syndrome after drug-induced toxic epidermal necrolysis. *Lancet* 1985; **i**: 609–11.

18 Westly ED, Wechsler HL. Toxic epidermal necrolysis. Granulocytic leukopenia as a prognostic indicator. *Arch Dermatol* 1984; **120**: 721–6.

19 Roujeau JC, Guillaume JC, Revuz J, *et al*. Granulocytes, lymphocytes and toxic epidermal necrolysis. *Arch Dermatol* 1985; **121**: 305.

20 Stratigos JD, Bartsokas SK, Capetanakis J. Further experiences of toxic epidermal necrolysis incriminating allopurinol, pyrazolone, and derivatives. *Br J Dermatol* 1972; **86**: 564–7.

21 Roujeau J-C, Guillaume J-C, Fabre J-D, *et al*. Toxic epidermal necrolysis (Lyell syndrome). Incidence and drug etiology in France, 1981–1985. *Arch Dermatol* 1990; **126**: 37–42.

22 Chan H-L, Stern RS, Arndt KA, *et al*. The incidence of erythema multiforme, Stevens–Johnson syndrome, and toxic epidermal necrolysis. A population-based study with particular reference to reactions caused by drugs among outpatients. *Arch Dermatol* 1990; **126**: 43–7.

23 Nanda A, Kaur S. Drug-induced toxic epidermal necrolysis in developing countries. *Arch Dermatol* 1990; **126**: 125.

24 Stern RS, Chan H-L. Usefulness of case report literature in determining drugs responsible for toxic epidermal necrolysis. *J Am Acad Dermatol* 1989; **21**: 317–22.

25 Strom BL, Carson JL, Halpern AC, *et al*. A population-based study of Stevens–Johnson syndrome. Incidence and antecedent drug exposures. *Arch Dermatol* 1991; **127**: 831–8.

26 Schöpf E, Stühmer A, Rzany B, *et al*. Toxic epidermal necrolysis and Stevens–Johnson syndrome. An epidemiologic study from West Germany. *Arch Dermatol* 1991; **127**: 839–42.

27 Taylor B, Duffill M. Toxic epidermal necrolysis from griseofulvin. *J Am Acad Dermatol* 1988; **19**: 565–7.

28 Mion G, Verdon G, Le Gulluche Y, *et al*. Fatal toxic epidermal necrolysis after griseofulvin. *Lancet* 1989; **ii**: 1331.

29 Kaftori JK, Abraham Z, Gilhar A. Toxic epidermal necrolysis after excretory pyelography. Immunologic-mediated contrast medium reaction? *Int J Dermatol* 1988; **27**: 346–7.

30 Prendiville JS, Hebert AA, Greenwald MJ, *et al*. Management of Stevens–Johnson syndrome and toxic epidermal necrolysis in children. *J Pediatr* 1989; **115**: 881–7.

31 Kelly DF, Hope DG. Fatal phenytoin-related toxic epidermal necrolysis: case report. *Neurosurgery* 1989; **25**: 976–8.

32 Roujeau JC, Albengres E, Moritz S, *et al*. Lymphocyte transformation test in drug-induced toxic epidermal necrolysis. *Int Arch Allergy Appl Immunol* 1985; **78**: 22–4.

33 Lever WF, Schaumburg-Lever G. *Histopathology of the Skin*, 7th edn. JB Lippincott, Philadelphia, 1990.

34 Goens J, Song M, Fondu P, *et al*. Haematological disturbances and immune mechanisms in toxic epidermal necrolysis. *Br J Dermatol* 1986; **114**: 255–9.

35 Roujeau J-C, Huynh TN, Bracq C, *et al*. Genetic susceptibility to toxic epidermal necrolysis. *Arch Dermatol* 1987; **123**: 1171–3.

36 Burge SM, Dawber RPR. Stevens–Johnson syndrome and toxic epidermal necrolysis in a patient with systemic lupus erythematosus. *J Am Acad Dermatol* 1985; **13**: 665–6.

37 Peck GL, Herzig GP, Elias PM. Toxic epidermal necrolysis in a patient with graft-vs-host reaction. *Arch Dermatol* 1972; **105**: 561–9.

38 Saurat JH. Cutaneous manifestations of graft-vs-host disease. *Int J Dermatol* 1981; **20**: 249–56.

39 Roujeau JC, Moritz S, Guillaume JC, *et al*. Lymphopenia and abnormal balance of T-lymphocyte subpopulations in toxic epidermal necrolysis. *Arch Dermatol* 1985; **277**: 24–7.

40 Merot Y, Gravallese E, Guillén FJ, Murphy GF. Lymphocyte subsets and Langerhans' cells in toxic epidermal necrolysis. Report of a case. *Arch Dermatol* 1986; **122**: 455–8.

41 Villada G, Roujeau J-C, Cordonnier C, *et al*. Toxic epidermal necrolysis after bone marrow transplantation: Study of nine cases. *J Am Acad Dermatol* 1990; **23**: 870–5.

42 Miyauchi H, Hosokawa H, Akaeda T, *et al*. T-cell subsets in drug-induced toxic epidermal necrolysis. *Arch Dermatol* 1991; **127**: 851–5.

43 Tagami H, Tatsuta K, Iwatsuki K, *et al*. Delayed hypersensitivity in ampicillin-induced toxic epidermal necrolysis. *Arch Dermatol* 1983; **119**: 910–13.

44 Schopf D, Schulz KH, Kessler R, *et al*. Allergologische Untersuchungen beim Lyell-Syndrome. *Z Hautkr* 1975; **50**: 865–73.

45 Stein KM, Schlappner OLA, Heaton CL, Decherd JW. Demonstration of basal cell immunofluorescence in drug-induced toxic epidermal necrolysis. *Br J Dermatol* 1972; **86**: 246–52.

46 Rasmussen JE. Toxic epidermal necrolysis, a review of 75 cases in children. *Arch Dermatol* 1975; **111**: 1135–9.

47 Amon RB, Dimond RL. Toxic epidermal necrolysis. Rapid differentiation between staphylococcal- and drug-induced disease. *Arch Dermatol* 1975; **111**: 1433–7.

48 Ochsendorf FR, Schöfer H, Milbradt R. Diagnostik des 'Lyell-Syndroms': SSSS oder TEN? *Dtsch Med Wochenschr* 1988; **113**: 860–3.

3.12 Fixed drug eruptions

Clinical features [1—11]

Fixed eruptions characteristically recur in the same site or sites each time the drug is administered; with each exposure, however, the number of involved sites may increase. Usually just one drug is involved, although independent lesions from more than one drug have been described [12,13]. Cross-sensitivity to related drugs may occur, such as between phenylbutazone and oxyphenbutazone and between tetracycline-type drugs, and there are occasional reports of recurrences at the same site induced by drugs which appear to be chemically unrelated, e.g. oxyphenbutazone and tetracycline [9,14]. Sometimes the inducing drug can be re-administered without exacerbation [5], and there may be a refractory period after the occurrence of a fixed eruption. Fixed drug eruption may occasionally occur only with a combination preparation, and not to the individual constituents [15].

Acute lesions are sharply marginated, round or oval plaques of erythema and oedema becoming dusky violaceous (Fig. 3.33) or brown in colour, and sometimes surmounted by vesiculation or bulla formation (Figs 3.34 & 3.35). They usually develop within 30 minutes to 8 hours of drug administration, and are associated with itching or burning. Local or constitutional symptoms are usually mild or absent; systemic symptoms are, however, recorded [9]. The eruption may initially be morbilliform, scarlatiniform, or erythema multiforme-like; urticarial, nodular or eczematous lesions are less common [9]. Lesions are sometimes solitary at first, but with repeated attacks new lesions usually appear and existing lesions may increase in size. A multifocal bullous fixed drug eruption due to mefenamic acid resembled erythema multiforme [16]. Occasionally, involvement is so extensive as to mimic TEN (see Fig. 4.7, p. 148) [17,18].

Lesions are commoner on the limbs than on the trunk; the hands and feet, genitalia (glans penis) (Fig. 3.36) and perianal areas are favoured sites. Perioral and periorbital lesions may occur. Genital [19] and oral mucous membranes [20] may be involved in association with skin lesions, or alone. In the case of isolated male genital fixed drug eruption (often affecting only the glans penis), the drugs most commonly implicated in one series were: co-trimoxazole (trimethoprim—sulphamethoxazole), tetracycline and ampicillin [19]. Pigmentation of the tongue may occur as a form of fixed drug eruption in heroin addicts [21]. A curious linear fixed drug eruption to intramuscular cephazolin has occurred [22].

As healing occurs, crusting and scaling are followed by pigmentation, which may be very persistent and occasionally extensive, especially in pigmented individuals [9]; pigmentation may be all that is visible between attacks (Fig. 3.37). Diffuse hypermelanosis of extensive areas of trunk, face or limbs is perhaps more common in the Negro [6]. Non-pigmenting fixed reactions have been reported

[72]

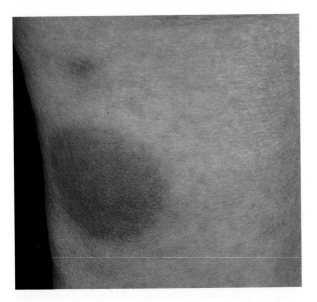

Figure 3.33 Well-defined dusky erythema in a fixed drug eruption due to co-trimoxazole (trimethoprim–sulphamethoxazole).

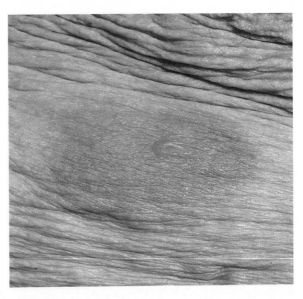

Figure 3.34 Erythema with overlying vesiculation in fixed drug eruption due to co-trimoxazole (trimethoprim–sulphamethoxazole).

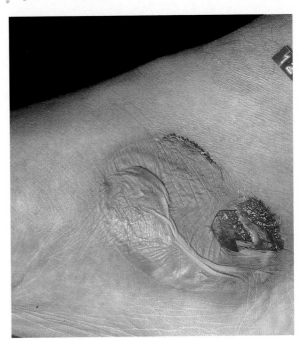

Figure 3.35 Marked blistering of a lesion in fixed drug eruption due to co-trimoxazole (trimethoprim–sulphamethoxazole).

in association with pseudoephedrine, tetrahydrozoline, piroxicam and the radiopaque contrast medium iothalamate [23–25].

Drug aetiology

The number of drugs capable of producing fixed eruptions is very large [9], and it is no longer possible to give a list of the most common causes that will remain valid for many years. However,

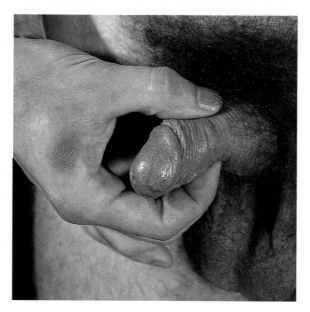

Figure 3.36 Fixed drug eruption due to sulphamethoxydiazine; typical involvement of the hand and glans penis.

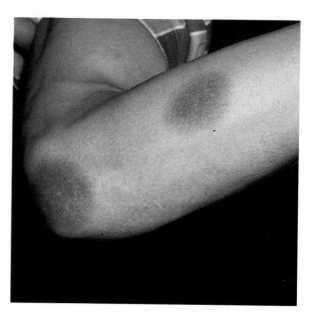

Figure 3.37 Postinflammatory hyperpigmentation in lesions of fixed drug eruption due to sulpha-methoxydiazine.

most fixed drug reactions are due to one or other of the substances listed in Table 3.8. Earlier series incriminated particularly analgesics, sulphonamides and tetracyclines [2,4]. In a recent report from Finland, phenazones caused most eruptions, with barbiturates, sulphonamides, tetracyclines and carbamazepine causing fewer reactions [26]. A series from India reported that acetylsalicylic acid was the drug most commonly implicated in children [27]. Even apparently innocuous preparations such as magnesium trisilicate given for relief of dyspepsia have been reported to cause fixed eruptions, in the latter case confirmed by challenge [28]. Dextro-methorphan, used as an antitussive, has also caused a fixed reaction [29]. Patch testing in a previously involved site, but not in normal skin, may yield a positive response in a proportion of cases of fixed drug eruption, especially with phenazone (pyrazolone) derivatives (e.g. phenylbutazone) [30].

Histology [9,31]

In the acute stage, the epidermal changes may be indistinguishable from those seen in erythema multiforme. Hydropic degeneration of epidermal basal cells results in pigmentary incontinence, and scattered individually necrotic keratinocytes may be seen. Subepidermal bulla formation may develop, with dermal oedema, vascular dilatation, and a conspicuous perivascular lymphohistiocytic infiltrate. There is increased melanin in the epidermis and within melanophages in the dermis, which persists between attacks.

[74]

Table 3.8 Drugs causing fixed eruptions [9]

Antibacterial substances
Sulphonamides (co-trimoxazole)
Tetracyclines
Penicillin
Ampicillin
Amoxycillin
Erythromycin
Trimethoprim
Nystatin
Griseofulvin
Dapsone
Arsenicals
Mercury salts
p-Aminosalicylic acid
Thiacetazone
Quinine
Metronidazole

Barbiturates and other tranquillizers
Barbiturate derivatives
Opium alkaloids
Chloral hydrate
Benzodiazepines
   Chlordiazepoxide
Anticonvulsants
Dextromethorphan

Non-steroidal anti-inflammatory agents
Aspirin (acetylsalicylic acid)
Oxyphenbutazone
Phenazone (antipyrine)
Metimazole
Paracetamol
Ibuprofen
Various non-proprietary analgesic combinations

Phenolphthalein and related compounds

Miscellaneous
Hydralazine
Oleoresins
Sympathomimetics
Sympatholytics
Parasympatholytics
   Hyoscine butylbromide
Magnesium hydroxide
Magnesium trisilicate
Anthralin
Chlorthiazone
Chlorphenesin carbamate
Food substitutes and flavours

Immunopathogenesis of fixed drug eruption

The results of graft autotransplantation investigations carried out in
the 1930s were conflicting [7,9], with two studies [32,33] reporting
that the epidermis is the primary site of cutaneous memory in fixed
drug eruption, while other reports suggested the importance of

[75]

dermal factors [34,35]. A role for serum factors has been postulated. Sustained inflammation occurred on injection of a thermolabile agent (not the drug itself), present in serum obtained during an acute episode of fixed drug reaction, into a previously involved site, but not into normal skin [36]. Furthermore, autologous serum from patients with fixed drug eruption produced lymphocyte blast transformation, which increased on addition of the causative drug, while the drug alone did not induce blast transformation [37]. A soluble cutaneous extract fractionated by gel filtration was as potent as autologous serum in inducing lymphocyte blastogenesis in another study [38].

Direct immunofluorescence revealed deposition of IgG and C3 in the epidermal intercellular cement substance of lesional skin only, in cases of fixed drug eruption to phenolphthalein [39] and paracetamol [40]. However, in other reports, immunofluorescence demonstrated only binding of fibrin to the dermo-epidermal junction [41], or showed basement membrane zone deposition of IgM and C3 in only one of five cases [42]. Thus, humoral immunity mediated by immunoreactants is not thought to play a major role in the development of lesions in this condition. It is thought more likely that cell-mediated immune reactions are involved.

Lesional skin contains increased numbers of T lymphocytes, of both helper and suppressor cell phenotypes [42−45]. Epidermal T suppressor/cytotoxic T cells may be seen adjacent to necrotic keratinocytes in well-formed lesions [43]. The persistence of T cells within lesional skin may be of significance to immunological memory [46], and thus to the recurrence of lesions at identical sites. In this regard, it is of interest that CD8$^+$ suppressor/cytotoxic T cells were observed in suprabasal epidermis in biopsies of involved skin 3 weeks after challenge [42]. The fact that keratinocytes in lesional skin of patients with fixed drug eruptions express the intercellular cell adhesion molecule (ICAM-1) (Fig. 3.38) [47], which is involved in interaction between keratinocytes and lymphocytes, HLA-DR (Fig. 3.39) [43], and the chemotactic protein IP-10 (especially in areas of blister formation) [45], may also be of relevance to the localized nature of the recurrent lesions in this condition [47]. These findings have been interpreted as evidence in support of a role for cytokines in the evolution of the histological changes, since keratinocyte IP-10 and HLA-DR may be induced by γ interferon, and since there is more intense keratinocyte IP-10 staining above collections of γ-gamma interferon-secreting HLA-DR$^+$ dermal lymphocytes [45].

1 Savin J. Current causes of fixed drug eruptions. *Br J Dermatol* 1970; **83**: 546−9.
2 Sehgal UN, Rege VL, Kharangate UN. Fixed drug eruptions caused by medications: a report from India. *Int J Dermatol* 1978; **17**: 78−81.
3 Pasricha JS. Drugs causing fixed eruptions. *Br J Dermatol* 1979; **100**: 183−5.
4 Shukla SR. Drugs causing fixed eruptions. *Dermatologica* 1981; **163**: 160−3.

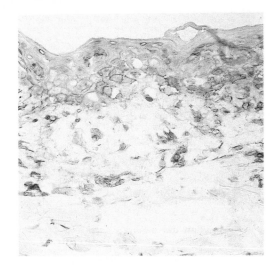 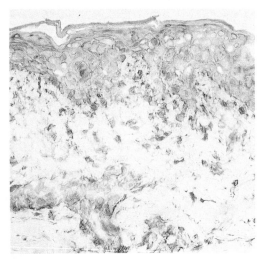

Figure 3.38 Expression of ICAM-1 by keratinocytes in lesional skin in fixed drug eruption.

Figure 3.39 Expression of HLA-DR by keratinocytes in lesional skin in fixed drug eruption.

5 Commens C. Fixed drug eruption. *Aust J Dermatol* 1983; **24**: 1−8.

6 Chan HL. Fixed drug eruptions. A study of 20 occurrences in Singapore. *Int J Dermatol* 1984; **23**: 607−9.

7 Korkij W, Soltani K. Fixed eruption. A brief review. *Arch Dermatol* 1984; **120**: 520−4.

8 Kauppinen K, Stubb S. Fixed eruptions: causative drugs and challenge tests. *Br J Dermatol* 1985; **112**: 575−8.

9 Sehgal VN, Gangwani OP. Fixed drug eruption. Current concepts. *Int J Dermatol* 1987; **26**: 67−74.

10 Kanwar AJ, Bharija SC, Singh M, Belhaj MS. Ninety-eight fixed drug eruptions with provocation tests. *Dermatologica* 1988; **177**: 279.

11 Sehgal VN, Gangwani OP. Fixed drug eruptions: A study of epidemiological, clinical and diagnostic aspects of 89 cases from India. *J Dermatol (Tokyo)* 1988; **15**: 50−4.

12 Pasricha JS, Shukla SR. Independent lesions of fixed eruption due to two unrelated drugs in the same patient. *Br J Dermatol* 1979; **101**: 361−2.

13 Kivity S. Fixed drug eruption to multiple drugs: clinical and laboratory investigation. *Int J Dermatol* 1991; **30**: 149−51.

14 Bhargava NC, Singh G. Fixed drug eruption due to two unrelated drugs. *Int J Dermatol* 1981; **20**: 435.

15 Verbov J. Fixed drug eruption due to a drug combination but not to its constituents. *Dermatologica* 1985; **171**: 60−1.

16 Sowden JM, Smith AG. Multifocal fixed drug eruption mimicking erythema multiforme. *Clin Exp Dermatol* 1990; **15**: 387−8.

17 Saiag P, Cordoliani F, Roujeau JC, *et al*. Érytheme pigmenté fixe bulleux disséminé simulant un syndrome de Lyell. *Ann Dermatol Vénéréol (Paris)* 1987; **114**: 1440−2.

18 Baird BJ, De Villez RL. Widespread bullous fixed drug eruption mimicking toxic epidermal necrolysis. *Int J Dermatol* 1988; **27**: 170−4.

19 Gaffoor PMA, George WM. Fixed drug eruptions occurring on the male genitals. *Cutis* 1990; **45**: 242−4.

20 Tagami H. Pigmented macules of the tongue following fixed drug eruption. *Dermatologica* 1973; **147**: 157−60.

21 Westerhof W, Wolters EC, Brookbakker JTW, *et al*. Pigmented lesions of the tongue in heroin addicts − fixed drug eruption. *Br J Dermatol* 1983; **109**: 605−10.

22 Sigal-Nahum M, Konqui A, Gauliet A, Sigal S. Linear fixed drug eruption. *Br J Dermatol* 1988; **118**: 849–51.

23 Shelly WB, Shelly ED. Nonpigmenting fixed drug reaction pattern: Examples caused by sensitivity to pseudoephedrine hydrochloride and tetrahydrozoline. *J Am Acad Dermatol* 1987; **17**: 403–7.

24 Valsecchi R, Cainelli T. Nonpigmenting fixed drug reaction to piroxicam. *J Am Acad Dermatol* 1989; **21**: 1300.

25 Benson PM, Giblin WJ, Douglas DM. Transient, nonpigmenting fixed drug eruption caused by radiopaque contrast media. *J Am Acad Dermatol* 1990; **23**: 379–81.

26 Stubb S, Alanko K, Reitamo S. Fixed drug eruptions: 77 cases from 1981 to 1985. *Br J Dermatol* 1989; **120**: 583.

27 Kanwar AJ, Bharija SC, Belhaj MS. Fixed drug eruptions in children: a series of 23 cases with provocative tests. *Dermatologica* 1986; **172**: 315–18.

28 Sehgal VN, Shyam Prasad AL, Gangwani OP. Magnesium trisilicate induced fixed drug eruptions. *Dermatologica* 1986; **172**: 123.

29 Stubb S, Reitamo S. Fixed drug eruption due to dextromethorphan. *Arch Dermatol* 1990; **126**: 970–1.

30 Alanko K, Stubb S, Reitamo S. Topical provocation of fixed drug eruption. *Br J Dermatol* 1987; **116**: 561–7.

31 Lever WF, Schaumburg-Lever G. *Histopathology of the Skin*, 7th edn. JB Lippincott, Philadelphia, 1990.

32 Naegeli O, De Quervain F, Stadler W. Nachweis des cellulären Sitzes der Allergie beim Fixen Antipyrin-exanthem (Autotransplantationenen Versuch *in vitro*). *Klin Wochenschr* 1930; **9**: 924–7.

33 Urbach E, Sidaravieius B. Zur Kritik der Methoden der Passiven Uebertragung der Ueberempfindlichkeit. *Klin Wochenschr* 1930; **9**: 2095–9.

34 Wise F, Sulzberger MB. Drug eruptions: I. Fixed phenolphthalein eruptions. *Arch Dermatol* 1933; **27**: 549–67.

35 Loveman AB. Experimental aspect of fixed eruption due to alurate, a compound of allonol. *JAMA* 1934; **102**: 97–101.

36 Wyatt E, Greaves M, Søndergaard J. Fixed drug eruption (phenolphthalein). *Arch Dermatol* 1972; **106**: 671–3.

37 Gimenez-Camarasa JM, Garcia-Calderon P, De Moragas JM. Lymphocyte transformation test in fixed drug eruption. *N Engl J Med* 1975; **292**: 819–21.

38 Suzuki S, Asai Y, Toshio H, *et al*. Drug-induced lymphocyte transformation in peripheral lymphocytes from patients with drug eruption. *Dermatologica* 1978; **157**: 146–53.

39 Shelley WB, Schlappner OLA, Heiss HB. Demonstration of intercellular immunofluorescence and epidermal hysteresis in bullous fixed drug eruption due to phenolphthalein. *Br J Dermatol* 1972; **86**: 118–25.

40 Duhra P, Porter DI. Paracetamol-induced fixed drug eruption with positive immunofluorescence findings. *Clin Exp Dermatol* 1990; **15**: 293–5.

41 Theodoridis A, Varezidis A, Sivenas C, *et al*. Fibrin deposition in fixed drug eruption. *Arch Dermatol Res* 1979; **264**: 73–6.

42 Hindsén M, Christensen OB, Gruic V, Löfberg H. Fixed drug eruption: an immunohistochemical investigation of the acute and healing phase. *Br J Dermatol* 1987; **116**: 351–6.

43 Murphy GF, Guillén FJ, Flynn TC. Cytotoxic T lymphocytes and phenotypically abnormal epidermal dendritic cells in fixed cutaneous eruption. *Hum Pathol* 1985; **16**: 1264–71.

44 Visa K, Käyhkö K, Stubb S, Reitamo S. Immunocompetent cells of fixed drug eruption. *Acta Derm Venereol (Stockh)* 1987; **67**: 30–5.

45 Smoller BR, Luster AD, Krane JF, *et al*. Fixed drug eruptions: evidence for a cytokine-mediated process. *J Cutan Pathol* 1991; **18**: 13–19.

46 Scheper RJ, Von Blomberg M, Boerrigter GH, *et al*. Induction of immunological memory in the skin. Role of local T cell retention. *Clin Exp Immunol* 1983; **51**: 141–8.

47 Shiohara T, Nickoloff BJ, Sagawa Y, *et al*. Fixed drug eruption. Expression of epidermal keratinocyte intercellular adhesion molecule-1 (ICAM–1). *Arch Dermatol* 1989; **125**: 1371–6.

[78]

3.13 Lichenoid eruptions

Clinical features

Lichenoid eruptions are so called because of their clinical and histological resemblance to idiopathic lichen planus, which characteristically presents as a violaceous papular eruption. Lichenoid drug eruptions tend to be extensive (Figs 3.40–3.43), and may be linked with, or develop into, an exfoliative dermatitis [1]. The eruption may develop weeks or months after initiation of therapy. Lesions may be rather more psoriasiform than in idiopathic lichen planus, and oral involvement is rare. Hyperpigmentation, alopecia, and skin atrophy with anhidrosis due to sweat gland atrophy, may develop. Resolution of the skin eruption may be slow after cessation of therapy.

Drug aetiology

Some of the drugs which induce this pattern of reaction are listed in Table 3.9. These include β-blockers [2], thiazide diuretics, gold, captopril [3,4], antimalarials, quinidine [5–8], *p*-aminosalicylic acid [9], penicillamine [10], tiopronin [11], chlorpropamide and tolazamide [12], the anabolic steroid nandrolone furylpropionate [13], cinnarazine (Figs 3.42 & 3.43) and cyanamide [14]. With pyritinol

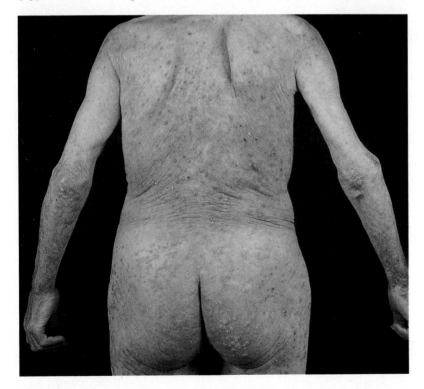

Figure 3.40 Widespread lichenoid drug eruption. (Courtesy of Professor K. Wolff, Vienna.)

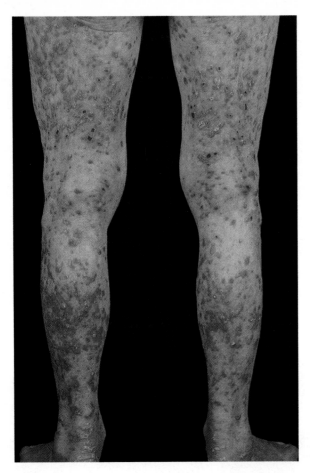

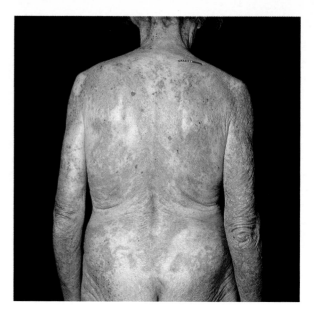

Figure 3.42 Widespread lichenoid drug eruption in a patient treated with cinnarazine and lorazepam.

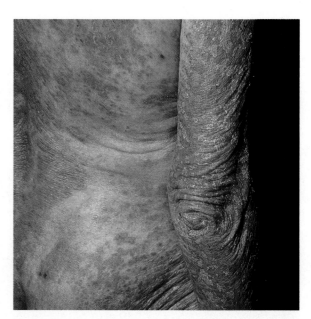

Figure 3.41 Widespread lichenoid drug eruption. (Courtesy of Professor K. Wolff, Vienna.)

Figure 3.43 Close-up of lichenoid drug eruption in a patient treated with cinnarazine and lorazepam.

[15–18] and thiazides [19,20], lesions may be preferentially distributed in light exposed areas. Unlike idiopathic lichen planus, the lichenoid eruption following quinacrine (mepacrine) may undergo malignant change [21]. In the case of cinnarazine, clinical and immunofluorescence features of lichen planus were combined with the presence of a circulating anti-basement membrane zone IgG antibody, i.e. the pattern of lichen planus pemphigoides [22]. A lichenoid eruption followed the occurrence of drug-induced lupus erythematosus secondary to procainamide [23]. Lichenoid eruptions may also result from contact dermatitis in photographic workers who handle certain *p*-phenylenediamines [24,25]. In one series, either eczematous or lichenoid eruptions were produced; even where lesions with a lichenoid clinical and histological appearance were produced, patch tests were eczematous [25].

Differential diagnosis: paraneoplastic pemphigus

The recently reported and newly recognized entity of paraneoplastic pemphigus may present with urticarial, papulosquamous, lichenoid, erythema multiforme-like or TEN-like lesions; mucosal erosions are usual [26]. The lichenoid variant of the eruption may mimic a lichenoid drug eruption (Fig. 3.44). Immunofluorescence shows the pattern of intercellular deposition of immunoreactants, but also of linear-granular complement deposition at the basement membrane zone.

Histology [27–31]

The changes may be non-specific or may resemble idiopathic lichen planus (Fig. 3.45), though the cellular infiltrate tends to be more pleomorphic and less dense, and the presence of focal parakeratosis, focal interruption of the granular layer, and cytoid bodies in the cornified and granular layers suggest a drug cause [28]. Later there may be scarring with destruction of the sweat glands. However, the histopathology of photodistributed, as opposed to non-photodistributed, lichenoid drug eruptions has been shown to be often indistinguishable from that of idiopathic lichen planus [30].

Table 3.9 Drugs causing lichenoid eruptions

β-Blockers
Captopril
Methyldopa
Thiazides
Frusemide
Gold
Antimalarials
   Mepacrine (quinacrine, atebrin)
   Chloroquine
   Quinine
Quinidine
Chlorpropamide
Penicillamine
Tiopronin
Pyritinol
Amiphenazole
Carbamazepine
Demeclocycline
Phenytoin
Ethambutol
Isoniazid
p-Aminosalicylic acid
Streptomycin
Phenothiazine
Phenylbutazone
Pyrimethamine
Levamisole
Cinnarazine
Flunarizine
Cyanamide
Nandrolone furylpropionate
Bismuth

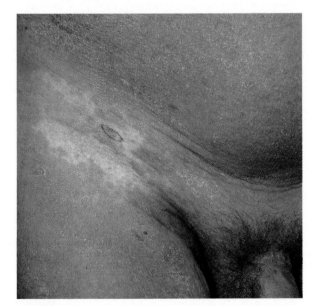

Fig. 3.44

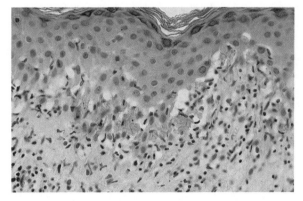

Figure 3.45 Histopathology of lichenoid drug eruption, showing band-like lymphocytic infiltrate at dermo-epidermal junction, liquefaction degeneration of the epidermal basal cell layer, and multiple colloid bodies.

Figure 3.44 Lichenoid eruption in a patient with paraneoplastic pemphigus and non-Hodgkin's lymphoma; skin biopsy revealed intercellular deposition of immunoreactants.

Immunopathogenesis

The mechanism by which lichenoid drug eruptions are produced is essentially unknown. However, it has been proposed that lichenoid drug eruptions may develop as a result of autoreactive cytotoxic T cell clones directed against a drug–class II MHC antigen complex, such that keratinocytes and Langerhans cells are viewed by the immune system as 'non-self'. In support of this is the fact that cloned murine autoreactive T cells may produce a lichenoid reaction in recipient animals following injection [32]. A correlation has been reported between the presence of epidermotropic T cells and class II MHC (HLA-DR) expressing keratinocytes and Langerhans cells [33].

1 Almeyda J, Levantine A. Drug reactions XVI. Lichenoid drug eruptions. *Br J Dermatol* 1971; **85**: 604–7.
2 Hödl S. Nebenwirkungen der Beta-Rezeptoren-blocker an der Haut. *Z Hautkr* 1983; **58**: 17–28.
3 Bravard P, Barbet M, Eich D, *et al.* Éruption lichénoide au captopril. *Ann Dermatol Venereol (Paris)* 1983; **110**: 433–8.
4 Reinhardt LA, Wilkin JK, Kirkendall WM. Lichenoid eruption produced by captopril. *Cutis* 1983; **31**: 98–9.
5 Anderson TE. Lichen planus following quinidine therapy. *Br J Dermatol* 1967; **79**: 500.
6 Maltz BL, Becker LE. Quinidine-induced lichen planus. *Int J Dermatol* 1980; **19**: 96–7.
7 Wolf R, Dorfman B, Krakowski A. Quinidine-induced lichenoid and eczematous photodermatitis. *Dermatologica* 1987; **174**: 285–9.
8 De Larrard G, Jeanmougin M, Moulonguet I, *et al.* Toxidermie lichénoide alopéciante a la quinidine. *Ann Dermatol Vénéréol (Paris)* 1988; **115**: 1172–4.
9 Shatin M, Canizares O, Worthington EL. Lichen planus-like drug eruption due to para-amino salicylic acid. Report of 5 cases, two showing mouth lesions. *J Invest Dermatol* 1953; **21**: 135–8.
10 Van Hecke E, Kint A, Temmerman L. A lichenoid eruption induced by penicillamine. *Arch Dermatol* 1981; **117**: 676–7.
11 Kurumaji Y, Miyazaki K. Tiopronin-induced lichenoid eruption in a patient with liver disease and positive patch test reaction to drugs with sulfhydryl group. *J Dermatol (Tokyo)* 1990; **17**: 176–81.
12 Barnett JH, Barnett SM. Lichenoid drug reactions to chlorpropamide and tolazamide. *Cutis* 1984; **34**: 542–4.
13 Aihara M, Kitamura K, Ikezawa Z. Lichenoid drug eruption due to nandrolone furylpropionate (Cemelon®). *J Dermatol (Tokyo)* 1989; **16**: 330–4.
14 Torrelo A, Soria C, Rocamora A, *et al.* Lichen planus-like eruption with esophageal involvement as a result of cyanamide. *J Am Acad Dermatol* 1990; **23**: 1168–9.
15 Dupré A, Carrère S, Launais B, Bonafé J-L. Lichen plan avec photosensibilisation après pyritinol et PUVA thérapie. *Ann Dermatol Vénéréol (Paris)* 1980; **107**: 557–9.
16 Duterque M, Crouzet J, Civatte J. Trois cas de lichen induit par le pyritinol. *Ann Dermatol Vénéréol (Paris)* 1983; **110**: 707–8.
17 Méraud J-P, Géniaux M, Tamisier M-M, *et al.* Eruption squamo-crouteuse a type histologique de lichen plan au cours d'un traitement par le pyritinol. *Ann Dermatol Vénéréol (Paris)* 1980; **107**: 561–4.
18 Ishibashi A, Hirano K, Nishiyama Y. Photosensitive dermatitis due to pyritinol. *Arch Dermatol* 1973; **107**: 427–8.
19 Robinson HN, Morison WL, Hood AF. Thiazide diuretic therapy and chronic photosensitivity. *Arch Dermatol* 1985; **121**: 522–4.

20 Addo HA, Ferguson J, Frain-Bell W. Thiazide-induced photosensitivity: a study of 33 subjects. *Br J Dermatol* 1987; **116**: 749−60.

21 Bauer F. Quinacrine hydrochloride drug eruption (tropical lichenoid dermatitis). Its early and late sequelae and its malignant potential. A review. *J Am Acad Dermatol* 1981; **4**: 239−48.

22 Miyagawa W, Ohi H, Muramatsu T, *et al*. Lichen planus pemphigoides-like lesions induced by cinnarizine. *Br J Dermatol* 1985; **112**: 607−13.

23 Sherertz EF. Lichen planus following procainamide-induced lupus erythematosus. *Cutis* 1988; **42**: 51−3.

24 Buckley WR. Lichenoid eruptions following contact dermatitis. *Arch Dermatol* 1958; **78**: 454−7.

25 Fry L. Skin disease from colour developers. *Br J Dermatol* 1965; **77**: 456−61.

26 Anhalt GJ, Kim S, Stanley JR, *et al*. Paraneoplastic pemphigus. An autoimmune mucocutaneous disease associated with neoplasia. *N Engl J Med* 1990; **323**: 1729−35.

27 Watanabe C, Hayashi T, Kawada A. Immunofluorescence study of drug-induced lichen planus-like lesions. *J Dermatol (Tokyo)* 1981; **8**: 473−7.

28 Van den Haute V, Antoine JL, Lachapelle JM. Histopathological discriminant criteria between lichenoid drug eruption and idiopathic lichen planus: retrospective study on selected samples. *Dermatologica* 1989; **179**: 10−13.

29 Lever WF, Schaumburg-Lever G. *Histopathology of the Skin*, 7th edn. JB Lippincott, Philadelphia, 1990.

30 West AJ, Berger TG, LeBoit PE. A comparative histopathologic study of photodistributed and nonphotodistributed lichenoid drug eruptions. *J Am Acad Dermatol* 1990; **23**: 689−93.

31 Patterson JW. The spectrum of lichenoid dermatitis. *J Cutan Pathol* 1991; **18**: 67−74.

32 Shiohara T. The lichenoid tissue reaction. An immunological perspective. *Am J Dermatopathol* 1988; **10**: 252−6.

33 Shiohara T, Moriya N, Tanaka Y, *et al*. Immunopathological study of lichenoid skin diseases: correlation between HLA-DR-positive keratinocytes or Langerhans cells and epidermotropic T cells. *J Am Acad Dermatol* 1988; **18**: 67−74.

3.14 Photosensitivity

Drug−light reactions, which cause eruptions on exposed areas of the skin, with sparing of upper eyelids, and submental and retro-auricular areas, may be phototoxic or photo-allergic; these reactions cannot always be distinguished clinically, and some drugs may produce cutaneous involvement by both mechanisms [1−10]. The main drugs which are implicated in causing photosensitivity reactions are listed in Table 3.10.

Phototoxic reactions

Phototoxic reactions are commoner, and can be produced in almost all individuals given a high enough dose of drug and sufficient light irradiation; they occur within 5−20 hours of the first exposure, and resemble exaggerated sunburn. Erythema, oedema, blistering, weeping, desquamation and residual hyperpigmentation occur on exposed areas; there may be photo-onycholysis. The following are well-recognized causes of phototoxicity: tetracyclines [11−15], especially demeclocycline, less frequently doxycycline, oxytetracycline, and tetracycline, and rarely minocycline and methacycline; pheno-

Table 3.10 Drugs causing photosensitivity

Frequent	*Less frequent: systemic*
Amiodarone	Ampicillin
Phenothiazines	Antidepressants: tricyclic
Chlorpromazine	Imipramine
Promethazine	Protriptyline
Psoralens	Antidepressants: MAOI
Sulphonamides	Phenelzine
Co-trimoxazole	Antifungal agents
Tetracyclines	Griseofulvin
Demeclocycline	Ketoconazole
Thiazides	β-Blockers
Non-steroidal anti-inflammatory drugs	Carbamazepine
Azapropazone	Cimetidine
Piroxicam	Cytotoxic agents
Carprofen	Dacarbazine
Tiaprofenic acid	Fluorouracil
Benoxaprofen (withdrawn)	Mitomycin
Nalidixic acid	Vinblastine
Coal tar	Diazepam
	Frusemide
Less frequent: topical	Methyldopa
	Oral contraceptives
Antihistamines	Quinine
Local anaesthetics	Quinidine
Benzydamine	Sulphonylureas
Hydrocortisone	Chlorpropamide
Sunscreens	Tolbutamide
PABA	Retinoids
Benzophenone	Isotretinoin
Halogenated salicylanilides	Etretinate
	Triamterene

thiazines, especially chlorpromazine, promethazine and less commonly thioridazine; sulphonamides; frusemide [16] and nalidixic acid [17−19], both of which produce a pseudoporphyria syndrome, with blistering of the exposed areas, especially on the lower legs and feet; non-steroidal anti-inflammatory agents (Fig. 3.46) [20,21] including piroxicam [21−23], carprofen and tiaprofenic acid [24] (and benoxaprofen, now withdrawn [25]); psoralens; amiodarone (which causes photosensitivity in greater than 50% of cases) [26−29]; certain anticancer drugs [30] including dacarbazine [30,31], 5-fluorouracil, mitomycin and vinblastine; coal tar and its derivatives.

1 Cronin E. Photosensitisers. In *Contact Dermatitis*. Churchill Livingstone, Edinburgh, 1980, pp 414−60.
2 Hawk JLM. Photosensitizing agents used in the United Kingdom. *Clin Exp Dermatol* 1984; **9**: 300−2.
3 Johnson BE. Light sensitivity associated with drugs and chemicals. In Jarrett

A (ed.) *The Physiology and Pathophysiology of the Skin*. Academic Press, New York, 1984, pp 2541–606.

4 Epstein JH, Wintroub BU. Photosensitivity to drugs. *Drugs* 1985; **30**: 42–57.

5 Frain-Bell W. Drug-induced photosensitivity. In *Cutaneous Photobiology*. Oxford University Press, Oxford, 1985, 74–7.

6 Ljunggren B, Bjellerup M. Systemic drug photosensitivity. *Photodermatol* 1986; **3**: 26–35.

7 Elmets CA. Drug-induced photoallergy. *Dermatol Clin* 1986; **4**: 231–41.

8 Lowe NJ. Cutaneous phototoxicity reactions. *Br J Dermatol*; 1986; **115** (Suppl 31): 86–92.

9 Harber LC, Bickers DR. Drug induced photosensitivity (phototoxic and photo-allergic drug reactions). In *Photosensitivity Diseases. Principles of Diagnosis and Treatment*, 2nd edn. BC Decker Inc, Toronto, 1989, pp 160–202.

10 Rosen C. Photo-induced drug eruptions. *Semin Dermatol* 1989; **8**: 149–57.

11 Blank H, Cullen SI, Catalano PM. Photosensitivity studies with demethyl-chlortetracycline and doxycycline. *Arch Dermatol* 1968; **97**: 1–2.

12 Ramsay CA. Longwave ultraviolet radiation sensitivity induced by oxytetra-cycline: a case report. *Clin Exp Dermatol* 1977; **2**: 255–8.

13 Cullen SI, Catalano PM, Helfmann RS. Tetracycline sun sensitivity. *Arch Dermatol* 1966; **93**: 77.

14 Frost P, Weinstein GP, Gomez EC. Phototoxic potential of minocycline and doxycycline. *Arch Dermatol* 1972; **105**: 681–3.

15 Wright AL, Colver GB. Tetracyclines — how safe are they? *Clin Exp Dermatol* 1988; **13**: 57–61.

16 Burry JN, Lawrence JR. Phototoxic blisters from high frusemide dosage. *Br J Dermatol* 1976; **94**: 495–9.

17 Baes H. Photosensitivity caused by nalidixic acid. *Dermatologica* 1968; **136**: 61–4.

18 Birkett DA, Garretts M, Stevenson CJ. Phototoxic bullous eruptions due to nalidixic acid. *Br J Dermatol* 1969; **81**: 342–4.

19 Ramsay CA, Obreshkova E. Photosensitivity from nalidixic acid. *Br J Dermatol* 1974; **91**: 523–8.

20 Przybilla B, Ring J, Schwab U, *et al*. Photosensibilisierende Eigenschaften nichtsteroidaler Antirheumatika im Photopatch-Test. *Hautarzt* 1987; **38**: 18–25.

21 Stern RS. Phototoxic reactions to piroxicam and other nonsteroidal anti-inflammatory agents. *N Engl J Med* 1983; **309**: 186–7.

22 Serrano G, Bonillo J, Aliaga A, *et al*. Piroxicam-induced photosensitivity. *In vivo* and *in vitro* studies of its photosensitizing potential. *J Am Acad Dermatol* 1984; **11**: 113–20.

23 Figueiredo A, Fontes Ribeiro CA, Conçalo S, *et al*. Piroxicam-induced photo-sensitivity. *Contact Dermatitis* 1987; **17**: 73–9.

24 Przybilla B, Ring J, Galosi A, Dorn M. Photopatch test reactions to tiaprofenic acid. *Contact Dermatitis* 1984; **1**: 55–6. .

25 Ferguson J, Addo HA, McGill PE, *et al*. A study of benoxaprofen-induced photosensitivity. *Br J Dermatol* 1982; **107**: 429–42.

26 Chalmers RJG, Muston HL, Srinivas V, Bennett DH. High incidence of amiodarone-induced photosensitivity in North-west England. *Br Med J* 1982; **285**: 341.

27 Zachary CB, Slater DN, Holt DW, *et al*. The pathogenesis of amiodarone-induced pigmentation and photosensitivity. *Br J Dermatol* 1984; **110**: 451–6.

28 Walter JF, Bradner H, Curtis GP. Amiodarone photosensitivity. *Arch Dermatol* 1984; **120**: 1591–4.

29 Ferguson J, Addo HA, Jones S, *et al*. A study of cutaneous photosensitivity induced by amiodarone. *Br J Dermatol* 1985; **113**: 537–49.

30 Kerker BJ, Hood AF. Chemotherapy-induced cutaneous reactions. *Semin Dermatol* 1989; **8**: 173–81.

31 Bonifazi E, Angelini G, Meneghini CL. Adverse photoreaction to dacarbazine (DITC). *Contact Dermatitis* 1981; **7**: 161.

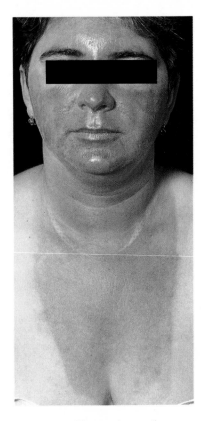

Figure 3.46 Phototoxic eruption due to the anti-inflammatory agent lonazolac-calcium.

Photo-allergic reactions

Photo-allergic reactions, by contrast, require a latent period during which sensitization occurs, and usually appear within 24 hours of re-exposure to drug and light in a sensitized individual; unlike phototoxic reactions, they may spread beyond irradiated areas. Most systemic drugs causing photo-allergy also cause phototoxicity. In patients with photo-allergy there may be cross-reactivity with chemically related substances. Various mechanisms may be involved in photo-allergic reactions; light may either alter the hapten, or the avidity with which it binds to a carrier protein [1].

Photo-allergic reactions may occur as a result of local photocontact dermatitis to a topical photo-allergen. Photocontact dermatitis is a relatively common cause of photosensitivity, accounting for 9% of cases in a multicentre study [2]. Topical photo-allergens include antihistamines, chlorpromazine, local anaesthetics [3], benzydamine, hydrocortisone, desoximetasone, and sunscreens containing *p*-aminobenzoic acid (PABA) and its derivatives. PABA-free sunscreens, and PABA-containing sunscreens with sun protection factor values of greater than 8, mostly contain benzophenones. Contact and photo-allergy to benzophenones is less well documented than that to PABA derivatives, but may be commoner than is realized [4,5]. Halogenated salicylanilides, previously used as a disinfectant in soaps, and related compounds also cause a photocontact dermatitis (Fig. 3.47).

Photo-allergic reactions may in addition occur as a result of systemically administered drugs [6], such as phenothiazines (chlorpromazine, promethazine), sulphonamides, aromatic sulphonamides such as thiazide diuretics [7,8] and oral hypoglycaemic agents (chlorpropamide and tolbutamide), griseofulvin [9] and quinidine [10,11]. Thiazide photo-eruptions may be characterized by erythema, dermatitis, or a lichenoid appearance; a subacute lupus erythematosus-like eruption may be precipitated. Griseofulvin photo-allergic reactions may be clinically eczematous, occasionally pellagra-like, or show pigmentary changes; there may be photo-cross-reactivity with penicillin [9]. Photopatch tests have been positive in some cases. The histology of griseofulvin photo-allergic reactions has been reported as non-specific; direct immuno-fluorescence showed immunoglobulin and complement at the dermo-epidermal junction and in a perivascular distribution in the papillary dermis [9]. Quinidine-induced photo-eruptions may be either eczematous or lichenoid; a persistent livedo reticularis-like eruption may be seen in severe cases of quinidine photosensitivity [10−12]. Tricyclic antidepressants may cause contact allergy as well as photosensitivity [13]. Non-steroidal anti-inflammatory drugs, disinfectants, sunscreens, phenothiazines and fragrances caused photo-allergic reactions most often in a 5-year survey by the German, Austrian, and Swiss photopatch test group [14].

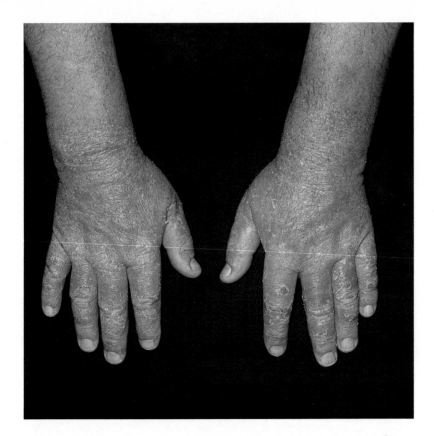

Figure 3.47 Photo-allergic contact dermatitis due to halogenated salicylanilide.

1 Harber LC, Baer RL. Pathogenic mechanisms of drug-induced photosensitivity. *J Invest Dermatol* 1972; **58**: 327–42.

2 Wennersten G, Thune P, Brodthagen H, *et al*. The Scandinavian multicenter photopatch study. Preliminary results. *Contact Dermatitis* 1984; **10**: 305–9.

3 Horio T. Photosensitivity reaction to dibucaine. Case report and experimental induction. *Arch Dermatol* 1979; **115**: 986–7.

4 Knobler E, Almeida L, Ruxkowski AM, *et al*. Photoallergy to benzophenone. *Arch Dermatol* 1989; **125**: 801–4.

5 Schauder S, Ippen H. Photoallergisches und allergisches Kontaktekzem durch Dibenzoylmethan-Verbindungen und andere Lichtschutzfilter. *Hautarzt* 1988; **39**: 435–40.

6 Giudici PA, Maguire HC. Experimental photoallergy to systemic drugs. *J Invest Dermatol* 1985; **85**: 207–11.

7 Robinson HN, Morison WL, Hood AF. Thiazide diuretic therapy and chronic photosensitivity. *Arch Dermatol* 1985; **121**: 522–4.

8 Addo HA, Ferguson J, Frain-Bell W. Thiazide-induced photosensitivity: a study of 33 subjects. *Br J Dermatol* 1987; **116**: 749–60.

9 Kojima T, Hasegawa T, Ishida H, *et al*. Griseofulvin-induced photodermatitis. Report of six cases. *J Dermatol (Tokyo)* 1988; **15**: 76–82.

10 De Groot WP, Wuite J. Livedo racemosa-like photosensitivity reaction during quinidine durettes medication. *Dermatologica* 1974; **148**: 371–6.

11 Bruce S, Wolf JE Jr. Quinidine-induced photosensitive livedo reticularis-like eruption. *J Am Acad Dermatol* 1985; **12**: 332–6.

12 Marion DF, Terrien CM Jr. Photosensitive livedo reticularis. *Arch Dermatol* 1973; **108**: 100–1.

13 Ljunggren B, Bojs G. A case of photosensitivity and contact allergy to systemic

tricyclic drugs, with unusual features. *Contact Dermatitis* 1991; **24**: 259—65.

14 Hölzle E, Neumann N, Hausen B, *et al*. Photopatch testing: The 5-year experience of the German, Austrian, and Swiss photopatch test group. *J Am Acad Dermatol* 1991; **25**: 59—68.

Chronic actinic dermatitis [1—4]

Following an episode of photo-allergy caused by contact with a photo-allergen such as halogenated salicylanilide, quinoxaline dioxide, or the fragrance musk ambrette, some subjects develop persistent photosensitivity of both exposed and covered skin, despite avoidance of the offending chemical; this condition is termed persistent light reactivity [1]. The action spectrum for the initiating photocontact reaction is in the long-wave ultraviolet band (UV-A, 315—400 nm); progression to persistent light reactivity is accompanied by a change in photosensitivity to the UV-B (280—315 nm) region. The term 'actinic reticuloid' was coined to describe a severe, chronic photodermatosis, mostly of elderly men, characterized by infiltrated plaques on an eczematous background in exposed areas, with histological features resembling those of cutaneous T cell lymphoma, and photosensitivity to UV-B and UV-A irradiation [3]. The term chronic actinic dermatitis (Fig. 3.48) has been introduced to encompass the spectrum of patients with persistent light reactivity, photosensitive eczema, photosensitivity dermatitis, and actinic reticuloid, now thought to be variants of a single condition, principally seen in elderly men [1—4].

In some patients, there appears to be a clear progression to chronic actinic dermatitis from a previous photo-allergic contact dermatitis, or persistent photosensitivity to systemic medication. It has been proposed that ultraviolet light irradiation alters a normal skin constituent such that it is no longer regarded as self, thus provoking a delayed hypersensitivity-like response. Evidence in support of this theory, at least in relation to progression of photo-allergic contact dermatitis to chronic actinic dermatitis, comes from an *in vitro* study in which phototoxic oxidation of histidine in albumin, which acts as the carrier protein for the photosensitizer tetrachlorosaliclylanilide, renders albumin weakly antigenic [5]. Several studies have suggested that chronic actinic dermatitis involves a T cell-mediated immunological reaction. Dermal infiltrates contain T lymphocytes, many of which express activation (HLA-DR, interleukin 2 receptor) or proliferation (Ki67 nuclear antigen, transferrin receptor) markers, in addition to Langerhans cells, and non-Langerhans cell macrophages [6—8]. CD8$^+$ suppressor/cytotoxic T cells tend to predominate in the dermal infiltrate where the histological changes are more florid. HLA-DR$^+$ non-Langerhans cell macrophages and other leucocytes invaded the epidermis, and focal HLA-DR expression by keratinocytes has been noted.

1 Wolf C, Hönigsmann H. Das Syndrom der chronisch-aktinischen Dermatitis.

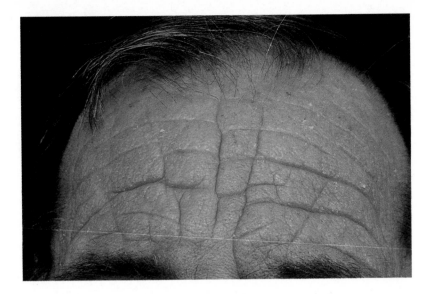

Figure 3.48 Marked lichenification of the exposed skin of the forehead, typical of chronic actinic dermatitis. (Courtesy of St John's Institute of Dermatology, London.)

Persistierende Lichtreaktion — aktinisches Retikuloid. *Hautarzt* 1988; **39**: 635—41.

2 Norris PG, Hawk JL. Chronic actinic dermatitis: A unifying concept. *Arch Dermatol* 1990; **126**: 376—8.

3 Ive FA, Magnus IA, Warin RP, Wilson Jones E. 'Actinic reticuloid'; a chronic dermatosis associated with severe photosensitivity and the histological resemblance to lymphoma. *Br J Dermatol* 1969; **81**: 469—85.

4 Lim HW, Buchness MR, Ashinoff R, Soter NA. Chronic actinic dermatitis: study of the spectrum of chronic photosensitivity in 12 patients. *Arch Dermatol* 1990; **126**: 317—23.

5 Kochevar IE, Harber LC. Photoreactions of 3,3',4',5-tetrachlorosalicylanilide with proteins. *J Invest Dermatol* 1977; **68**: 151—6.

6 Ralfkiaer E, Lange Wantzin G, Stein H, Mason DY. Photosensitive dermatitis with actinic reticuloid syndrome: an immunohistological study of the cutaneous infiltrate. *Br J Dermatol* 1986; **114**: 47—56.

7 Norris PG, Morris J, Smith NP, *et al*. Chronic actinic dermatitis: An immuno-histologic and photobiologic study. *J Am Acad Dermatol* 1989; **21**: 966—71.

8 Toonstra H, van der Putte SCJ, van Wichen DF, *et al*. Actinic reticuloid: immunohistochemical analysis of the cutaneous infiltrate in 13 patients. *Br J Dermatol* 1989; **120**: 779—86.

Porphyria and pseudoporphyria

A number of drugs may precipitate porphyria cutanea tarda with resultant photosensitivity, or cause a pseudoporphyria syndrome with bulla formation. The reader is referred to section 3.19 for details (p. 100).

Photo-recall reactions

A curious photo-recall-like eruption occurred, restricted to an area of sunburn sustained 1 month previously, in a patient treated with cefazolin and gentamicin [1]. A recurrent cutaneous reaction localized to the site of pelvic radiotherapy for adenocarcinoma of the prostate followed sun exposure in one patient [2]. Methotrexate is associated with severe reactivation of sunburn [3,4].

1 Flax SH, Uhle P. Photo recall-like phenomenon following the use of cefazolin and gentamicin sulfate. *Cutis* 1990; **46**: 59–61.
2 Del Guidice SM, Gerstley JK. Sunlight-induced radiation recall. *Int J Dermatol* 1988; **27**: 415–16.
3 Mallory SB, Berry DH. Severe reactivation of sunburn following methotrexate use. *Pediatrics* 1986; **78**: 514–15.
4 Westwick TJ, Sherertz EF, McCarley D, Flowers FP. Delayed reactivation of sunburn by methotrexate: sparing of chronically sun-exposed skin. *Cutis* 1987; **39**: 49–51.

Photo-onycholysis

Photo-onycholysis may be caused by tetracycline, PUVA therapy, and the fluoroquinolone antibiotics pefloxacine and ofloxacine.

3.15 Pigmentary abnormalities

Hyperpigmentation (Table 3.11)

Drug-induced alteration in skin colour [1–3] may result from increased (or more rarely decreased) melanin synthesis, increased lipofuscin synthesis, cutaneous deposition of drug-related material, or most commonly as a result of postinflammatory hyper-pigmentation (e.g. fixed drug eruption). Oral contraceptives may induce chloasma [4]. Other drugs implicated in cutaneous hyper-pigmentation include minocycline [5,6], antimalarials [7–10], chlorpromazine [11], imipramine [12], amiodarone [13], carotene, and heavy metals. Long-term (more than 4 months) antimalarial therapy may result in brownish or blue–black pigmentation, especially on the shin, face, and hard palate or subungually with chloroquine [7,8], or hydroxychloroquine [8], which is usually temporary. Chloroquine has an affinity for melanin [9]. Yellowish discoloration may occur with mepacrine (quinacrine) or amodiaquin. Pigmentation appears to result from melanin, haemosiderin and quinacrine-containing complexes, since ultrastructural micro-analysis has demonstrated the presence of sulphur [10]. Long-term high dose phenothiazine (especially chlorpromazine) therapy results in a blue–grey or brownish pigmentation of sun-exposed areas, the result of a phototoxic reaction. The cancer chemotherapeutic agents may be associated with pigmentation as follows [14]. Skin pigmentation may be caused by bleomycin, busulphan, topical carmustine, cyclophosphamide, daunorubicin, fluorouracil, hydroxyurea, topical mechlorethamine, methotrexate, mithramycin, mitomycin, and thio-TEPA. Busulphan and doxorubicin cause mucous membrane pigmentation. Nail pigmentation may result from bleomycin, cyclophosphamide, daunorubicin, doxorubicin, and fluorouracil. Methotrexate may induce pigmentation of the hair, and cyclophosphamide of teeth.

Table 3.11 Drugs causing pigmentation

Oral contraceptives
Minocycline
Antimalarials
  Chloroquine
  Hydroxychloroquine
  Mepacrine
Chlorpromazine
Imipramine
Heavy metals
  Gold
  Lead
  Silver
Chemotherapeutic agents
Amiodarone
Carotene
Clofazimine

Gold may cause blue–grey pigmentation in light-exposed areas (chrysiasis) [15] and silver may cause a similar discoloration (argyria) (Fig. 3.49) [16,17]. Lead poisoning can cause a blue–black line at the gingival margin and grey discoloration of the skin. Clofazimine produces red–brown discoloration of exposed skin and the conjunctivae, together with red sweat, urine and faeces [18]. Rarely an acanthosis nigricans-like reaction can occur, e.g. with nicotinic acid. Slate-grey to blue–black pigmentation may occur after long-term topical application of hydroquinone, causing ochronosis [19]. Topical application of red azo dye applied as a cosmetic by Hindu women ('kumkum') may result in pigmentation [20].

Hypopigmentation

Topical thiotepa has produced periorbital leucoderma [21]. Hypopigmentation has occurred as a result of occupational exposure to: monobenzyl ether of hydroquinone, *p-tert* butyl catechol, *p-tert* butyl phenol, *p-tert* amylphenol, monomethyl ether of hydroquinone, and hydroquinone [22,23]. In addition, hypopigmentation may result from phenolic detergent germicides [24], and following use of diphencyprone for alopecia areata [25].

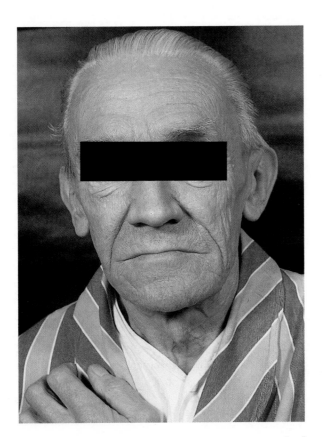

Figure 3.49 Slate-grey pigmentation due to argyria.

1 Levantine A, Almeyda J. Drug reactions: XXII. Drug induced changes in pigmentation. *Br J Dermatol* 1973; **89**: 105–12.
2 Granstein RD, Sober AJ. Drug- and heavy metal-induced hyperpigmentation. *J Am Acad Dermatol* 1981; **5**: 1–18.
3 Ferguson J, Frain-Bell W. Pigmentary disorders and systemic drug therapy. *Clin Dermatol* 1989; **7**: 44–54.
4 Smith AG, Shuster S, Thody AJ, *et al*. Chloasma, oral contraceptives, and plasma immunoreactive beta-melanocyte-stimulating hormone. *J Invest Dermatol* 1977; **68**: 169–70.
5 McGrae JD, Zelickson AS. Skin pigmentation secondary to minocycline therapy. *Arch Dermatol* 1980; **116**: 1262–5.
6 Layton AM, Cunliffe WJ. Minocycline induced pigmentation in the treatment of acne — a review and personal observations. *J Dermatol Treat* 1989; **1**: 9–12.
7 Doll JLC, Keane JA. Disturbances of pigmentation with chloroquine. *Br Med J* 1959; **i**: 1387–9.
8 Tuffanelli D, Abraham RK, Dubois EJ. Pigmentation from antimalarial therapy. Its possible relationship to the ocular lesions. *Arch Dermatol* 1963; **88**: 419–26.
9 Sams WM, Epstein JH. The affinity of melanin for chloroquine. *J Invest Dermatol* 1965; **45**: 482–8.
10 Leigh IM, Kennedy CTC, Ramsey JD, Henderson WJ. Mepacrine pigmentation in systemic lupus erythematosus. New data from an ultrastructural, biochemical and analytical electron microscope investigation. *Br J Dermatol* 1979; **101**: 147–53.
11 Benning TL, McCormack KM, Ingram P, *et al*. Microprobe analysis of chlorpromazine pigmentation. *Arch Dermatol* 1988; **124**: 1541–4.
12 Hashimoto K, Joselow SA, Tye MJ. Imipramine hyperpigmentation: A slate-gray discoloration caused by long-term imipramine administration. *J Am Acad Dermatol* 1991; **25**: 357–61.
13 Zachary CB, Slater DN, Holt DW, *et al*. The pathogenesis of amiodarone-induced pigmentation and photosensitivity. *Br J Dermatol* 1984; **110**: 451–6.
14 Kerker BJ, Hood AF. Chemotherapy-induced cutaneous reactions. *Semin Dermatol* 1989; **8**: 173–81.
15 Leonard PA, Moatamed F, Ward JR, *et al*. Chrysiasis: the role of sun exposure in dermal hyperpigmentation secondary to gold therapy. *J Rheumatol* 1986; **13**: 58–64.
16 Marshall JP II, Schneider RP. Systemic argyria secondary to topical silver nitrate. *Arch Dermatol* 1977; **113**: 1077–9.
17 Gherardi R, Brochard P, Chamak B, *et al*. Human generalized argyria. *Arch Pathol Lab Med* 1984; **108**: 181–2.
18 Thomsen K, Rothenborg HW. Clofazimine in the treatment of pyoderma gangrenosum. *Arch Dermatol* 1979; **115**: 851–2.
19 Hull PR, Procter LR. The melanocyte: An essential link in hydroquinone-induced ochronosis. *J Am Acad Dermatol* 1990; **22**: 529–31.
20 Goh CL, Kozuka T. Pigmented contact dermatitis from 'kumkum'. *Clin Exp Dermatol* 1986; **11**: 603–6.
21 Harben DJ, Cooper PH, Rodman OG. Thiotepa-induced leukoderma. *Arch Dermatol* 1979; **115**: 973–4.
22 James O, Mayes RW, Stevenson CJ. Occupational vitiligo induced by *p-tert*-butyl phenol, a systemic disease? *Lancet* 1977; **ii**: 1217–19.
23 Stevenson CJ. Occupational vitiligo: clinical and epidemiological aspects. *Br J Dermatol* 1981; **105** (Suppl 21): 51–6.
24 Kahn G. Depigmentation caused by phenolic detergent germicides. *Arch Dermatol* 1970; **102**: 177–87.
25 Hatzis J, Gourgiotou K, Tosca A, *et al*. Vitiligo as a reaction to topical treatment with diphencyprone. *Dermatologica* 1988; **177**: 146–8.

3.16 Acneiform and pustular eruptions

The term acneiform is applied to drug eruptions which resemble acne vulgaris [1,2]. Lesions are papulopustular, but comedones are usually absent. Adrenocorticotrophic hormone (ACTH), corticosteroids [3], as with dexamethasone in neurosurgical patients (Figs 3.50 & 3.51), anabolic steroids for body-building [4], androgens (in females), oral contraceptives, iodides and bromides may produce acneiform eruptions. Isoniazid may induce acne, especially in slow inactivators of the drug [5]. Other drugs implicated in the production of acneiform rashes include dantrolene [6], danazol [7], quinidine [8], lithium [9], and azathioprine [10].

In addition, pustular reactions have been reported in association with a number of drugs as follows [11–14]: pyrimethamine, frusemide, piperazine ethionamate, iodides and bromides, carbamazepine [15], naproxen [16], chloramphenicol succinate, norfloxacin [17], streptomycin sulphate [18], ampicillin, amoxycillin (Fig. 3.52), cephalosporins (cephalexin and cephadrine) [19,20], imipinem [21], co-trimoxazole [22], isoniazid, the mucolytic agent eprazinone [23], hydroxychloroquine [24], and diltiazem [25]. A generalized pustular eruption probably due to penicillin was associated with a histological pattern of a leucocytoclastic vasculitis [26]. A recent series of 63 patients with an acute generalized exanthematous pustulosis reported that adverse drug eruptions were responsible for 87% of cases, with antibiotics being implicated as the causative agent in 80% of individuals [27]. The latter included particularly ampicillin, amoxycillin, spiramycin, erythromycin, and cyclins. Hypersensitivity to mercury was also recorded as a precipitating cause. The

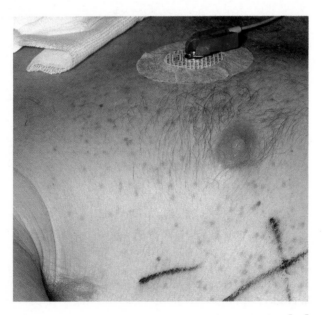

Figure 3.50 Steroid acne in a neurosurgical patient treated with 50 mg dexamethasone daily for 17 days.

[93]

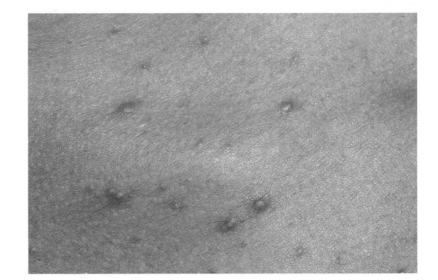

Figure 3.51 Papulopustular eruption due to systemic steroid therapy. (Courtesy of Professor H. Kerl, University of Graz.)

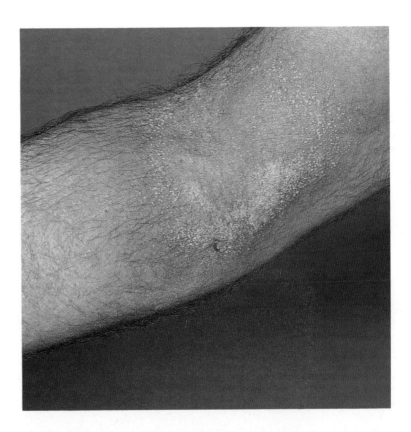

Figure. 3.52 Pustular eruption at the antecubital fossa in a patient treated with epicillin.

pustulosis developed within 24 hours of drug administration, often started on the face or in flexural areas, rapidly becoming disseminated, was accompanied by fever, and settled spontaneously with desquamation. Facial oedema, purpura, vesicles, blisters and erythema multiforme-like lesions were also seen. Histological features included spongiform superficial pustules, papillary oedema, peri-

[94]

vascular neutrophil infiltration with leucocytoclastic vasculitis and fibrin deposition. Neutrophil leucocytosis was recorded frequently, and transient renal failure was noted in 32% of cases. The authors suggested that cases previously reported as 'drug-induced pustular psoriasis' may have represented this condition. Cases of generalized pustulation in association with the anticonvulsant hypersensitivity syndrome caused by phenytoin have been recorded [28].

1 Hitch JM. Acneform eruptions induced by drugs and chemicals. *JAMA* 1967; **200**: 879–80.

2 Bedane C, Souyri N. Les acnés induites. *Ann Dermatol Vénéréol (Paris)* 1990; **117**: 53–8.

3 Hurwitz RM. Steroid acne. *J Am Acad Dermatol* 1989; **21**: 1179–81.

4 Merkle T, Landthaler M, Braun-Falco O. Acne-conglobata-artige Exazerbation einer Acne vulgaris nach Einnahme von Anabolika und Vitamin-B-Komplex-haltigen Präparaten. *Hautarzt* 1990; **41**: 280–2.

5 Cohen LK, George W, Smith R. Isoniazid-induced acne and pellagra. Occurrence in slow inactivators of isoniazid. *Arch Dermatol* 1974; **109**: 377–81.

6 Pembroke AC, Saxena SR, Kataria M, Zilkha KD. Acne induced by dantrolene. *Br J Dermatol* 1981; **104**: 465–8.

7 Greenberg RD. Acne vulgaris associated with antigonadotrophic (Danazol) therapy. *Cutis* 1979; **24**: 431–2.

8 Burkhart CG. Quinidine-induced acne. *Arch Dermatol* 1981; **117**: 603–4.

9 Heng MCY. Cutaneous manifestations of lithium toxicity. *Br J Dermatol* 1982; **106**: 107–9.

10 Schmoeckel C, von Liebe V. Akneiformes Exanthem durch Azathioprin. *Hautarzt* 1983; **34**: 413–15.

11 McMillan AL. Generalized pustular drug rash. *Dermatologica* 1973; **146**: 285–91.

12 Ogino A, Tagami H, Takahashi C, Higuchi T. Generalized pustular toxic erythema: Pathogenetic relationship between pustule and epidermal appendage (hair follicle or sweat duct). *Acta Derm Venereol (Stockh)* 1978; **58**: 257–61.

13 Staughton RCD, Harper JI, Rowland Payne CME, *et al.* Toxic pustuloderma: a new entity? *J R Soc Med* 1984; **77** (Suppl 4): 6–8.

14 Bernard P, Amici JM, Catanzano G, *et al.* Toxicodermie pustuleuse aigüe generalisée. A propos d'un cas induit par la josamycine. *Ann Dermatol Vénéréol (Paris)* 1989; **116**: 31–3.

15 Commens CA, Fischer GO. Toxic pustuloderma following carbamazepine therapy. *Arch Dermatol* 1988; **124**: 178–9.

16 Grattan CEH. Generalized pustular drug rash due to naproxen. *Dermatologica* 1989; **179**: 57–8.

17 Shelley ED, Shelley WB. The subcorneal pustular drug eruption: an example induced by norfloxacin. *Cutis* 1988; **42**: 24–7.

18 Kushimoto H, Aoki T. Toxic erythema with generalized follicular pustules caused by streptomycin. *Arch Dermatol* 1981; **117**: 444–5.

19 Kalb RE, Grossman ME. Pustular eruption following administration of cephadrine. *Cutis* 1986; **38**: 58–60.

20 Jackson H, Vion B, Levy PM. Generalized eruptive pustular drug rash due to cephalexin. *Dermatologica* 1988; **177**: 292–4.

21 Escallier F, Dalac S, Foucher JL, *et al.* Pustulose exanthématique aigüe généralisée imputabilité a l'imipéneme (Tienam®). *Ann Dermatol Vénéréol (Paris)* 1989; **116**: 407–9.

22 MacDonald KJS, Green CM, Kenicer KJA. Pustular dermatosis induced by co-trimoxazole. *Br Med J* 1986; **293**: 1279–80.

23 Faber M, Maucher OM, Stengel R, Goerttler E. Epraxinonenexanthem mit subkornealer Pustelbildung. *Hautarzt* 1984; **35**: 200–3.

24 Lotem M, Ingber A, Segal R, Sandbank M. Generalized pustular drug rash induced by hydroxychloroquine. *Acta Derm Venereol (Stockh)* 1990; **70**: 250–1.

25 Lambert DG, Dalac S, Beer F, *et al.* Acute generalized exanthematous pustular dermatitis induced by diltiazem. *Br J Dermatol* 1988; **118**: 308–9.
26 Röckl H. Medikamentenallergische Vasculitis leucocytoclastica unter dem Bild eines generalisierten pustulösen Exanthems. *Hautarzt* 1981; **32**: 467–70.
27 Roujeau J-C, Bioulac-Sage P, Bourseau C, *et al.* Acute generalized exanthematous pustulosis. Analysis of 63 cases. *Arch Dermatol* 1991; **127**: 1333–8.
28 Kleier RS, Breneman DL, Boiko S. Generalized pustulation as a manifestation of the anticonvulsant hypersensitivity syndrome. *Arch Dermatol* 1991; **127**: 1361–4.

3.17 Eczematous eruptions

The topic of contact dermatitis, both irritant and allergic forms, will not be discussed here, since it is a very broad subject, and has been widely reviewed in a number of excellent texts, to which the reader is referred for further information [1–5]. This section will, however, discuss the entity termed 'systemic contact-type dermatitis medicamentosa' [6–10].

Drug aetiology

A patient whose initial sensitization to a drug has been induced as a result of allergic contact dermatitis may develop an eczematous reaction when the same, or a chemically related substance, is subsequently administered systemically. The eruption tends to be symmetrical, but may involve first, or most severely, the sites affected by the original dermatitis. Continued administration may lead to generalization of the eruption. For example, patients with a contact allergy to ethylenediamine may develop urticaria or systemic eczema following injection of aminophylline preparations containing ethylenediamine as a solubilizer for theophylline [11,12]. Patients who are contact allergic to parabens and who receive a medicament containing parabens as a preservative may develop systemic eczema [13]. Similarly, sensitized patients may develop eczema following oral ingestion of neomycin [14,15] or hydroxyquinolines [15], and eczema after apresoline and isoniazid has been linked to cross-sensitivity with a hydrazine derivative in a stain remover, to which the patient had become contact allergic [16]. Diabetic patients who become sensitized by topical preparations containing *p*-amino compounds, such as *p*-phenylenediamine hair dyes, *p*-aminobenzoic acid sunscreens, and certain local anaesthetic agents (e.g. benzocaine), may acquire a systemic contact dermatitis following ingestion of the hypoglycaemic agents tolbutamide or chlorpropamide. Sulphonylureas may also induce eczematous eruptions in sulphanilamide-sensitive patients as a result of cross-reactivity. Phenothiazines can produce allergic contact dermatitis, photoallergic reactions, and eczematous contact-type dermatitis, and may cross-react with certain antihistamines. Tetraethylthiuram disulphide (Antabuse) for the management of alcoholism can cause eczematous reactions in patients sensitized to thiurams via rubber gloves. 'Systemic contact-type dermatitis' reactions have also been described with [8]: acetylsalicylic acid, codeine, phenobarbital, dimethyl sulphoxide, hydroxyquinone, nystatin, vitamin B_1, vitamin C, parabens, butylated hydroxyanisole, and hydroxytoluene.

The descriptive term 'baboon syndrome' has been applied to denote a characteristic pattern of systemic allergic contact dermatitis, provoked by ampicillin, nickel and mercury, in which there is diffuse erythema of the buttocks, upper inner thighs, and axillae [17]. Patch tests are commonly positive and usually vesicular, although histology of the eruption itself may show leucocytoclastic vasculitis; oral challenge with the suspected antigen may be required to substantiate the diagnosis. Antabuse therapy of a nickel-sensitive alcoholic patient may induce this syndrome, since this drug leads to an initial acute increase in the blood nickel concentration [17]. Cases have been described from Japan under the name 'mercury exanthem' following inhalation of mercury vapour from crushed thermometers in patients with a history of mercury allergy.

Recently, allergic eczematous reactions to endogenous or exogenous systemic corticosteroids have been documented in patients who are patch test positive to topical corticosteroids [18]. *In vitro*, enriched Langerhans cells, but not peripheral blood mononuclear antigen-presenting cells, are capable of presenting corticosteroid to T cells of corticosteroid-sensitive subjects [19]. This may explain why systemic provocation testing with hydrocortisone results in a reaction confined to the skin in such patients. Another possible explanation is that antigen-specific T cell clones persist in the skin only, and are responsible for the local nature of flare reactions [20].

The reverse situation to that occurring in 'systemic contact-type dermatitis medicamentosa' may also occur, namely primary sensitization by oral therapy can sometimes induce an eczematous drug reaction, or a patient with a drug-related exanthem may later develop localized dermatitis due to topical therapy with the drug. The latter condition has been termed 'endogenic contact eczema' [21]. Thus eczematous eruptions may develop following therapy with penicillin [22], methyldopa, allopurinol, indomethacin and sulphonamides, gold therapy, quinine, chloramphenicol, clonidine, or bleomycin [23]. The alkylating agent mitomycin C administered intravesically for carcinoma of the bladder has been associated with an eczematous eruption, particularly on the face, palms and soles in some patients; these may have positive patch tests to the drug [24,25].

Some of the more important causes of eczematous drug reactions are listed in Table 3.12. Sensitivity to the suspected drug may be confirmed by subsequent patch testing, when the skin reaction has settled.

1 Cronin E. *Contact Dermatitis*. Churchill Livingstone, Edinburgh, 1980.
2 Nater JP, de Groot AC. *Unwanted Effects of Cosmetics and Drugs Used in Dermatology*, 2nd edn. Elsevier, Amsterdam, 1985.
3 Fisher AA. *Contact Dermatitis*. Lea & Febiger, Philadelphia, 1986.

Table 3.12 Systemic drugs which can reactivate allergic contact eczema to chemically related topical medicaments [3]

Systemic drug	Topical medicament
Ethylenediamine antihistamines Aminophylline Piperazine	Aminophylline suppositories Ethylenediamine hydrochloride
Organic and inorganic mercury compounds	Ammoniated mercury
Tr. Benzoin inhalation	Balsam of Peru
Procaine Acetohexamide p-Aminosalicylic acid Azo dyes in foods and drugs Chlorothiazide Chlorpropamide Tolbutamide	Benzocaine (p-amino compound) Glyceryl PABA sunscreens
Chloral hydrate	Chlorobutanol
Iodochlorhydroxyquinoline	Halogenated hydroxyquinoline creams (Vioform)
Iodides, iodinated organic compounds, radiographic contrast media	Iodine
Streptomycin, kanamycin, paromycin, gentamicin	Neomycin sulphate
Nitroglycerine tablets	Nitroglycerine ointment
Disulfiram (Antabuse)	Thiuram

4 Frosch PJ, Dooms-Goossens A, Lachapelle J-M, *et al.* (eds) *Current Topics in Contact Dermatitis*. Springer-Verlag, Berlin, 1989.
5 Rycroft RJG, Menné T, Frosch PJ, Benezra CM (eds) *Textbook of Contact Dermatitis*. Springer-Verlag, Berlin, 1992.
6 Cronin E. Contact dermatitis XVII. Reactions to contact allergens given orally or systemically. *Br J Dermatol* 1972; **86**: 104–7.
7 Truchetet F, Grosshans E, Brandenburger M. Les tests cutanés dans l'allergie médicamenteuse endogene. *Ann Dermatol Vénéréol (Paris)* 1987; **114**: 989–97.
8 Menné T, Veien NK, Maibach HI. Systemic contact-type dermatitis due to drugs. *Semin Dermatol* 1989; **8**: 144–8.
9 Menné T, Maibach HI. Systemic contact allergy reactions. *Immunol Allergy Clin North Am* 1989; **9**: 507–22.
10 Aquilina C, Sayag J. Eczéma par réactogenes internes. *Ann Dermatol Vénéréol (Paris)* 1989; **116**: 753–65.
11 Berman BA, Ross RN. Ethylenediamine: systemic eczematous contact-type dermatitis. *Cutis* 1983; **31**: 594–8.
12 Hardy C, Schofield O, George CF. Allergy to aminophylline. *Br Med J* 1983; **286**: 2051–2.
13 Aeling JL, Nuss DD. Systemic eczematous 'contact-type' dermatitis medicamentosa caused by parabens. *Arch Dermatol* 1974; **110**: 640.
14 Menné T, Weismann K. Hämatogenes Kontaktekzem nach oraler Gabe von Neomyzin. *Hautarzt* 1984; **35**: 319–20.
15 Ekelund E-G, Möller H. Oral provocation in eczematous contact allergy to neomycin and hydroxy-quinolines. *Acta Derm Venereol (Stockh)* 1969; **49**: 422–6.

16 van Ketel WG. Contact dermatitis from a hydrazine-derivative in a stain remover. Cross sensitization to apresoline and isoniazid. *Acta Derm Venereol (Stockh)* 1964; **44**: 49–53.

17 Andersen KE, Hjorth N, Menné. The baboon syndrome: systemically-induced allergic contact dermatitis. *Contact Dermatitis* 1984; **10**: 97–100.

18 Lauerma AI, Reitamo S, Maibach HI. Systemic hydrocortisone/cortisol induces allergic skin reactions in presensitized subjects. *J Am Acad Dermatol* 1991; **24**: 182–5.

19 Lauerma AI, Räsänen L, Reunala T, Reitamo S. Langerhans cells but not monocytes are capable of antigen presentation *in vitro* in corticosteroid contact hypersensitivity. *Br J Dermatol* 1991; **123**: 699–705.

20 Scheper RJ, Von Blomberg M, Boerrigter GH, *et al*. Induction of immunological memory in the skin. Role of local T cell retention. *Clin Exp Immunol* 1983; **51**: 141–8.

21 Pirilä V. Endogenic contact eczema. *Allerg Asthma* 1970; **16**: 15–19.

22 Girard JP. Recurrent angioneurotic oedema and contact dermatitis due to penicillin. *Contact Dermatitis* 1978; **4**: 309.

23 Lincke-Plewig H. Bleomycin-Exantheme. *Hautarzt* 1980; **31**: 616–18.

24 Colver GB, Inglis JA, McVittie E, *et al*. Dermatitis due to intravesical mitomycin C: a delayed-type hypersensitivity reaction? *Br J Dermatol* 1990; **122**: 217–24.

25 De Groot AC, Conemans JMH. Systemic allergic contact dermatitis from intravesical instillation of the antitumor antibiotic mitomycin C. *Contact Dermatitis* 1991; **24**: 201–9.

3.18 Bullous eruptions

Bullous drug eruptions encompass many different clinical reactions, and a correspondingly large number of pathomechanisms are involved. Isolated blisters, often located preferentially on the extremities, may be caused by a wide variety of chemically distinct drugs [1]. Fixed drug eruptions (Fig. 3.53), erythema multiforme, and drug-induced vasculitis, may have a bullous component; drug-induced toxic epidermal necrolysis (TEN) is associated with widespread blistering. The specific drug-induced entities of porphyria and pseudoporphyria, bullous pemphigoid, and pemphigus are discussed separately below.

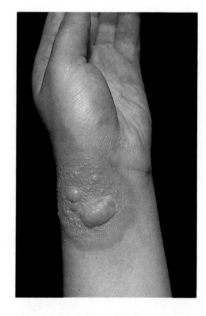

Bullous eruption in drug overdosage

Bullae, often at pressure areas, may be seen in patients comatose after overdosage with barbiturates, methadone, meprobamate, imipramine, nitrazepam or glutethimide [1–5].

1 Bork K. *Cutaneous Side Effects of Drugs*. WB Saunders, Philadelphia, 1988.

2 Brehmer-Andersson E, Pedersen NB. Sweat gland necrosis and bullous skin changes in acute drug intoxication. *Acta Derm Venereol (Stockh)* 1969; **49**: 157–62.

3 Mandy S, Ackerman AB. Characteristic traumatic skin lesions in drug-induced coma. *JAMA* 1970; **213**: 253–6.

4 Arndt KA, Mihm MC Jr, Parrish JA. Bullae: A cutaneous sign of a variety of neurologic diseases. *J Invest Dermatol* 1973; **60**: 312–20.

5 Herschtal D, Robinson MJ. Blisters of the skin in coma induced by amitriptyline and chlorazepate dipotassium. Report of a case with underlying sweat gland necrosis. *Arch Dermatol* 1979; **115**: 499.

Figure 3.53 Bullous fixed drug eruption due to sulphamethoxydiazine.

3.19 Porphyria and pseudoporphyria

Drug-induced porphyria

Clinical features of drug-induced porphyria

A large number of drugs (Table 3.13) have been reported to exacerbate the acute hepatic porphyrias; these either cause excess destruction of haem, or else inhibit haem synthesis [1,2]. Drugs implicated in precipitating porphyria cutanea tarda include especially barbiturates, griseofulvin (which inhibits ferrochelatase), sulphonamides, oestrogens either given to men for prostatic carcinoma, or to women either alone or in the contraceptive pill [3–7], and rifampicin [8]. Clinical features consist of photosensitivity, blistering or erosions, scarring and hirsutism of exposed areas, especially on the dorsal aspect of the hands (Fig. 3.54). Porphyria cutanea tarda was precipitated by ingestion of wheat seed accidentally impregnated with hexachlorobenzene in Turkey; children were affected more severely than adults [9]. Industrial exposure to other polyhalogenated hydro-

Table 3.13 Drugs which are unsafe to use in patients with acute intermittent porphyria, porphyria cutanea tarda or variegate porphyria [1]

Aminoglutethimide
Barbiturates
Carbamazepine
Carbromal
Chlorpropamide
Danazol
Diclofenac
Diphenylhydantoin
Ergot preparations
Glutethimide
Griseofulvin
Meprobamate
Novobiocin
Oestrogens
Primadone
Progestagens
Pyrazolone derivatives
Sulphonamides
Tolbutamide
Trimethadione
Valproic acid

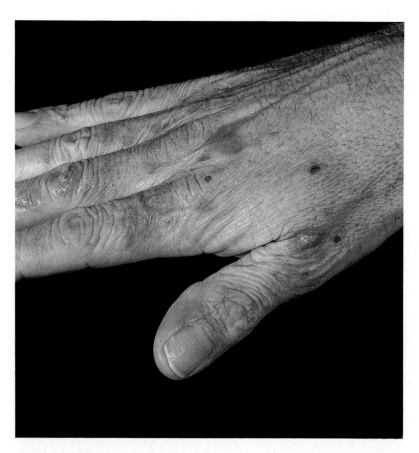

Figure 3.54 Erythema, haemorrhagic crusting and scarring related to previous blisters in porphyria cutanea tarda.

[100]

carbons, including dichlorophenols, trichlorophenols, dioxin, and polychlorinated and polybrominated biphenyls, have also caused this condition [1,10].

Histology

Histological examination reveals subepidermal bulla formation, thickened blood vessel walls, readily identifiable in periodic acid–Schiff (PAS)-stained sections, and very little in the way of a dermal inflammatory infiltrate (Fig. 3.55). Subepidermal blistering, with splitting at the level of the lamina lucida, occurs in both porphyria cutanea tarda and drug-induced porphyria [11]. Direct tissue immunofluorescence reveals the deposition of immunoglobulins and complement on blood vessels and along the dermo-epidermal junction (Fig. 3.56).

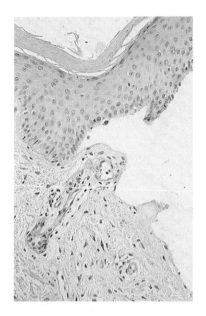

Figure 3.55 Subepidermal blister with thickening of blood vessel walls in porphyria cutanea tarda; PAS stain.

1 Targovnick SE, Targovnik JH. Cutaneous drug reactions in porphyrias. *Clin Dermatol* 1986; **4**: 111–17.
2 Köstler E, Seebacher C, Riedel H, Kemmer C. Therapeutische und pathogenetische Aspekte der Porphyria cutanea tarda. *Hautarzt* 1986; **37**: 210–16.
3 Becker FT. Porphyria cutanea tarda induced by estrogens. *Arch Dermatol* 1965; **92**: 252–6.
4 Vail JT. Porphyria cutanea tarda and estrogens. *JAMA* 1967; **20**: 671–4.
5 Roenigk HH, Gottlob ME. Estrogen-induced porphyria cutanea tarda. Report of three cases. *Arch Dermatol* 1970; **102**: 260–6.
6 Behm AR, Unger WP. Oral contraceptives and porphyria cutanea tarda. *Can Med Assoc J* 1974; **110**: 1052–4.
7 Byrne JPH, Boss JM, Dawber RPR. Contraceptive pill-induced porphyria cutanea tarda presenting with onycholysis of the finger nails. *Postgrad Med J* 1976; **52**: 535–8.
8 Millar JW. Rifampicin-induced porphyria cutanea tarda. *Br J Dis Chest* 1980; **74**: 405–8.
9 Cam C, Nigogosyan G. Acquired toxic porphyria cutanea tarda due to hexachlorobenzene. *JAMA* 1963; **183**: 88–91.
10 Bleiberg J, Wallen M, Brodken R, *et al*. Industrially acquired porphyria. *Arch Dermatol* 1964; **89**: 793–7.
11 Dabski C, Beutner EH. Studies of laminin and type IV collagen in blisters of porphyria cutanea tarda and drug-induced pseudoporphyria. *J Am Acad Dermatol* 1991; **25**: 28–32.

Pseudoporphyria

Pseudoporphyria, in which porphyria-like blistering of exposed areas on the extremities occurs in the absence of abnormal porphyrin metabolism, may be caused by high dose frusemide [1], naproxen [2], nalidixic acid [3], tetracyclines [4,5], sulphonylurea drugs, and non-steroidal anti-inflammatory agents [6,7]. Phototoxic mechanisms have been implicated in some cases. A similar syndrome has been reported in a patient taking very large doses of pyridoxine (vitamin B_6) [8]. Use of UV-A sunbeds may result in a pseudoporphyria syndrome [9–12]. A pseudoporphyria syndrome has been described in patients treated with dialysis for renal failure; porphyrin levels may or may not be abnormal [13–15].

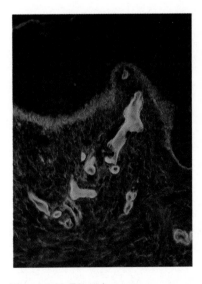

Figure 3.56 Direct immunofluorescence with anti-IgG in porphyria cutanea tarda; note fluorescence of thickened vessel walls and along the dermo-epidermal junction.

1 Burry JN, Lawrence JR. Phototoxic blisters from high frusemide dosage. *Br J Dermatol* 1976; **94**: 495−9.
2 Judd LE, Henderson DW, Hill DC. Naproxen-induced pseudoporphyria: a clinical and ultrastructural study. *Arch Dermatol* 1986; **122**: 451−4.
3 Keane JT, Pearson RW, Malkinson FD. Nalidixic acid-induced photosensitivity in mice: a model for pseudoporphyria. *J Invest Dermatol* 1984; **82**: 210−13.
4 Epstein JH, Tuffanelli DL, Seibert JS, Epstein WL. Porphyria-like cutaneous changes induced by tetracycline hydrochloride photosensitization. *Arch Dermatol* 1976; **112**: 661−6.
5 Hawk JLM. Skin changes resembling hepatic cutaneous porphyria induced by oxytetracycline photosensitization. *Clin Exp Dermatol* 1980; **5**: 321−5.
6 Stern RS. Phototoxic reactions to piroxicam and other nonsteroidal anti-inflammatory agents. *N Engl J Med* 1983; **309**: 186−7.
7 Taylor BJ, Duffill MB. Pseudoporphyria from nonsteroidal anti-inflammatory drugs. *N Z Med J* 1987; **100**: 322−3.
8 Baer R, Stilman MA. Cutaneous skin changes probably due to pyridoxine abuse. *J Am Acad Dermatol* 1984; **10**: 527−8.
9 Farr PM, Marks JM, Diffey BL, Ince P. Skin fragility and blistering due to use of sunbeds. *Br Med J* 1988; **296**: 1708−9.
10 Murphy GM, Wright J, Nicholls DSH, *et al*. Sunbed-induced pseudoporphyria. *Br J Dermatol* 1989; **120**: 555−62.
11 Poh-Fitzpatrick MB, Ellis DL. Porphyria like bullous dermatosis after chronic intense tanning bed and/or sunlight exposure. *Arch Dermatol* 1989; **125**: 1236−8.
12 Sternberg A. Pseudoporphyria and sunbeds. *Acta Derm Venereol (Stockh)* 1990; **70**: 354−6.
13 Gilchrest B, Rowe JW, Mihm ME Jr. Bullous dermatosis of hemodialysis. *Ann Intern Med* 1975; **83**: 480−3.
14 Poh-Fitzpatrick MB, Bellet N, DeLeo VA, *et al*. Porphyria cutanea tarda in two patients treated with hemodialysis for chronic renal failure. *N Engl J Med* 1978; **299**: 292−4.
15 Gupta AK, Gupta MA, Cardella CJ, Haberman HF. Cutaneous complications of chronic renal failure and dialysis. *Int J Dermatol* 1986; **25**: 498−504.

3.20 Drug-induced bullous pemphigoid

Idiopathic bullous pemphigoid

Idiopathic bullous pemphigoid is an autoimmune condition chiefly restricted to elderly patients, in which large tense bullae develop on an erythematous, urticated base. Blistering is subepidermal, direct tissue immunofluorescence reveals deposition of immunoglobulins and complement along the dermo-epidermal basement membrane zone, and patients have circulating IgG autoantibodies which bind to an antigen of M_r 220−240 kDa (bullous pemphigoid antigen) located in the lamina lucida of the basement membrane zone [1].

Drug aetiology

Drug-induced bullous pemphigoid has been reported with a number of medications [2,3], especially with frusemide [4,5], but also with penicillamine [6,7], the penicillamine analogue tiobutarit [8], penicillin [9] and its derivatives [10], sulphasalazine, salicylazo-sulphapyridine, phenacetin [11], novoscabin, topical fluorouracil, and PUVA therapy [12]. Several of the drugs implicated have sulphur within the molecule, and it has been postulated that thiol formation plays a role in the pathogenesis of drug-induced bullous pemphigoid. We have seen bullous pemphigoid induced by flupenthixol (Figs 3.57 & 3.58). In the case induced by phenacetin, indirect immunofluorescence binding of circulating autoantibody to the basement membrane zone could not be completely blocked by preincubation of substrate with bullous pemphigoid serum, unlike the case for idiopathic bullous pemphigoid [11]. This suggested that the antigenic site(s) within the lamina lucida for the drug-induced case differed from that in idiopathic bullous pemphigoid. A blistering skin disease similar to bullous pemphigoid, both clinically and by immunofluorescence, developed in a man after injections of human placental extracts; his serum did not, however, react with the classical 220−240 kDa bullous pemphigoid antigen on immunoblotting [13].

Clinico-pathological features of drug-induced pemphigoid

There is a broad spectrum of clinical presentation in drug-induced bullous pemphigoid [3], encompassing widely scattered classical large tense bullae, classical but fewer lesions, scarring plaques, an erythema multiforme-like picture, and a pemphigus-like picture. Affected patients tend to be younger than the average age of onset of idiopathic bullous pemphigoid. There may be perivascular lymphocytes with eosinophils and neutrophils, intra-epidermal vesicles with focal keratinocyte necrosis, and thrombi in deep dermal blood vessels. Tissue-bound and circulating anti-basement membrane zone IgG antibodies may be absent [6], or additional antibodies such as intercellular [7] or anti-epidermal cytoplasmic antibodies [11] may be detected. Some cases of drug-induced bullous pemphigoid

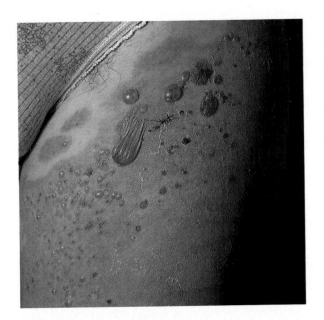

Figure 3.57 Bullous pemphigoid due to flupenthixol-melitracen in a 26-year-old patient.

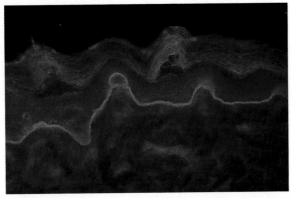

Figure 3.58 Indirect immunofluorescence in drug-induced bullous pemphigoid, demonstrating the presence of circulating anti-basement membrane zone antibodies.

are short-lived, whereas others become chronic. Cicatricial pemphigoid has been described in association with clonidine [14], and was also associated with practolol (no longer commercially available) [15].

1 Stanley JR, Hawley-Nelson P, Yuga SH, *et al.* Characterization of bullous pemphigoid antigen: a unique basement membrane protein of stratified squamous epithelia. *Cell* 1981; **24**: 897−903.
2 Ahmed AR, Newcomer VD. Drug-induced bullous pemphigoid. *Clin Dermatol* 1987; **5**: 8−10.
3 Ruocco V, Sacerdoti G. Pemphigus and bullous pemphigoid due to drugs. *Int J Dermatol* 1991; **30**: 307−12.
4 Fellner MJ, Katz JM. Occurrence of bullous pemphigoid after furosemide therapy. *Arch Dermatol* 1976; **112**: 75−7.
5 Castel T, Gratacos R, Castro J, *et al.* Bullous pemphigoid induced by furosemide. *Clin Exp Dermatol* 1981; **6**: 635−8.
6 Brown MD, Dubin HV. Penicillamine-induced bullous pemphigoid-like eruption. *Arch Dermatol* 1987; **123**: 1119−20.
7 Rasmussen HB, Jepsen LV, Brandrup F. Penicillamine-induced bullous pemphigoid with pemphigus-like antibodies. *J Cutan Pathol* 1989; **16**: 154−7.
8 Yamaguchi R, Oryu F, Hidano A. A case of bullous pemphigoid induced by tiobutarit (D-penicillamine analogue). *J Dermatol (Tokyo)* 1989; **16**: 308−11.
9 Alcalay J, David M, Ingber A, *et al.* Bullous pemphigoid mimicking bullous erythema multiforme: an untoward side effect of penicillins. *J Am Acad Dermatol* 1988; **18**: 345−9.
10 Hodak E, Ben-Shetrit A, Ingber A, Sandbank M. Bullous pemphigoid: an adverse effect of ampicillin. *Clin Exp Dermatol* 1990; **15**: 50−2.
11 Kashihara M, Danno K, Miyachi Y, *et al.* Bullous pemphigoid-like lesions induced by phenacetin: report of a case and an immunopathologic study. *Arch Dermatol* 1984; **120**: 1196−9.
12 Abel EA, Bennett A. Bullous pemphigoid. Occurrence in psoriasis treated with psoralens plus long-wave ultraviolet radiation. *Arch Dermatol* 1979; **115**: 988−9.
13 Saurat J-H, Didierjean L, Mérot Y, Salomon D. Blistering skin disease in a man after injections of human placental extracts. *Br Med J* 1988; **297**: 775.
14 Van Joost T, Faber WR, Manuel HR. Drug-induced anogenital cicatricial pemphigoid. *Br J Dermatol* 1980; **102**: 715−18.
15 Van Joost T, Crone RA, Overdijk AD. Ocular cicatricial pemphigoid associated with practolol therapy. *Br J Dermatol* 1976; **94**: 447−50.

3.21 Drug-induced pemphigus

Idiopathic pemphigus

Idiopathic pemphigus erythematosus, foliaceus and vulgaris are autoimmune bullous disorders in which the level of blister formation is more superficial than in bullous pemphigoid. In the erythematosus and foliaceus variants, blisters may not be evident, and erythema, crusting and scaling may be the major clinical features. In pemphigus vulgaris, erosions rather than intact blisters may be seen; ulceration of the buccal mucous membranes is common. In all variants, the histology is characterized by intra-epidermal splitting and acantholysis (occurring at a subcorneal level in pemphigus foliaceus, and a suprabasal level in pemphigus vulgaris); direct tissue, and indirect, immunofluorescence reveals the presence of circulating

IgG autoantibodies which bind to the intercellular region of the epidermis in a 'chicken-wire' pattern. These autoantibodies mediate the blistering, since pemphigus may be induced in neonatal mice by passive transfer of IgG from patients with the disease [1]. In idiopathic pemphigus foliaceus, autoantibodies bind to a characteristic complex of epidermal polypeptides of M_r 260, 160 (the desmosomal core protein, desmoglein) and 85 kDa, while in pemphigus foliaceus they bind to another characteristic complex of epidermal polypeptides of M_r 210, 130 (pemphigus vulgaris antigen) and 85 kDa [2]. The common 85 kDa polypeptide present in both complexes is the desmosomal and adherens junction-associated molecule, plakoglobin [3].

Drug aetiology

A number of drugs have been implicated in the production of a disorder closely resembling idiopathic pemphigus (Table 3.14) [4–13]. About 80% of cases are caused by drugs associated with a thiol group. These include drugs with a thiol group in the molecule, penicillamine (Fig. 3.59) especially (about 7% of those receiving the drug for more than 6 months develop pemphigus) [14–19] and the structurally related drug captopril [19–22], gold sodium thiomalate, drugs with disulphide bonds such as pyritinol [23], *S*-thiopyridoxine, thiopronine which is chemically related to penicillamine and used as an alternative therapy in penicillamine intolerance [24], and mercapto-propionylglycine [25], as well as those with a sulphur-containing ring that may undergo metabolic change to the thiol form, such as piroxicam [26]. Penicillin [27–29] and its derivatives ampicillin [29], procaine penicillin and amoxycillin [12], may also cause pemphigus; traces of penicillamine are detectable as penicillin metabolic degradation products in the plasma of patients with penicillin-induced pemphigus [27], so that these cases may also belong to the thiol group. Rifampicin [30,31], cephalexin [32], cefadroxil [12], pyrazolone derivatives [33], propranolol, optalidon, pentachlorophenol, phenobarbital [34], phosphamide, hydantoin, combinations of indomethacin and aspirin [35], and propranolol and meprobamate [36], as well as heroin [37], have all been established as rare causes of pemphigus-like reaction.

Clinico-pathological patterns of drug-induced pemphigus

In drug-induced pemphigus, the clinical pattern is most often that of pemphigus foliaceus (Fig. 3.59), but the erythematosus, herpetiformis (with annular or gyrate lesions) [35,38], and urticaria-like forms of pemphigus also occur. Drug-induced pemphigus vulgaris [26,27,29] is rare. The oral mucosa is involved in 50% of cases. The level of intra-epidermal splitting (Fig. 3.60) is variable both within the same and different lesions of individual patients.

Table 3.14 Drugs implicated in the development of pemphigus

Thiol drugs
Penicillamine
Captopril
Gold sodium thiomalate
Pyritinol
Thiamazole
Thiopronine
Mercapto-propionylglycine

Non-thiol drugs
Antibiotics
    Penicillin and derivatives
    Rifampicin
    Cephalexin
    Cefadroxil
Pyrazolone derivatives
    Aminophenazone
    Aminopyrine
    Azapropazone
    Oxyphenylbutazone
    Phenylbutazone
Miscellaneous
    Hydantoin
    Levodopa
    Lysine acetylsalicylate
    Phenobarbital
    Piroxicam
    Progesterone
    Propranolol
    Heroin

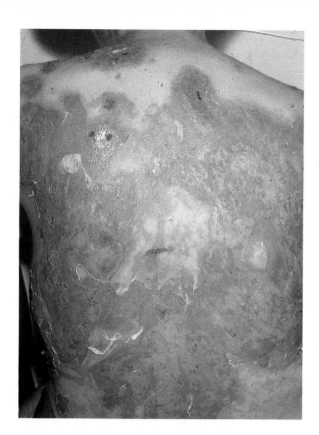

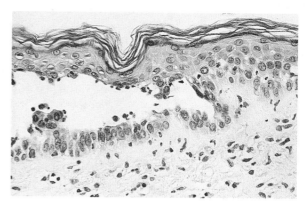

Figure 3.60 Suprabasal splitting and acantholysis in drug-induced pemphigus vulgaris.

Figure 3.59 Extensive superficial erosion in pemphigus foliaceus induced by D-penicillamine. (Courtesy of Dr M.M. Black, St John's Institute of Dermatology, London.)

The majority of patients with drug-induced pemphigus have tissue bound and/or low titre circulating autoantibodies directed against epidermal cell surface antigens (Fig. 3.61) [5,19]. Immunoprecipitation studies have shown that three patients with drug-induced pemphigus foliaceus (two due to penicillamine, and one due to captopril), and one patient with drug-induced pemphigus vulgaris (due to captopril), had circulating autoantibodies with the same antigenic specificity at a molecular level as autoantibodies from patients with the corresponding subtype of idiopathic pemphigus [19]. However, in the case of penicillamine-induced pemphigus, 10% of patients do not have tissue-bound, and more than 30% do not have circulating, autoantibodies [9]. Patch testing [27], and a lymphocyte transformation test to the drug [39], may occasionally be positive.

Prognosis of drug-induced pemphigus

The reaction usually regresses within weeks of cessation of therapy, but it may persist for years, and the occasional fatal outcome of drug-induced pemphigus has been recorded [15,26]. Patients with pemphigus induced by a drug containing a sulphydryl radical show spontaneous recovery, following drug withdrawal, in 39% of cases

[106]

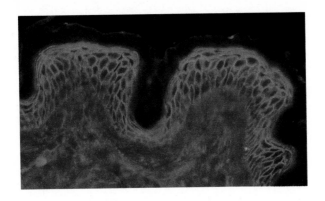

Figure 3.61 Indirect immunofluorescence in drug-induced pemphigus foliaceus demonstrating intercellular binding of circulating IgG antibodies.

induced by penicillamine and 53% of cases caused by other drugs in the group, compared with a spontaneous recovery rate of only 15% for non-sulphydryl radical-containing drugs [12,13]. It has been proposed that a tendency for drug-induced pemphigus to resolve soon after withdrawal of the drug is correlated with a lack of circulating or tissue-bound autoantibodies. However, disease resolution may occur despite the presence of circulating and tissue bound autoantibodies [19].

Pathomechanisms of drug-induced pemphigus

Since only a very few patients develop pemphigus following drug exposure, it has been argued that genetic factors must be of importance; the phenotype HLA-A26, B38, DR4 has been reported in several drug-induced pemphigus patients [11]. However, the existence of haplotypes with predisposition to drug-induced pemphigus has been disputed [9].

The active sulphydryl group common to many drugs which induce pemphigus [40] could bind to the pemphigus antigen complexes, interfering with their cell adhesion function. Drugs with thiol groups in their molecule, such as penicillamine, captopril and thiopronine, as well as piroxicam, have in fact been recently reported to cause acantholysis *in vitro* in the absence of autoantibody [9,41–44]. This may explain in part the faster recovery following removal of drugs with a thiol group. Alternatively, binding of an active thiol group to the pemphigus antigen complex might render it immunogenic, with resultant autoantibody production. Since penicillamine therapy is known to be associated with development of other autoimmune diseases such as myasthenia gravis [40], penicillamine may result in immune dysregulation, with an increased tendency to develop autoantibodies. Penicillamine does have immunomodulatory properties [45], and drug-specific antibodies may be found in patients treated with penicillamine [46,47] and captopril [48]. Serum IgG antibody from patients with idiopathic pemphigus induces epidermal acantholysis in organ culture [49]. It has been proposed that in sporadic pemphigus, binding of autoantibody to the keratin-ocyte cell surface induces proteinase activity with resultant acantholysis [50]; a similar mechanism has been postulated for penicillamine-induced pemphigus [51].

1 Anhalt GJ, Labib KS, Voorhees JS, *et al.* Induction of pemphigus in neonatal mice by passive transfer of IgG from patients with the disease. *N Engl J Med* 1982; **306**: 1189−92.

2 Eyre RW, Stanley JR. Identification of pemphigus vulgaris antigen extracted from normal human epidermis and comparison with pemphigus foliaceus antigen. *J Clin Invest* 1988; **81**: 807−12.

3 Korman NJ, Eyre RW, Klaus-Kovtun V, Stanley JR. Demonstration of an adhering-junction molecule (plakoglobin) in the autoantigens of pemphigus foliaceus and pemphigus vulgaris. *N Engl J Med* 1989; **321**: 631−5.

4 Fellner MJ, Moshell A, Mont MA. Pemphigus vulgaris and drug reactions. *Int J Dermatol* 1980; **20**: 115−18.

5 Kaplan RP, Callen JP. Pemphigus associated diseases and induced pemphigus. *Clin Dermatol* 1983; **1**: 42−71.

6 Ruocco V, Pisani M. Induced pemphigus. *Arch Dermatol Res* 1984; **274**: 123−40.

7 Pisani M, Ruocco V. Drug-induced pemphigus. *Clin Dermatol* 1986; **4**: 118−32.

8 Enjolras O, Sedel D, Leibowitch M, Escande J-P. Pemphigus induits. *Ann Dermatol Vénéréol (Paris)* 1987; **114**: 25−37.

9 Anhalt GJ. Drug-induced pemphigus. *Semin Dermatol* 1989; **8**: 166−72.

10 Civatte J. Durch Medikamente induzierte Pemphigus-Erkrankungen. *Dermatol Monatschr* 1989; **175**: 1−7.

11 Ruocco V, Sacerdoti G. Pemphigus and bullous pemphigoid due to drugs. *Int J Dermatol* 1991; **30**: 307−12.

12 Wolf R, Tamir A, Brenner S. Drug-induced versus drug-triggered pemphigus. *Dermatologica* 1991; **182**: 207−10.

13 Wolf R, Brenner S Arzneimittelbedingter Pemphigus − Übersicht. *Z Hautkr* 1991; **66**: 289−93.

14 Marsden RA, Ryan TJ, Van Hegan RI, *et al.* Pemphigus foliaceus induced by penicillamine. *Br Med J* 1976; **iv**: 1423−4.

15 Matkaluk RM, Bailin PL. Penicillamine-induced pemphigus foliaceus. A fatal outcome. *Arch Dermatol* 1981; **117**: 156−7.

16 Yung CW, Hambrick GW Jr. D-Penicillamine-induced pemphigus syndrome. *J Am Acad Dermatol* 1982; **6**: 317−24.

17 Zone J, Ward J, Boyce E, Schupbach C. Penicillamine induced pemphigus. *JAMA* 1982; **247**: 2705−7.

18 Kind P, Goerz G, Gleichmann E, Plewig G. Penicillamininduzierter Pemphigus. *Hautarzt* 1987; **38**: 548−52.

19 Korman NJ, Eyre RW, Stanley JR. Drug-induced pemphigus: autoantibodies directed against the pemphigus antigen complexes are present in penicillamine and captopril-induced pemphigus. *J Invest Dermatol* 1991; **96**: 273−6.

20 Parfrey PS, Clement M, Vandenburg MJ, Wright P. Captopril-induced pemphigus. *Br Med J* 1980; **281**: 194.

21 Clement M. Captopril-induced eruptions. *Arch Dermatol* 1981; **117**: 525−6.

22 Katz RA, Hood AF, Anhalt GJ. Pemphigus-like eruption from captopril. *Arch Dermatol* 1987; **123**: 20−1.

23 Civatte J, Duterque M, Blanchet P, *et al.* Deux cas de pemphigus superficiel induit par le pyritinol. *Ann Dermatol Vénéréol (Paris)* 1978; **105**: 573−7.

24 Alinovi A, Benoldi D, Manganelli P. Pemphigus erythematosus induced by thiopronin. *Acta Derm Venereol (Stockh)* 1982; **62**: 452−4.

25 Lucky PA, Skovby F, Thier SO. Pemphigus foliaceus and proteinuria induced by α-mercapto-propionylglycine. *J Am Acad Dermatol* 1983; **8**: 667−72.

26 Martin RL, McSweeny GW, Schneider J. Fatal pemphigus vulgaris in a patient taking piroxicam. *N Engl J Med* 1983; **309**: 795−6.

27 Ruocco V, Rossi A, Pisani M, *et al*. An abortive form of pemphigus vulgaris probably induced by penicillin. *Dermatologica* 1979; **159**: 266–73.

28 Duhra PL, Foulds IS. Penicillin-induced pemphigus vulgaris. *Br J Dermatol* 1988; **118**: 307.

29 Fellner MJ, Mark AS. Penicillin- and ampicillin-induced pemphigus vulgaris. *Int J Dermatol* 1980; **19**: 392–3.

30 Gange RW, Rhodes EL, Edwards CO, Powell MEA. Pemphigus induced by rifampicin. *Br J Dermatol* 1976; **95**: 445–8.

31 Lee CW, Lim JH, Kang HJ. Pemphigus foliaceus induced by rifampicin. *Br J Dermatol* 1984; **111**: 619–22.

32 Wolf R, Dechner E, Ophir J, Brenner S. Cephalexin. A nonthiol drug that may induce pemphigus vulgaris. *Int J Dermatol* 1991; **30**: 213–15.

33 Chorzelski TP, Jablonska S, Blaszczyk M. Autoantibodies in pemphigus. *Acta Derm Venereol (Stockh)* 1966; **46**: 26.

34 Dourmishev AL, Rahman MA. Phenobarbital-induced pemphigus vulgaris. *Dermatologica* 1986; **173**: 256–8.

35 DeMento FJ, Grover RW. Acantholytic herpetiform dermatitis. *Arch Dermatol* 1973; **107**: 883–7.

36 Goddard W, Lambert D, Gavanou J, Chapius JL. Pemphigus acquit apres traitement par l'association propranolol-meprobamate. *Ann Dermatol Vénéréol (Paris)* 1980; **107**: 1213–16.

37 Fellner MJ, Winiger J. Pemphigus erythematosus and heroin addiction. *Int J Dermatol* 1978; **17**: 308–11.

38 Morioka S, Ogawa H. Herpetiform pemphigus-like skin lesions induced by D-penicillamine. *J Dermatol (Tokyo)* 1980; **7**: 425–9.

39 Stewart W-M, Lauret P, Boullie M-C, *et al*. A propos de deux cas d'accidents bulleux, dont un cas de pemphigus, dus a la pénicillamine. *Ann Dermatol Vénéréol (Paris)* 1977; **104**: 542–8.

40 Jaffe IA. Adverse effects profile of sulfhydryl compounds in man. *Am J Med* 1986; **80**: 471–6.

41 Ruocco V, de Angelis E, Lombardi ML, Pisani M. *In vitro* acantholysis by captopril and thiopronine. *Dermatologica* 1988; **176**: 115–23.

42 Yokel BK, Hood AF, Anhalt GJ. Induction of acantholysis in organ explant culture by penicillamine and captopril. *Arch Dermatol* 1989; **125**: 1367–70.

43 De Dobbeleer G, Godfrine S, De Graef C, *et al*. Reproduction d'acantholyse *in vitro* par l'addition de piroxicam, de captopril et de D-pénicillamine au milieu de culture de kératinocytes humains cultivés sur derme dévitalisé. *Ann Dermatol Vénéréol (Paris)* 1989; **116**: 279–80.

44 Ruocco V, Pisani M, de Angelis E, Lombardi ML. Biochemical acantholysis provoked by thiol drugs. *Arch Dermatol* 1990; **126**: 965–6.

45 Chen DM, Di Sabato G, Field L, *et al*. Some immunological effects of penicillamine. *Clin Exp Immunol* 1977; **30**: 317–22.

46 Sparrow GP. Penicillamine pemphigus and the nephrotic syndrome occurring simultaneously. *Br J Dermatol* 1978; **98**: 103–4.

47 Storch WB. Clinical significance of penicillamine antibodies. *Lancet* 1988; **ii**: 214.

48 Coleman JW, Yeung JHK, Roberts DH, *et al*. Drug-specific antibodies in patients receiving captopril. *Br J Clin Pharmacol* 1986; **22**: 161–5.

49 Schiltz JR, Michel B. Production of epidermal acantholysis in normal human skin *in vitro* by the IgG fraction from pemphigus serum. *J Invest Dermatol* 1976; **67**: 254–60.

50 Hashimoto K, Shafran KM, Webber PS, *et al*. Anti-cell surface pemphigus autoantibody stimulates plasminogen activator activity of human epidermal cells; a mechanism for the loss of epidermal cohesion and blister formation. *J Exp Med* 1983; **157**: 259–72.

51 Hashimoto K, Singer K, Lazarus GS. Penicillamine-induced pemphigus. Immunoglobulin from this patient induces plasminogen activator synthesis by human epidermal cells in culture: mechanism for acantholysis in pemphigus. *Arch Dermatol* 1984; **120**: 762–4.

Table 3.15 Drugs recorded as inducing vasculitis

Allopurinol
Aminosalicylic acid
Amiodarone
Amphetamine
Ampicillin
Aspirin
Arsenic
Captopril
Cimetidine
Coumadin
Erythromycin
Ethacrynic acid
Fluoroquinolone antibiotics
Frusemide
Griseofulvin
Guanethidine
Hydralazine
Iodides
Levamisole
Maprotiline
Methotrexate
Penicillin
Phenacetin
Phenothiazines
Phenylbutazone
Phenytoin
Procainamide
Propylthiouracil
Quinidine
Radiocontrast media
Streptomycin
Sulphonamides
Trazodone
Tetracycline
Thiazides
Vaccination

3.22 Vasculitis

Clinical features

Drug-induced cutaneous necrotizing vasculitis presents with palpable purpuric lesions on the legs; urticarial lesions, ulcerated areas, and haemorrhagic blisters may also be present (Figs 3.62 & 3.63). Drug-induced vasculitis may involve not only the skin, but also internal organs, including the heart, liver and kidneys, with fatal results [2]. The patterns of polyarteritis nodosa, Henoch–Schönlein vasculitis and hypocomplementaemic vasculitis do not seem to be caused by drugs commonly. The vasculitis may be a manifestation of immune complex disease [1–13].

Drug aetiology

Drugs which have been implicated are listed in Table 3.15. These include: ampicillin, thiazide diuretics, phenylbutazone, sulphonamides, quinidine [13], hydralazine [14], frusemide [15], propylthiouracil [16–18], non-steroidal anti-inflammatory agents, cimetidine [19], coumadin [20], amiodarone [21], hyposensitization therapy [22,23], BCG vaccination (which may cause a papulonecrotic type of vasculitis) [24], radiographic contrast media [25], food and drug additives [26], and vitamin B$_6$ [27]. Leucocytoclastic vasculitis and necrotizing angiitis have also been documented in drug abusers [28–30].

Histology and immunopathology

The histology has been reported to be characterized by either a lymphocytic or a leucocytoclastic perivascular infiltrate [2,7,12,13,31].

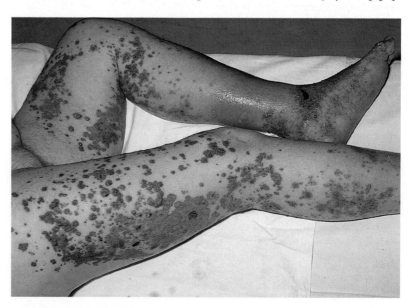

Figure 3.62 Extensive leucocytoclastic vasculitis with purpura and haemorrhagic bulla formation.

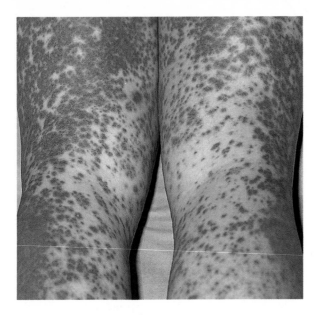

Figure 3.63 Palpable purpura in leucocytoclastic vasculitis.

In the case of a lymphocytic drug-induced vasculitis, there is an infiltrate of mononuclear cells and eosinophils in the walls of, and around, involved small cutaneous blood vessels, without evidence of fibrinoid deposits. In leucocytoclastic vasculitis, there is fibrinoid degeneration of upper dermal blood vessel walls, with neutrophil and variable eosinophil and mononuclear cell infiltration of the vessel wall and the surrounding dermis (Fig. 3.64). Leucocytoclasis, with nuclear dust resulting from disintegration of neutrophils, is prominent (Fig. 3.65). A histological study of a case of quinidine-induced leucocytoclastic vasculitis demonstrated a progressive change from a neutrophilic-predominant to a mononuclear-predominant infiltrate with time, suggesting the dynamic nature of the inflammatory process [13].

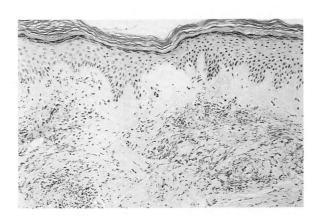

Figure 3.64 Histopathology of leucocytoclastic vasculitis affecting postcapillary venules in the upper dermis.

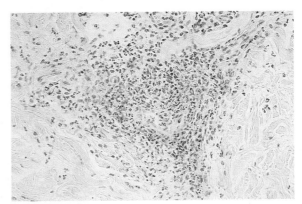

Figure 3.65 Higher power view of involved upper dermal vessel in leucocytoclastic vasculitis showing neutrophil extravasation and leucocytoclasis.

In keeping with the immune complex-mediated mechanisms operative in some cases of drug-induced vasculitis, direct tissue immunofluorescence may reveal deposition of immunoreactants including C3, IgM, and IgA in the walls of upper dermal blood vessels (Fig. 3.66).

1 Fauci AS, Haynes EF, Katz P. The spectrum of vasculitis; clinical, pathologic, immunologic and therapeutic considerations. *Ann Intern Med* 1978; **89**: 660–76.
2 Mullick FG, McAllister HA Jr, Wagner BM, Fenoglio JJ Jr. Drug-related vasculitis. Clinicopathologic correlations in 30 patients. *Hum Pathol* 1979; **10**: 313–25.
3 Sams WM Jr. Necrotizing vasculitis. *J Am Acad Dermatol* 1980; **3**: 1–13.
4 Herrmann WA, Kauffmann RH, van Es LA, *et al*. Allergic vasculitis. A histological and immunofluorescent study of lesional and non-lesional skin in relation to circulating immune complexes. *Arch Dermatol Res* 1980; **269**: 179–87.
5 Mackel SE, Jordon RE. Leukocytoclastic vasculitis. A cutaneous expression of immune complex disease. *Arch Dermatol* 1983; **118**: 296–301.
6 Wenner NP, Safai B. Circulating immune complexes in Henoch–Schönlein purpura. *Int J Dermatol* 1983; **22**: 383–5.
7 Massa MC, Su WPD. Lymphocytic vasculitis: is it a specific clinicopathologic entity? *J Cutan Pathol* 1984; **11**: 132–9.
8 Sanchez NP, Van Hale HM, Su WPD. Clinical and histopathologic spectrum of necrotizing vasculitis. Report of findings in 101 cases. *Arch Dermatol* 1985; **121**: 220–4.
9 Van Hale HM, Gibson LE, Schroeter AL. Henoch–Schönlein vasculitis; Direct immunofluorescence study of uninvolved skin. *J Am Acad Dermatol* 1986; **15**: 665–70.
10 Sams WM Jr. Immunologic aspects of cutaneous vasculitis. *Semin Dermatol* 1988; **7**: 140–8.
11 Sams WM Jr. Hypersensitivity angiitis. *J Invest Dermatol* 1989; **93**: 78S–81S.
12 Smoller BR, McNutt NS, Contreras F. The natural history of vasculitis. What the histology tells us about pathogenesis. *Arch Dermatol* 1990; **126**: 84–9.
13 Zax RH, Hodge SJ, Callen JP. Cutaneous leucocytoclastic vasculitis. Serial

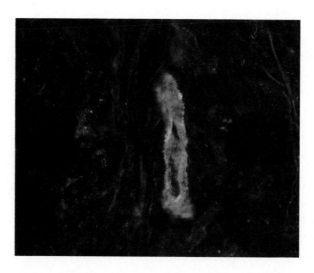

Figure 3.66 Direct immunofluorescence in leucocytoclastic vasculitis demonstrating C3 deposition in the wall of a dermal blood vessel.

histopathologic evaluation demonstrates the dynamic nature of the infiltrate. *Arch Dermatol* 1990; **126**: 69−72.

14 Peacock A, Weatherall D. Hydralazine-induced necrotizing vasculitis. *Br Med J* 1981; **282**: 1121−2.

15 Hendricks WM, Ader RS. Furosemide-induced cutaneous necrotizing vasculitis. *Arch Dermatol* 1977; **113**: 375−6.

16 Vasily DB, Tyler WB. Propylthiouracil-induced cutaneous vasculitis. Case presentation and review of literature. *JAMA* 1980; **243**: 458−61.

17 Gammeltoft M, Kristensen JK. Propylthio-uracil-induced cutaneous vasculitis. *Acta Derm Venereol (Stockh)* 1982; **62**: 171−3.

18 Cassorla FG, Finegold DN, Parks JS, *et al*. Vasculitis, pulmonary cavitation and anemia during antithyroid therapy. *Am J Dis Child* 1983; **137**: 118−22.

19 Mitchell GG, Magnusson AR, Weiler JM. Cimetidine-induced cutaneous vasculitis. *Am J Med* 1983; **75**: 875−6.

20 Tanay A, Yust I, Brenner S, *et al*. Dermal vasculitis due to coumadin hypersensitivity. *Dermatologica* 1982; **165**: 178−85.

21 Staubli M, Zimmerman A, Bircher J. Amiodarone-induced vasculitis and polyserositis. *Postgrad Med J* 1985; **61**: 245−7.

22 Phanuphak P, Kohler PF. Onset of polyarteritis nodosa during allergic hyposensitisation treatment. *Am J Med* 1980; **68**: 479−85.

23 Merk H, Kober ML. Vasculitis nach spezifischer Hyposensibilisierung. *Z Hautkr* 1982; **57**: 1682−5.

24 Lübbe D. Vasculitis allergica vom papulonekrotischen Typ nach BCG-Impfung. *Dermatol Monatsschr* 1982; **168**: 186−92.

25 Kerdel FA, Fraker DL, Haynes HA. Necrotizing vasculitis from radiographic contrast media. *J Am Acad Dermatol* 1984; **10**: 25−9.

26 Michäelsson G, Petterson L, Juhlin L. Purpura caused by food and drug additives. *Arch Dermatol* 1974; **109**: 49−52.

27 Ruzicka T, Ring J, Braun-Falco O. Vasculitis allergica durch Vitamin B₆. *Hautarzt* 1984; **35**: 197−9.

28 Citron BP, Halpern M, McCarron M, *et al*. Necrotizing angiitis associated with drug abuse. *N Engl J Med* 1970; **283**: 1003−11.

29 Lignelli GJ, Bucheit WA. Angiitis in drug abusers. *N Engl J Med* 1971; **284**: 112−13.

30 Gendelman H, Linzer M, Barland P, *et al*. Leukocytoclastic vasculitis in an intravenous heroin abuser. *N Y State J Med* 1983; **83**: 984−6.

31 Lever WF, Schaumburg-Lever G. *Histopathology of the Skin*, 7th edn. JB Lippincott, Philadelphia, 1990.

3.23 Lupus erythematosus (LE)-like syndrome induced by drugs

Clinical features

A reaction resembling idiopathic LE has been reported in association with a large variety of drugs [1−8], although only about 5% of cases of systemic lupus erythematosus are drug-induced. Cutaneous manifestations are in general rare in drug-induced lupus; 18% and 26% respectively of patients with procainamide- and hydralazine-induced LE had skin changes in one series [8]. An erythemato-squamous eruption localized especially to exposed areas on the face (in a 'butterfly' distribution), neck and chest may be seen (Fig. 3.67). Photosensitivity may be prominent. Some patients develop lesions of discoid LE, with erythema, scaling, atrophy, follicular plugging, and pigmentary changes. Urticarial or erythema multiforme-like

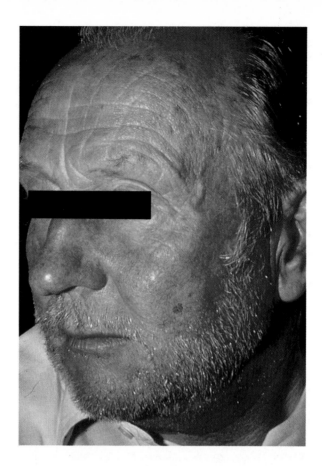

Figure 3.67 Erythema of the nose and malar area in drug-induced lupus erythematosus.

lesions may also be seen, Constitutional symptoms including malaise, fever, myalgia, and arthralgia may be present, and there may be evidence of Raynaud's disease, arthritis or polyserositis. Renal involvement is rare, although recorded [9], as is central nervous system involvement. The condition usually, but not always, resolves after discontinuation of the drug; there have, however, been occasional reports of fatalities [9].

Drug aetiology

A partial list of drugs reported to induce a systemic LE-like syndrome or exacerbate idiopathic LE is given in Table 3.16. Drugs most commonly implicated in inducing LE include especially hydralazine [10–15] and procainamide [9,16–18], and less commonly β-blockers [18], phenytoin, isoniazid [19], quinidine [20,21], and methyldopa [22,23]. LE following penicillamine therapy [24,25], and subacute LE with positive Ro/SS-A antibodies in association with hydrochlorothiazide [26,27] or with hydrochlorothiazide and triamterene [28], have also been reported. A gyrate subacute LE has been described in association with captopril [29], and a lupus-like syndrome with 2-mercaptopropionylglycine [30]. In addition, a number of drugs may exacerbate a pre-existing systemic LE, such as griseofulvin, β-blockers, sulphonamides, testosterone and oestrogens. The oral contraceptive induced LE lesions on the palms and feet of a patient [31].

Histology and immunopathology

Well-developed lesions may show evidence of a patchy lymphoid cell infiltrate which tends to be centred round cutaneous appendages, oedema of the upper dermis, hydropic change of the epidermal basal layer, and variable hyperkeratosis, follicular plugging, and epidermal atrophy [32].

Abnormal laboratory findings are common. These include the presence of LE cells, and of antinuclear antibodies (Fig. 3.68) directed against ribonucleoprotein, single-stranded DNA, and especially against histones [33−36]. Antibodies against native double-stranded DNA are rarely found in drug-induced LE (as opposed to idiopathic systemic LE) [4,6,33]; complement levels are normal. While deposition of immunoglobulins and complement in involved skin is seen on direct tissue immunofluorescence (Fig. 3.69), deposition of immunoreactants in uninvolved skin is rare [37]. Laboratory findings are common in otherwise asymptomatic patients [9,33], especially with hydralazine, isoniazid, procainamide and methyldopa. Autoantibody titres may decline despite continued therapy, and it has been stated that it is not necessary to stop therapy unless patients are symptomatic [12]. Patients with drug-induced lupus may have the lupus anticoagulant [38,39].

Pathomechanisms operative in drug-induced lupus erythematosus

Susceptibility to drug-induced LE is to a degree under genetic control. Both hydralazine and procainamide are inactivated by acetylation; there is genetic polymorphism of N-acetyltransferase, and there is increased risk of development of an LE-like syndrome

Table 3.16 Drugs inducing lupus erythematosus-like syndromes

Allopurinol
Aminoglutethimide
p-Aminosalicylic acid
β-Blockers
Chlorpromazine
Clonidine
Co-trimoxazole
Ethosuximide
Gold salts
Griseofulvin
Hydantoins
Hydralazine
Ibuprofen
Isoniazid
Lithium
Methyldopa
Methysergide
Nitrofurantoin
Oral contraceptives
Penicillin
Penicillamine
Phenothiazine
Phenylbutazone
Primidone
Procainamide
Thiouracils
Quinidine
Streptomycin
Sulphasalazine
Sulphonamides
Tetracycline
Thionamide
Trimethadione

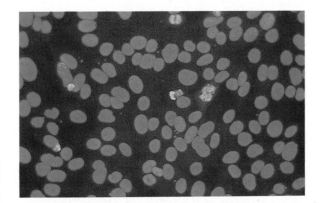

Figure 3.68 Homogeneous antinuclear antibody fluorescence in lupus erythematosus; Hep-2 cell line substrate.

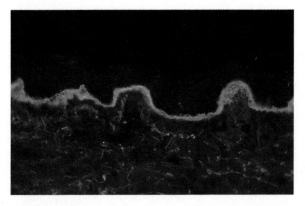

Figure 3.69 Direct immunofluorescence demonstrating basement membrane zone deposition of C3 in lesional skin in drug-induced lupus erythematosus: ('LE band').

[115]

with the slow acetylator phenotype [11,13,40]. Hydralazine-induced lupus is commonest in female patients with the HLA-DRw4 haplotype [11,13]. One theory derived to explain the occurrence of drug-induced lupus, with production of antihistone antibodies, is that interaction between the drug and nuclear material produces a drug—nucleoprotein complex which is immunogenic [35]. Alternatively, it has been suggested that drugs may alter immunoregulation in such a way that autoantibody production is favoured [4,14,35,41,42]. Procainamide and hydralazine modulate lymphocyte function directly [41−43] and may induce autoreactivity [43]. Thus it has been proposed that drugs may cause a systemic LE-like condition by a mechanism analogous to that in immunostimulatory graft-versus-host disease [44]. A further possible mechanism by which drugs may produce an LE-like syndrome is by inhibiting the complement cascade. Hydralazine, isoniazid, and the hydroxylamine metabolites of procainamide and practolol, inhibit covalent binding of complement component C_4 to immune complexes, thus blocking binding of C_3 to the complexes [15,18,19]. This in turn prevents complement-mediated clearance of immune complexes by solubilization and opsonization, and predisposes to development of an LE-like syndrome [45].

1 Harpey JP. Lupus-like syndromes induced by drugs. *Ann Allergy* 1974; **33**: 256−61.
2 Lee SL, Chase PH. Drug-induced systemic lupus erythematosus: a critical review. *Semin Arthritis Rheum* 1975; **5**: 83−103.
3 Reidenberg MM. The chemical induction of systemic lupus erythematosus and lupus-like illnesses. *Arthritis Rheum* 1981; **24**: 1004−9.
4 Schoen RT, Trentham DE. Drug-induced lupus: An adjuvant disease? *Am J Med* 1981; **71**: 5−8.
5 Harmon CE, Portonova JP. Drug-induced lupus: clinical and serological studies. *Clin Rheum Dis* 1982; **8**: 121−35.
6 Stratton MA. Drug-induced systemic lupus erythematosus. *Clin Pharm* 1985; **4**: 657−63.
7 Totoritis MC, Rubin RL. Drug-induced lupus. Genetic, clinical, and laboratory features. *Postgrad Med* 1985; **78**: 149−52.
8 Dubois EL. Serologic abnormalities in spontaneous and drug-induced systemic lupus erythematosus. *J Rheumatol* 1975; **2**: 204−14.
9 Whittle TS Jr, Ainsworth SK. Procainamide-induced systemic lupus erythematosus. Renal involvement with deposition of immune complexes. *Arch Pathol Lab Med* 1976; **100**: 469−74.
10 Alarcón-Segovia D, Wakim KG, Worthington JW, Ward LE. Clinical and experimental studies on the hydralazine syndrome and its relationship to systemic lupus erythematosus. *Medicine* 1967; **46**: 1−33.
11 Batchelor JR, Welsh KI, Mansilla Tinoco R, *et al*. Hydralazine-induced systemic lupus erythematosus: influence of HLA-DR and sex on susceptibility. *Lancet* 1980; **i**: 1107−9.
12 Mansilla Tinoco R, Harland SJ, Ryan PJ, *et al*. Hydralazine, antinuclear antibodies, and the lupus syndrome. *Br Med J* 1982; **284**: 936−9.
13 Russell GI, Bing RF, Jones JA, *et al*. Hydralazine sensitivity: clinical features, autoantibody changes and HLA-DR phenotype. *Q J Med* 1987; **65**: 845−52.
14 Dubroff LM, Reid R Jr, Papalian M. Molecular models for hydralazine-related systemic lupus erythematosus. *Arthritis Rheum* 1981; **24**: 1082−5.
15 Sim E, Law S-KA. Hydralazine binds covalently to complement component C_4. Different reactivity of C_4A and C_4B gene products. *FEBS Lett* 1985; **184**: 323−7.

16 Dubois EL. Procainamide induction of a systemic lupus erythematosus-like syndrome. Presentation of six cases, review of the literature, and analysis and follow up of reported cases. *Medicine* 1969; **48**: 217–28.

17 Blomgren SE, Condemi JJ, Vaughan JH. Procainamide-induced lupus erythematosus. Clinical and laboratory observations. *Am J Med* 1972; **52**: 338–48.

18 Sim E, Stanley L, Gill EW, Jones A. Metabolites of procainamide and practolol inhibit complement components C3 and C4. *Biochem J* 1988; **251**: 323–6.

19 Sim E, Gill EW, Sim RB. Drugs that induce systemic lupus erythematosus inhibit complement component C4. *Lancet* 1984; **ii**: 422–4.

20 McCormack GD, Barth WF. Quinidine induced lupus syndrome. *Semin Arthritis Rheum* 1985; **15**: 73–9.

21 Cohen MG, Kevat S, Prowse MV, *et al*. Two distinct quinidine-induced rheumatic syndromes. *Ann Intern Med* 1988; **108**: 369–71.

22 Harrington TM, Davis DE. Systemic lupus-like syndrome induced by methyldopa therapy. *Chest* 1981; **79**: 696–7.

23 Dupont A, Six R. Lupus-like syndrome induced by methyldopa. *Br Med J* 1982; **285**: 693–4.

24 Chalmers A, Thompson D, Stein HE, *et al*. Systemic lupus erythematosus during penicillamine therapy for rheumatoid arthritis. *Ann Intern Med* 1982; **97**: 659–63.

25 Tsankov NK, Lazarov AZ, Vasileva S, Obreshkova EV. Lupus erythematosus-like eruption due to D-penicillamine in progressive systemic sclerosis. *Int J Dermatol* 1990; **29**: 571–4.

26 Reed BR, Huff JC, Jones SK, *et al*. Subacute cutaneous lupus erythematosus associated with hydrochlorothiazide therapy. *Ann Intern Med* 1985; **103**: 49–51.

27 Berbis P, Vernay-Vaisse C, Privat Y. Lupus cutané subaigu observé au cours d'un traitement par diurétiques thiazidiques. *Ann Dermatol Vénéréol (Paris)* 1986; **113**: 1245–8.

28 Darken M, McBurney EI. Subacute cutaneous lupus erythematosus-like drug eruption due to combination diuretic hydrochlorothiazide and triamterene. *J Am Acad Dermatol* 1988; **18**: 38–42.

29 Patri P, Nigro A, Rebora A. Lupus erythematosus-like eruption from captopril. *Acta Derm Venereol (Stockh)* 1985; **65**: 447–8.

30 Katayama I, Nishioka K. Lupus like syndrome induced by 2-mercaptopropionylglycine. *J Dermatol (Tokyo)* 1986; **13**: 151–3.

31 Furukawa F, Tachibana T, Imamura S, Tamura T. Oral contraceptive-induced lupus erythematosus in a Japanese woman. *J Dermatol (Tokyo)* 1991; **18**: 56–8.

32 Lever WF, Schaumburg-Lever G. *Histopathology of the Skin*, 7th edn. JB Lippincott, Philadelphia, 1990.

33 Fritzler MJ, Tan EM. Antibodies to histones in drug-induced idiopathic lupus erythematosus. *J Clin Invest* 1978; **62**: 560–7.

34 Rubin RL, Nusinow SR, Johnson AD, *et al*. Serologic changes during induction of lupus-like disease by procainamide. *Am J Med* 1986; **80**: 999–1002.

35 Hobbs RN, Clayton AL, Bernstein RM. Antibodies to the five histones and poly(adenosine diphosphate-ribose) in drug induced lupus: implications for pathogenesis. *Ann Rheum Dis* 1987; **46**: 408–16.

36 Totoritis MC, Tan EM, McNally EM, *et al*. Association of antibody to histone complex H2A-H2B with symptomatic procainamide-induced lupus. *N Engl J Med* 1988; **318**: 1431–6.

37 Grossman J, Callerame ML, Condemi JJ. Skin immunofluorescence studies on lupus erythematosus and other antinuclear antibody-positive diseases. *Ann Intern Med* 1974; **80**: 496–500.

38 Bell WR, Boss GR, Wolfson JS. Circulating anticoagulant in the procainamide-induced lupus syndrome. *Arch Intern Med* 1977; **137**: 1471–3.

39 Canoso RT, Sise HS. Chlorpromazine-induced lupus anticoagulant and associated immunologic abnormalities. *Am J Hematol* 1982; **13**: 121–9.

40 Perry HM Jr, Sakamoto A, Tan EM. Relationship of acetylating enzyme to hydralazine toxicity. *J Lab Clin Med* 1967; **70**: 1020–1.

41 Adams LE, Sanders CE, Budinsky RA, *et al.* Immunomodulatory effects of procainamide metabolites: their implications in drug-related lupus. *J Lab Clin Med* 1989; **113**: 482−92.

42 Schopf RE, Hanauske-Abel HM, Tschank G, *et al.* Effects of hydrazyl group containing drugs on leukocyte functions: an immunoregulatory model for the hydralazine-induced lupus-like syndrome. *J Immunopharmacol* 1985; **7**: 385−401.

43 Cornacchia E, Golbus J, Maybaum J, *et al.* Hydralazine and procainamide inhibit T-cell DNA methylation and induce autoreactivity. *J Immunol* 1988; **140**: 2197−200.

44 Gleichman E, Pals ST, Rolinck AG, *et al.* Graft-versus-host reactions: clues to the etiopathogenesis of a spectrum of immunological diseases. *Immunol Today* 1984; **5**: 324−32.

45 Sim E. Drug-induced immune complex disease. *Complement Inflamm* 1989; **6**: 119−26.

3.24 Drug-induced dermatomyositis

The clinical features of dermatomyositis include lilac (heliotrope) discoloration around the eyes, malar erythema and oedema, streaks of erythema over the extensor tendons of the hands, lilac slightly atrophic papules over the knuckles (Gottron's papules), peri-ungual telangiectasia, and muscle weakness, especially of the proximal limb girdles. Dermatomyositis has been reported to be precipitated by a variety of drugs, including penicillamine [1−3], non-steroidal anti-inflammatory agents (niflumic acid and diclofenac) [4], carbamazepine [5], and vaccination, as with BCG [6]. Acral skin lesions simulating chronic dermatomyositis have been reported during long-term hydroxyurea therapy [7].

1 Simpson NB, Golding JR. Dermatomyositis induced by penicillamine. *Acta Derm Venereol (Stockh)* 1979; **59**: 543−4.

2 Wojnorowska F. Dermatomyositis induced by penicillamine. *J R Soc Med* 1980; **73**: 884−6.

3 Carroll GC, Will RK, Peter JB, *et al.* Penicillamine induced polymyositis and dermatomyositis. *J Rheumatol* 1987; **14**: 995−1001.

4 Grob JJ, Collet AM, Bonerandi JJ. Dermatomyositis-like syndrome induced by nonsteroidal anti-inflammatory agents. *Dermatologica* 1989; **178**: 58−9.

5 Simpson JR. 'Collagen disease' due to carbamazepine (Tegretol). *Br Med J* 1966; **ii**: 1434.

6 Kass E, Staume S, Mellbye OJ, *et al.* Dermatomyositis associated with BCG vaccination. *Scand J Rheumatol* 1979; **8**: 187−91.

7 Richard M, Truchetet F, Friedel, *et al.* Skin lesions simulating chronic dermatomyositis during long-term hydroxyurea therapy. *J Am Acad Dermatol* 1989; **21**: 797−9.

3.25 Scleroderma-like reactions

Clinico-pathological features of idiopathic morphea, scleroderma and eosinophilic fasciitis

Morphea is a localized form of scleroderma which presents with scattered pale indurated sclerotic plaques, often with a slightly violaceous border. Systemic sclerosis comprises sclerosis of the skin, especially of the hands, resulting in shiny, indurated, tethered skin (acrosclerosis or sclerodactyly) but also of the trunk, calcinosis of the fingers, Raynaud's phenomenon, mat-like telangiectasia of the face, a beaked nose, and radial furrowing around the mouth. There may be associated oesophageal and gastrointestinal dysmotility, malabsorption, pulmonary fibrosis, congestive cardiac failure, and kidney involvement leading to hypertension and renal failure. In eosinophilic fasciitis, tender swelling, usually of one or more limbs, with accompanying cutaneous induration, is associated with peripheral blood eosinophilia.

The histology of morphea and systemic sclerosis [1] is characterized in the early stages by an inflammatory (predominantly lymphoid) infiltrate between collagen bundles, and in a perivascular distribution, in the dermis and especially the subcutaneous fat, with extensive fibrosis and new collagen deposition. In later stages, the inflammatory infiltrate disappears. In eosinophilic fasciitis, the fascia is markedly thickened, and permeated by a chronic inflammatory infiltrate, with an admixture of eosinophils; the subcutaneous fat and underlying muscle may be involved [1,2]. It has been postulated that the cytokine transforming growth factor-β (TGF-β) may be implicated in mediating the fibrosis seen in these conditions [3], since mRNA and/or protein expression is elevated in generalized morphea and diffuse fasciitis [4] as well as in progressive systemic sclerosis [5]. TGF-β is released from activated lymphocytes and from fibroblasts [6] and has been shown to stimulate various fibroblast activities, including synthesis and incorporation into the extracellular matrix of fibronectin and collagen types I and III [7,8].

1 Lever WF, Schaumburg-Lever G. *Histopathology of the Skin*, 7th edn. JB Lippincott, Philadelphia, 1990.
2 Hintner H, Tappeiner G, Egg D, *et al*. Fasziitis mit Eosinophilie. Das Shulman Syndrom. *Hautarzt* 1981; **32**: 75–9.
3 Smith EA, LeRoy EC. A possible role for transforming growth factor-β in systemic sclerosis. *J Invest Dermatol* 1990; **95**: 125S–127S.
4 Peltonen J, Kähari L, Jaakkola S, *et al*. Evaluation of transforming growth factor β and type I procollagen gene expression in fibrotic skin diseases by *in situ* hybridization. *J Invest Dermatol* 1990; **94**: 365–71.
5 Gruschwitz M, Müller PU, Sepp N, *et al*. Transcription and expression of transforming growth factor type beta in the skin of progressive systemic sclerosis: A mediator of fibrosis? *J Invest Dermatol* 1990; **94**: 197–203.
6 van Obberghen-Schilling E, Roche NS, Flanders KC, *et al*. Transforming growth factor β$_1$ positively regulates its own expression in normal and transformed cells. *J Biol Chem* 1988; **263**: 7741–6.
7 Ignotz RA, Massague J. Transforming growth factor-β stimulates the expression of fibronectin and collagen and their incorporation into the extracellular matrix. *J Biol Chem* 1986; **261**: 4337–45.
8 Varga J, Rosenbloom J, Jimenez SA. Transforming growth factor β (TGFβ) causes a persistent increase in steady-state amounts of type I and type III collagen and fibronectin mRNAs in normal human dermal fibroblasts. *Biochem J* 1987; **247**: 597–604.

Drug aetiology

Penicillamine [1,2], bleomycin [3–5], bromocriptine [6,7], vitamin

K (phytomenadione) [8−10], sodium valproate [11] and 5-hydroxy-tryptophan combined with carbidopa [12−15] (see also the eosinophilia−myalgia syndrome below) have all been implicated in either localized or generalized morphea-like, or systemic sclerosis-like, reactions. Carbidopa, an aromatic L-amino acid decarboxylase inhibitor, binds pyridoxal phosphate and can produce a pyridoxal deficiency with elevated kynurenine levels; sclerodermatous changes developed in patients with elevated serotonin and kynurenine levels who had also received 5-hydroxytryptophan. Eosinophilic fasciitis has been associated with tryptophan ingestion in some cases [16], as well as with phenytoin [17]. Paradoxically, D-penicillamine has also been reported to be helpful in the treatment of localized scleroderma [18].

1 Bernstein RM, Hall MA, Gostelow BE. Morphea-like reaction to D-penicillamine therapy. *Ann Rheum Dis* 1981; **40**: 42−4.
2 Miyagawa S, Yoshioka A, Hatoko M, *et al*. Systemic sclerosis-like lesions during long-term penicillamine therapy for Wilson's disease. *Br J Dermatol* 1987; **116**: 95−100.
3 Finch WR, Rodnan GP, Buckingham RB, *et al*. Bleomycin-induced scleroderma. *J Rheumatol* 1980; **7**: 651−9.
4 Bork K, Korting GW. Symptomatische Sklerodermie durch Bleomyzin. *Hautarzt* 1983; **34**: 10−12.
5 Snauwaert J, Degreef H. Bleomycin-induced Raynaud's phenomenon and acral sclerosis. *Dermatologica* 1984; **169**: 172−4.
6 Dupont E, Olivarius B, Strong MJ. Bromocriptine-induced collagenosis-like symptomatology in Parkinson's disease. *Lancet* 1982; **i**: 850−1.
7 Leshin B, Piette WW, Caplin RM. Morphea after bromocriptine therapy. *Int J Dermatol* 1989; **28**: 177−9.
8 Janin-Mercier A, Mosser C, Souteyrand P, Bourges M. Subcutaneous sclerosis with fasciitis and eosinophilia after phytonadione injections. *Arch Dermatol* 1985; **121**: 1421−3.
9 Brunskill NJ, Berth-Jones J, Graham-Brown RAC. Pseudosclerodermatous reaction to phytomenadione injection (Texier's syndrome). *Clin Exp Dermatol* 1988; **13**: 276−8.
10 Pujol RM, Puig L, Moreno A, *et al*. Pseudoscleroderma secondary to phyto-nadione (vitamin K_1) injections. *Cutis* 1989; **43**: 365−8.
11 Goihman-Yahr M, Leal G, Essenfeld-Yahr E. Generalized morphea: a side effect of valproate sodium? *Arch Dermatol* 1980; **116**: 621.
12 Sternberg EM, Van Woert MH, Young SN, *et al*. Development of a scleroderma-like illness during therapy with L-5-Hydroxytryptophan and Carbidopa. *N Engl J Med* 1980; **303**: 782−7.
13 Auffranc JC, Berbis P, Fabre JF, *et al*. Syndrome sclérodermiforme et poïkilo-dermique observé au cours d'un traitement par carbidopa et 5-hydroxy-tryptophanne. *Ann Dermatol Vénéréol (Paris)* 1985; **112**: 691−2.
14 Chamson A, Périer C, Frey J. Syndrome sclérodermiforme et poïkilodermique observé au cours d'un traitement par carbidopa et 5-hydroxytryptophanne. Culture de fibroblastes avec analyse biochimique du métabolisme du col-lagene. *Ann Dermatol Vénéréol (Paris)* 1986; **113**: 71.
15 Joly P, Lampert A, Thomine E, Lauret P. Development of pseudobullous morphea and scleroderma-like illness during therapy with L-5-hydroxy-tryptophan and carbidopa. *J Am Acad Dermatol* 1991; **25**: 332−3.
16 Gordon ML, Lebwohl MG, Phelps RG, *et al*. Eosinophilic fasciitis associated with tryptophan ingestion. A manifestation of eosinophilia-myalgia syn-drome. *Arch Dermatol* 1991; **127**: 217−20.
17 Buchanan RR, Gordon DA, Muckle TJ, *et al*. The eosinophilic fasciitis syndrome after phenytoin (Dilantin) therapy. *J Rheumatol* 1980; **7**: 733−6.

18 Falanga V, Medsger TA Jr. D-Penicillamine in the treatment of localized scleroderma. *Arch Dermatol* 1990; **126**: 609–12.

Chemical and industrial causes of scleroderma-like reactions

Scleroderma-like changes formed part of the clinical spectrum of the Spanish 'toxic oil syndrome', which resulted from contamination of rapeseed cooking oil with acetanilide [1]. Scleroderma-like changes have been induced by industrial exposure to vinyl chloride [2], epoxy resins [3], organic solvents [4] including trichlorethylene, perchlorethylene [5] and trichlorethane [6], and in coal-miners due to silica exposure [7,8].

1 Rush PJ, Bell MJ, Fam AG. Toxic oil syndrome (Spanish oil disease) and chemically induced scleroderma-like conditions. *J Rheumatol* 1984; **11**: 262–4.
2 Harris DK, Adams WGF. Acroosteolysis occurring in men engaged in the polymerisation of vinyl chloride. *Br Med J* 1967; **3**: 712–24.
3 Yamakage A, Ishikawa H, Saito Y, Hattori A. Occupational scleroderma-like disorders occurring in men engaged in the polymerization of epoxy resins. *Dermatologica* 1980; **161**: 33–44.
4 Yamakage A, Ishikawa H. Generalized morphea-like scleroderma occurring in people exposed to organic solvents. *Dermatologica* 1982; **165**: 186–93.
5 Sparrow GP. A connective tissue disease similar to vinyl chloride disease in a patient exposed to perchlorethylene. *Clin Exp Dermatol* 1977; **2**: 17–22.
6 Flindt-Hansen H, Isager H. Scleroderma after occupational exposure to trichlorethylene and trichlorethane. *Acta Derm Venereol (Stockh)* 1987; **67**: 263–4.
7 Rodnan GP, Benedek TG, Medsger TA Jr, Cammarata RJ. The association of progressive systemic sclerosis (scleroderma) with coalminers' pneumoconiosis and other forms of silicosis. *Ann Intern Med* 1967; **66**: 323–4.
8 Rustin MHA, Bull HA, Ziegler V, *et al*. Silica-associated systemic sclerosis is clinically, serologically and immunologically indistinguishable form idiopathic systemic sclerosis. *Br J Dermatol* 1990; **123**: 725–34.

Scleroderma-like and other connective tissue reactions caused by silicone or paraffin augmentation mammoplasty

Direct injection of silicone into the breast, or use of silicone gel-filled elastomer envelope-type prostheses, for augmentation mammoplasty has been linked to development of morphea or scleroderma [1–9]. Considering that an estimated 2 million American women have received the silicone gel-filled breast implant [7], the risk of this complication is not very high. Characteristically, scleroderma-like changes develop after a delay of 2–21 years. Marked improvement in progressive systemic sclerosis followed removal of the implants in two cases [4]. Resolution of scleroderma occurred following removal of the silicone implants and their replacement with saline-filled implants in a further case [6]; there was evidence of leakage of silicone from the implant [6]. In other patients, implant removal has not led to improvement of scleroderma [3,5]. Mechanisms proposed for scleroderma production include: conversion of silicone to highly immunogenic silica by tissue macrophages, stimulation of macrophage release of TGF-β (with resultant increased collagen formation by fibroblasts), and induction of autoimmunity via an adjuvant effect [6,7]. In a Japanese series, the incidence of progressive systemic sclerosis was three times greater than expected, and the incidence of mixed connective tissue disease was elevated, in women following breast augmentation surgery; in the majority of cases paraffin rather than silicone was used [10].

Although scleroderma is the most frequently reported associated condition, other connective tissue diseases reported after implantation of silicone gel-filled prostheses include systemic lupus erythematosus, mixed connective tissue disease, and rheumatoid arthritis with Sjögren's syndrome [1]. Human adjuvant disease, consisting of arthralgia, lymphadenopathy, positive tests for serum rheumatoid factor and antinuclear antibody, and foreign body granulomas in lymph nodes, has also been reported [7].

1 van Nunen SA, Gatenby PA, Basten A. Post-mammoplasty connective tissue disease. *Arthritis Rheum* 1982; **25**: 694–7.
2 Endo LP, Edwards NL, Longley S, *et al*. Silicone and rheumatic diseases. *Semin Arthritis Rheum* 1987; **17**: 112–18.
3 Spiera F. Scleroderma after silicone augmentation mammoplasty. *JAMA* 1988; **260**: 236–8.
4 Brozena SJ, Fenske NA, Cruse CW, *et al*. Human adjuvant disease following augmentation mammoplasty. *Arch Dermatol* 1988; **124**: 1383–6.
5 Varga J, Schumacher HR, Jimenez SA. Systemic sclerosis after augmentation mammoplasty with silicone implants. *Ann Intern Med* 1989; **111**: 277–83.
6 Sahn EE, Garen PD, Silver RM, Maize JC. Scleroderma following augmentation mammoplasty. Report of a case and review of the literature. *Arch Dermatol* 1990; **126**: 1198–202.
7 Varga J, Jimenez SA. Augmentation mammoplasty and scleroderma. Is there an association? *Arch Dermatol* 1990; **126**: 1220–2.
8 Vasey FB, Espinoza LR, Martinez-Osuna P, *et al*. Silicone and rheumatic disease: replace implants or not? *Arch Dermatol* 1991; **127**: 907.
9 Lazar AP, Lazar P. Localized morphea after silicone gel breast implantation: more evidence for a cause-and-effect relationship. *Arch Dermatol* 1991; **127**: 263.
10 Kumagai Y, Shiokawa Y, Medsger TA Jr, Rodnan GP. Clinical spectrum of connective tissue disease after cosmetic surgery. Observations on eighteen patients and a review of the Japanese literature. *Arthritis Rheum* 1984; **27**: 1–12.

3.26 Eosinophilia–myalgia syndrome

Ingestion of tryptophan, taken as a mild antidepressant, a 'natural hypnotic', or by athletes to increase pain tolerance, has been associated with the eosinophilia–myalgia syndrome [1–8]. This is characterized by acute features as follows: eosinophilia of greater than $1 \times 10^9/l$, myalgia, arthralgia, limb swelling, fever, weakness and fatigue, respiratory complaints (cough, dyspnoea and eosinophilic pneumonitis), pulmonary hypertension, arrhythmias, ascending polyneuropathy, and a variety of cutaneous manifestations. The latter include diffuse morbilliform erythema, urticaria, angioedema, dermatographism, livedo reticularis and alopecia. Cutaneous papular mucinosis has been reported [9–11]. In a substantial proportion of cases, there is progression into a chronic multisystem disease despite discontinuation of L-tryptophan.

A subset of patients taking high dose tryptophan developed a more chronic condition, with muscle weakness, diffuse scleroderma-like or fasciitis-like skin changes, most commonly affecting the proximal extremities and trunk, with sparing of the hands, feet and face. The histology showed inflammation and fibrosis of the fascia, occasionally extending to the lower dermis and subjacent muscle, with tissue eosinophil infiltration, and glycosaminoglycans deposition in the dermis. Pseudoxanthoma elasticum-like papules within sclerodermatous skin of the neck and medial aspects of the arms have been reported in two patients; there were fragmented elastic fibres but calcification was absent [12].

The eosinophilia—myalgia syndrome is now thought to have been caused by a contaminant of levotryptophan, possibly 1,1'-ethylidene-*bis*(tryptophan), introduced following a change in the manufacturing process at a single Japanese company between October 1988 and June 1989 [13 – 15]. The change in the manufacturing process involved use of a new strain of a genetically modified *Bacillus amyloliquefaciens*, and of reduced quantities of powdered carbon in the purification procedure. However, it has been pointed out that cases of levotryptophan-induced morphea and eosinophilic fasciitis were recognized before the episode of contamination [16,17]. Similar cardiopulmonary, neuropathic and cutaneous lesions were seen in the Spanish 'toxic oil syndrome' due to adulterated rapeseed oil [17,18]; it is of interest that similar alterations in tryptophan metabolism were seen in the acute phase in both conditions [17]. Increased levels of TGF-β, type VI collagen, and fibronectin, and of mRNA for types I and VI collagen and TGF-β, have been reported in the extracellular matrix and/or fibroblasts of the fascia in L-tryptophan associated eosinophilia—myalgia syndrome [19,20]. The fact that there have been very few cases in Japan [21], and that by no means all of the US consumers of the drug developed the syndrome, suggests the importance of other, perhaps genetic, factors in the development of the eosinophilia—myalgia syndrome.

1 Varga J, Heiman-Patterson D, Emery D, *et al.* Clinical spectrum of the systemic manifestations of the eosinophilia—myalgia syndrome. *Semin Arthritis Rheum* 1990; **19**: 313—28.
2 Lacour JP, Ortonne JP. Syndrome myalgies-hyperéosinophile lié au L-tryptophanne. *Ann Dermatol Vénéréol (Paris)* 1990; **117**: 991—8.
3 Silver R, Heyes P, Maize J, *et al.* Scleroderma, fasciitis, and eosinophilia associated with the ingestion of tryptophan. *N Engl J Med* 1990; **322**: 874—8.
4 Kaufman LD, Seidman RJ, Phillips ME, Gruber BL. Cutaneous manifestations of the L-tryptophan-associated eosinophilia—myalgia syndrome: A spectrum of sclerodermatous skin disease. *J Am Acad Dermatol* 1990; **23**: 1063—9.
5 Philen RM, Eidson M, Kilbourne EM, *et al.* Eosinophilia—myalgia syndrome. A clinical case series of 21 patients. *Arch Intern Med* 1991; **151**: 533—7.
6 Reinauer S, Plewig G. Das Eosinophilie—Myalgie Syndrom. *Hautarzt* 1991; **42**: 137—9.
7 Gordon ML, Lebwohl MG, Phelps RG, *et al.* Eosinophilic fasciitis associated

with tryptophan ingestion. A manifestation of eosinophilia−myalgia syndrome. *Arch Dermatol* 1991; **127**: 217−20.

8 Connolly SM, Quimby SR, Griffing WL, Winkelmann RK. Scleroderma and L-tryptophan: A possible explanation of the eosinophilia−myalgia syndrome. *J Am Acad Dermatol* 1991; **23**: 451−7.

9 Dubin DB, Kwan TH, Morse DMA, Case DC. Cutaneous mucinosis in a patient with eosinophilia−myalgia syndrome associated with L-tryptophan ingestion. *Arch Dermatol* 1990; **126**: 1517−18.

10 Farmer KL, Hebert AA, Rapini RP, Jordan RE. Dermal mucinosis in the eosinophilia−myalgia syndrome. *Arch Dermatol* 1990; **126**: 1518−20.

11 Valicenti JMK, Fleming MG, Pearson RW, *et al.* Papular mucinosis in L-tryptophan-induced eosinophilia−myalgia syndrome. *J Am Acad Dermatol* 1991; **25**: 54−8.

12 Mainetti C, Masouyé I, Saurat J-H. Pseudoxanthoma elasticum-like lesions in the L-tryptophan-induced eosinophilia−myalgia syndrome. *J Am Acad Dermatol* 1991; **24**: 657−8.

13 Slutsker L, Hoesly FC, Miller LM, *et al.* Eosinophilia−myalgia syndrome associated with exposure to tryptophan from a single manufacturer. *JAMA* 1990; **264**: 213−17.

14 Belongia EA, Hedberg CW, Gleich GJ, *et al.* An investigation of the cause of the eosinophilia−myalgia syndrome associated with tryptophan use. *N Engl J Med* 1990; **323**: 357−65.

15 Mayeno AN, Lin F, Foote CS, *et al.* Characterization of 'peak E', a novel amino acid associated with eosinophilia−myalgia syndrome. *Science* 1990; **250**: 1707−8.

16 Blauvelt A, Falanga V. Idiopathic and L-tryptophan-associated eosinophilic fasciitis before and after L-tryptophan contamination. *Arch Dermatol* 1991; **127**: 1159−66.

17 Silver RM. Unraveling the eosinophilia−myalgia syndrome. *Arch Dermatol* 1991; **127**: 1214−16.

18 Kilbourne EM, Rigau-Perez JG, Heath CW Jr, *et al.* Clinical epidemiology of toxic-oil syndrome: manifestations of a new illness. *N Engl J Med* 1983; **309**: 1408−14.

19 Varga J, Petonen J, Uitto J, Jimenez SA. Development of diffuse fasciitis with eosinophilia during L-tryptophan treatment: demonstration of elevated type 1 collagen gene expression in affected tissues: a clinicopathological study of four patients. *Ann Intern Med* 1990; **112**: 344−52.

20 Peltonen J, Varga J, Sollberg S, *et al.* Elevated expression of the genes for transforming growth factor-β_1 and type VI collagen in diffuse fasciitis associated with the eosinophilia−myalgia syndrome. *J Invest Dermatol* 1991; **96**: 20−5.

21 Mizutani T, Mizutani H, Hashimoto K, *et al.* Simultaneous development of two cases of eosinophilia−myalgia syndrome with the same lot of L-tryptophan in Japan. *J Am Acad Dermatol* 1991; **25**: 512−17.

3.27 Erythema nodosum

This reaction consists of tender subcutaneous nodules usually distributed on the anterior aspect of the lower legs (Figs 3.70 & 3.71). Sulphonamides, and a variety of analgesics, antipyretics and anti-infectious agents have been implicated in the aetiology of erythema nodosum [1]. The contraceptive pill may play a role, perhaps as a result of an elevated oestrogen level [2,3].

1 Bork K. *Cutaneous Side Effects of Drugs.* WB Saunders, Philadelphia, 1988.
2 Posternal F, Orusco MMM, Laugier P. Eythème noueux et contraceptifs oraux. *Bull Derm* 1974; **81**: 642−5.
3 Bombardieri S, Di Munno O, Di Punzio C, Pasero G. Erythema nodosum associated with pregnancy and oral contraceptives. *Br Med J* 1977; **i**: 1509−10.

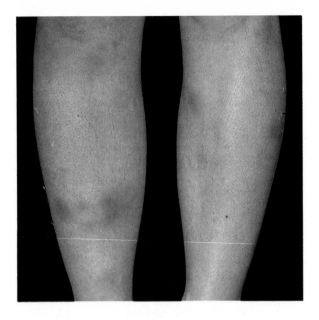

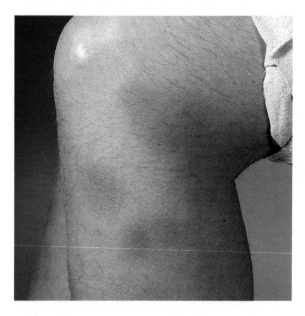

Figure 3.70 Erythema nodosum in a patient taking an oral contraceptive (norethisterone−ethinyloestradiol), penicillin, and propyphenazone−paracetamol.

Figure 3.71 Erythema nodosum due to oral contraceptive (desogestrel−ethinyloestradiol).

3.28 Pseudolymphomatous eruptions

A number of drugs may produce a reaction pattern which simulates a lymphoma [1]. The pseudolymphoma syndrome associated with a number of anticonvulsant drugs comprises fever, a generalized rash and lymphadenopathy, with variable hepatosplenomegaly, abnormal liver function, arthralgia, eosinophilia, and blood dyscrasias. Phenytoin especially, but also mephytoin, trimethadione, phenobarbital and carbamazepine, have been implicated [1−5]. Cutaneous lesions in patients with reactions to phenytoin or carbamazepine may show histological features of mycosis fungoides [6−11]; cutaneous lesions resembling those of mycosis fungoides in the absence of fever have been reported with phenytoin and carbamazepine [10].

A number of non-anticonvulsant drugs have been associated with mycosis fungoides-like drug eruptions [1], including angiotensin-converting enzyme inhibitors [12], atenolol [13], mexiletine, thioridazine, D-penicillamine and Moduretic (amiloride hydrochloride with hydrochlorothiazide). An erythema annulare centrifugum-like pseudolymphomatous eruption was associated with levomepromazin therapy [14]. The pseudolymphoma syndrome usually responds to drug withdrawal; failure to recognize this syndrome has resulted in use of antitumour therapy, sometimes with fatal outcome. Occasionally a true lymphoma may develop.

High molecular weight polyvinylpyrrolidone, used in depot preparations of subcutaneously or intramuscularly administered medications, has been associated with pseudotumours distant from the site of injection [15,16].

1 Kardaun SH, Scheffer E, Vermeer BJ. Drug-induced pseudolymphomatous skin reactions. *Br J Dermatol* 1988; **118**: 545−52.
2 Gams RA, Neal JA, Conrad FG. Hydantoin-induced pseudolymphoma. *Ann Intern Med* 1968; **69**: 557−68.
3 Charlesworth EN. Phenytoin-induced pseudolymphoma syndrome. *Arch Dermatol* 1977; **113**: 477−80.
4 Shuttleworth D, Graham-Brown RAC, Williams AJ, *et al.* Pseudo-lymphoma associated with carbamazepine. *Clin Exp Dermatol* 1984; **9**: 421−3.
5 Yates P, Stockdill G, McIntyre M. Hypersensitivity to carbamazepine presenting as pseudolymphoma. *J Clin Pathol* 1986; **39**: 1224−8.
6 Rosenthal CJ, Noguera CA, Coppola A, *et al.* Pseudolymphoma with mycosis fungoides manifestations, hyperresponsiveness to diphenylhydantoin and lymphocyte disregulation. *Cancer* 1982; **49**: 2305−14.
7 Cooke LE, Hardin TC, Hendrickson DJ. Phenytoin-induced pseudolymphoma with mycosis fungoides manifestations. *Clin Pharm* 1988; **7**: 153−7.
8 Souteyrand P, D'Incan M. Drug induced mycosis fungoides-like lesions. *Curr Probl Dermatol* 1990; **19**: 176−82.
9 Wolf R, Kahane E, Sandbank M. Mycosis fungoides-like lesions associated with phenytoin therapy. *Arch Dermatol* 1985; **121**: 1181−2.
10 Rijlaarsdam U, Scheffer E, Meijer CJLM, *et al.* Mycosis fungoides-like lesions associated with phenytoin and carbamazepine therapy. *J Am Acad Dermatol* 1991; **24**: 216−20.
11 Welykyj S, Gradini R, Nakao J, Massa M. Carbamazepine-induced eruption histologically mimicking mycosis fungoides. *J Cutan Pathol* 1990; **17**: 111−16.
12 Furness PN, Goodfield MJ, MacLennan KA, *et al.* Severe cutaneous reactions to captropril and enalapril: histological study and comparison with early mycosis fungoides. *J Clin Pathol* 1986; **39**: 902−7.
13 Henderson CA, Shamy HK. Atenolol-induced pseudolymphoma. *Clin Exp Dermatol* 1990; **15**: 119−20.
14 Blazejak T, Hölzle E. Phenothiazin-induziertes Pseudolymphom. *Hautarzt* 1990; **41**: 161−3.
15 Oehlschlaegel G, Marquart K-H, Steuer G, Burg G. Iatrogener, durch Polyvinylpyrrolidon (PVP) induzierter 'Pseudotumor' der Haut. *Hautarzt* 1983; **34**: 555−60.
16 Bork K. Multiple Lymphozytome an den Einstichstellen als Komplikation einer Akupunkturbehandlung. Zur traumatischen Entstehung des Lymphozytoms. *Hautarzt* 1983; **34**: 496−9.

3.29 Erythromelalgia

Erythromelalgia is characterized by burning pain, erythema, swelling and warmth in the feet or hands, which is aggravated by dependency, warming or exercise, and often relieved by cooling or elevation of the limb [1]. Drugs implicated include nicardipine [2], nifedipine [3], bromocriptine [4], and pergolide [5].

1 Healsmith MF, Graham-Brown RAC, Burns DA. Erythromelalgia. *Clin Exp Dermatol* 1991; **16**: 46−8.
2 Levesque H, Moore N, Wolfe LM, Courtoid H. Erythromelalgia induced by nicardipine (inverse Raynaud's phenomenon?). *Br Med J* 1989; **298**: 1252−3.
3 Fisher JR, Padnick MB, Olstein S. Nifedipine and erythromelalgia. *Ann Intern Med* 1983; **98**: 671−2.
4 Eisler T, Hall RP, Kalavar KAR, Calne DB. Erythromelalgia-like eruption in Parkinsonian patients treated with bromocriptine. *Neurology* 1981; **37**: 1368−70.

5 Monk BE, Parkes JD, Du Vivier A. Erythromelalgia following pergolide administration. *Br J Dermatol* 1984; **111**: 97–9.

3.30 Drug-induced alopecia

Drug aetiology

A considerable number of drugs have been reported to cause hair loss [1–6]; the most important causes are listed in Table 3.17. Cytotoxic drugs may cause alopecia by either anagen or telogen effluvium. Chemotherapeutic agents implicated in the production of alopecia include: amsacrine, bleomycin, cyclophosphamide, cytarabine, dactinomycin, daunorubicin, doxorubicin, etoposide, fluorouracil, methotrexate, and the nitrosoureas [4]. Telogen alopecia has been caused by anticoagulants (heparin and coumarin anticoagulants), thyrostatic drugs (carbimazole and thiouracils), levodopa, propranolol, albendazole, and oral contraceptives. Retinoids cause alopecia by disrupting keratinization. Hydantoins may cause scalp alopecia and hypertrichosis elsewhere, and retinoids and clofibrate may cause alopecia by interfering with keratinization. Temporary hair loss has been described after 5-aminosalicylic acid enemas [7] and the use of bromocriptine [8] and danazol has induced generalized alopecia [9]. Certain β-blockers have caused increased hair loss [10,11]; topical ophthalmic β-blockers, especially timolol, and occasionally betaxolol or levobunolol [12] are also linked with alopecia [12]. Alopecia associated with conjunctivitis and ichthyosis has been attributed to dixyrazine [13]. Ibuprofen is recorded as causing alopecia [14].

Table 3.17 Drugs causing alopecia

Anticoagulants
  Coumarins
  Dextran
  Heparin
  Heparinoids
Anticonvulsants
  Carbamazepine
  Valproic acid
Cytotoxic agents
Drugs acting on the CNS
  Amitriptyline
  Doxepin
  Haloperidol
  Lithium
Hypocholesterolaemic agents
  Clofibrate
  Nicotinic acid
  Triparanol
Antithyroid drugs
  Carbimazole
  Thiouracils
Retinoids
  Etretinate
  Isotretinoin
Miscellaneous
  Albendazole
  Allopurinol
  Amphetamine
  Antithyroid drugs
  Bromocriptine
  Captopril
  Cholestyramine
  Cimetidine
  Dixyrazine
  Gentamicin
  Gold
  Ibuprofen
  Levodopa
  Metoprolol
  Oral contraceptives
  Propranolol
  Trimethadione

1 Levantine A, Almeyda J. Drug reactions XXIII. Drug induced alopecia. *Br J Dermatol* 1973; **89**: 549–53.
2 Blankenship ML. Drugs and alopecia. *Australas J Dermatol* 1983; **24**: 100–4.
3 Brodin MB. Drug-related alopecia. *Dermatol Clinics* 1987; **5**: 571–9.
4 Kerker BJ, Hood AF. Chemotherapy-induced cutaneous reactions. *Semin Dermatol* 1989; **8**: 173–81.
5 Rook A, Dawber R. *Diseases of the Hair and Scalp*, 2nd edn. Blackwell Scientific Publications, Oxford, 1990.
6 Merk HF. Drugs affecting hair growth. In Orfanos CE, Happle R (eds) *Hair and Hair Diseases*. Springer-Verlag, Berlin, 1990; pp 601–9.
7 Kutty PK, Raman KRK, Hawken K, Barrowman JA. Hair loss and 5-aminosalicylic acid enemas. *Ann Intern Med* 1982; **97**: 785–6.
8 Blum I, Leiba S. Increased hair loss as a side effect of bromocriptine treatment. *N Engl J Med* 1980; **303**: 1418.
9 Duff P, Mayer AR. Generalized alopecia: an unusual complication of danazol therapy. *Am J Obstet Gynecol* 1981; **141**: 349–50.
10 England JR, England JD. Alopecia and propranolol therapy. *Aust Fam Physician* 1982; **11**: 225–6.
11 Graeber CW, Lapkin RA. Metoprolol and alopecia. *Cutis* 1981; **28**: 633–4.
12 Fraunfelder FT, Meyer SM, Menacker SJ. Alopecia possibly secondary to topical ophthalmic β-blockers. *JAMA* 1990; **263**: 1493–4.
13 Poulsen J. Hair loss, depigmentation of hair, ichthyosis, and blepharoconjunctivitis produced by dixyrazine. *Acta Derm Venereol (Stockh)* 1981; **61**: 85–8.
14 Meyer HC. Alopecia associated with ibuprofen. *JAMA* 1979; **242**: 142.

3.31 Drug-induced hypertrichosis

The hirsutism induced in women by corticosteroids, androgens and certain progestogens is well recognized. Other drugs which may cause hypertrichosis, especially phenytoin (Figs 3.72 & 3.73) are listed in Table 3.18. Up to 50% of children treated with diazoxide, and up to 40% of patients on cyclosporin A, develop hirsutism. Zidovudine has caused excessive growth of eyelashes [3].

1 Rook A, Dawber R. *Diseases of the Hair and Scalp*, 2nd edn. Blackwell Scientific Publications, Oxford, 1990.
2 Merk HF. Drugs affecting hair growth. In: Orfanos CE, Happle R (eds) *Hair and Hair Diseases*. Springer-Verlag: Berlin, 1990; pp 601−9.
3 Klutman NE, Hinthorn DR. Excessive growth of eyelashes in a patient with AIDS being treated with zidovudine. *N Engl J Med* 1991; **324**: 1896.

3.32 Drug-induced nail abnormalities

Drug-induced nail abnormalities have been the subject of several reviews [1−6]. Heavy metals may induce changes as follows: arsenic causes transverse broad white lines (Mee's lines), silver causes blue discoloration of the lunulae, gold results in thin and brittle nails with longitudinal streaking, yellow−brown discoloration, and onycholysis, and lead produces partial leuchonychia. D-Penicillamine therapy is associated with the yellow nail syndrome and nail dystrophy. Cytotoxic agents may produce transverse or longitudinal pigmentation, splinter haemorrhages, Beau's lines, which are horizontal notches in the nail plate, corresponding to a period of disrupted nail growth (Fig. 3.74), leuchonychia, Mee's lines, onycholysis, shortening of lunulae, pallor, atrophy, nail shedding and slow

Table 3.18 Drugs causing hypertrichosis

Androgens
Benoxaprofen (withdrawn)
Corticosteroids
Cyclosporin A
Diazoxide
Minoxidil
Penicillamine
Phenytoin
Psoralens
Streptomycin

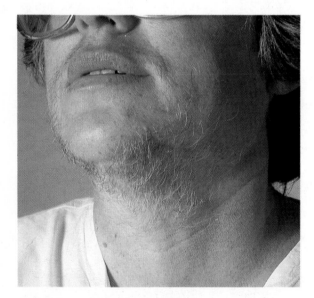

Figure 3.72 Hypertrichosis due to phenytoin taken for 14 years.

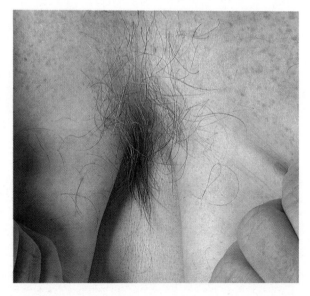

Figure 3.73 Intermammary hypertrichosis due to phenytoin taken for 14 years.

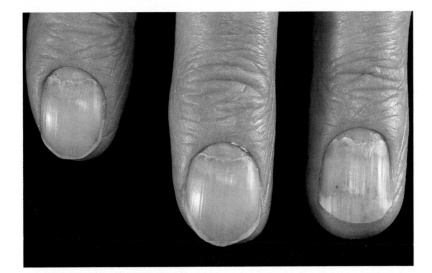

Figure 3.74 Beau's lines of nails.

Table 3.19 Drugs causing onycholysis

Antibiotics
  Cephaloridine
  Cloxacillin
  Chloramphenicol
  Chlortetracycline
  Demethylchlortetracycline
  Doxycycline
  Fluoroquinolones
  Minocycline
  Tetracycline hydrochloride
Chemotherapeutic agents
  Adriamycin
  Bleomycin
  5-Fluorouracil
  Mitozantrone
Miscellaneous
  Acridine
  Benoxaprofen (withdrawn)
  Captopril
  Norethindrone and mestranol
  Practolol
  Psoralens
  Phenothiazines
  Retinoids
  Sulpha-related drugs
  Thiazides

Photo-onycholysis
Oral contraceptives
Psoralens
Fluoroquinolones
Tetracyclines

growth; acute paronychia has occurred with methotrexate. β-Blockers may induce a psoriasiform nail dystrophy with onycholysis and subungual hyperkeratosis. Thiazide diuretics may result in onycholysis. Discoloration or pigmentation occurs with antimalarials (blue–brown discoloration), lithium (golden discoloration), phenolphthalein (dark-blue discoloration), phenothiazines (blue–black or purple pigmentation), phenytoin (pigmentation), psoralens, and tetracyclines (yellow pigmentation). Oral contraceptives may induce photo-onycholysis and onycholysis, and are associated with an increased growth rate and reduced splitting and fragility. By contrast, heparin reduces nail growth and causes transverse banding and subungual haematomas. Retinoids cause thinning and increased fragility, onychoschizia, onycholysis, temporary nail shedding, onychomadesis, ingrowing nails, periungual granulation tissue and paronychia.

Onycholysis

Drugs causing onycholysis [6,7], which refers to focal yellowish discoloration due to separation of the nail plate from the nail bed (Fig. 3.75), and photo-onycholysis, are listed in Table 3.19.

1 Daniel CR III, Scher RK. Nail changes secondary to systemic drugs or ingestants. *J Am Acad Dermatol* 1984; **10**: 250–8.
2 Fenton DA. Nail changes due to drugs. In Samman PD, Fenton DA. *The Nails in Disease*, 4th edn. William Heinemann Medical Books, London, 1986; pp 121–5.
3 Fenton DA, Wilkinson JD. The nail in systemic diseases and drug-induced changes. In Baran R, Dawber RPR (eds) *Diseases of the Nails and their Management*. Blackwell Scientific Publications, Oxford, 1984; pp 205–65.
4 Daniel CR III, Scher RK. Nail changes secondary to systemic drugs or ingestants. In Scher RK, Daniel CR III (eds) *Nails: Therapy, Diagnosis, Surgery*. W.B. Saunders, Philadelphia, 1990; pp 192–201.

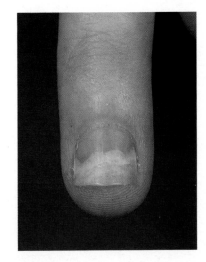

Figure 3.75 Onycholysis of nails.

5 Zaias N. *The Nail in Health and Disease*, 2nd edn. Appleton Lange, East Norwalk, Connecticut, 1990.
6 Baran R, Juhlin L. Drug-induced photo-onycholysis. Three subtypes identified in a study of 15 cases. *J Am Acad Dermatol* 1987; **17**: 1012−16.
7 Daniel CR. Onycholysis: an overview. *Semin Dermatol* 1991; **10**: 34−40.

3.33 Drug-induced oral conditions

Adverse drug reactions affecting the mouth are less common than those affecting the skin, and have been extensively reviewed [1]. Disturbance of taste has been reported with a wide variety of drugs, including captopril, griseofulvin, and metronidazole.

Xerostomia

Dryness of the mouth (xerostomia) may result from anticholinergic side-effects of drugs. Xerostomia has been recorded in association with antidepressants, tranquillizers, anti-Parkinsonian drugs, anti-hypertensives, and gastrointestinal antispasmodics (Table 3.20). Parotitis with salivary sialadenitis has been reported in up to 15% of patients taking phenylbutazone, and may be associated with fever, and a rash [2]. A similar syndrome may occur with repeated administration of iodinated contrast media [3], and with nitrofurantoin [4].

Stomatitis

Stomatitis (an inflammatory, bullous or ulcerative condition of the buccal mucosa) may form a part of drug-induced lichenoid reactions, fixed drug reactions, or erythema multiforme, but may also arise separately from these conditions as a side-effect of a number of drugs (Table 3.21). Chemotherapeutic agents causing stomatitis or buccal ulceration include [5]: actinomycin D, adriamycin, amsacrine, bleomycin, busulphan, chlorambucil, cyclophosphamide, dactinomycin, daunorubicin, doxorubicin, fluorouracil, interleukin-2, mercaptopurine, methotrexate, mithramycin, mitomcyin, nitrosoureas, procarbazine, and vincristine. Penicillamine may induce stomatitis or ulceration as part of drug-induced pemphigus [6] or a lichenoid drug eruption. Gold therapy is another well-recognized cause of stomatitis [7]. Allergic reactions to dental materials and therapy may cause stomatitis, and also contact dermatitis in dental personnel [8]. Stomatitis due to irritant or allergic contact dermatitis may be caused by topical anaesthetics, antibiotic-containing lozenges, cough drops, mouthwashes, toothpastes, perfumed lipsticks, dental adhesives, and acrylic resin dental prostheses [1]. Gold causes allergic contact stomatitis only very rarely [9].

Hyperpigmentation

Hyperpigmentation of the buccal mucosa may occur with chemo-

Table 3.20 Drugs associated with xerostomia [1]

Antidepressants
  Tricylic
    Amitriptyline
    Doxepin
    Imipramine
  Monoamine oxidase inhibitors
    Isocarboxazid
    Phenelzine
Psychotropic agents
  Chlorpromazine
  Thioridazine
  Haloperidol
  Prochlorperazine
Minor tranquillizers
  Diazepam
  Chordiazepoxide
  Hydroxyzine
Anti-Parkinsonian drugs
Antihypertensives (ganglion blockers)
Gastrointestinal antispasmodics
  Atropine
  Propantheline bromide
  Phenobarbital

therapeutic agents [10]. Oestrogen is associated with gingival hyper-melanosis [11]. Amalgam tattoos with localized hyperpigmentation of the buccal mucosa (Fig. 3.76) result from implantation of amalgam in soft tissues, especially of the gingival or alveolar mucosa [12].

Reactions caused by antibacterial, antifungal and immunosuppressive therapy

Systemic antibiotics or immunosuppressive medication [13], and corticosteroids administered by aerosol [14], may lead to development of candidiasis of the buccal mucosa (Fig. 3.77). Black hairy tongue (Fig. 3.78) may be associated with broad-spectrum antibiotic therapy and with griseofulvin treatment.

Gingival hyperplasia

Gingival hyperplasia (Fig. 3.79) may be caused by phenytoin [15], nifedipine [16], diltiazem [17], and cyclosporin A [18].

Table 3.21 Drugs causing stomatitis or buccal ulceration

Chemotherapeutic agents
Antirheumatic drugs
  Gold
  Naproxen
  Indomethacin
  Penicillamine
  Zomepirac
Antidepressants
  Amitriptyline
  Doxepin
  Imipramine
Antihypertensive agents
  Captopril
  Hydralazine
  Methyldopa (rare)
Miscellaneous
  Chlorpromazine
  Valproic acid

1 Zelickson BD, Rogers RS III. Drug reactions involving the mouth. *Clin Dermatol* 1986; **4**: 98–109.
2 Speed BR, Spelman DW. Sialadenitis and systemic reactions associated with phenylbutazone. *Aust N Z J Med* 1982; **12**: 261–4.
3 Chohen JC, Roxe DM, Said R, *et al*. Iodide mumps after repeated exposure to iodinated contrast media. *Lancet* 1980; **i**: 762–3.
4 Meyboom RH, van Gent A, Zinkstok DJ. Nitrofurantoin-induced parotitis. *Br Med J* 1982; **285**: 1049.
5 Kerker BJ, Hood AF. Chemotherapy-induced cutaneous reactions. *Semin Dermatol* 1989; **8**: 173–81.

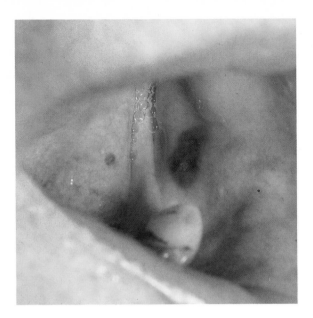

Figure 3.76 Hyperpigmentation of buccal mucosa related to mercury in dental amalgam.

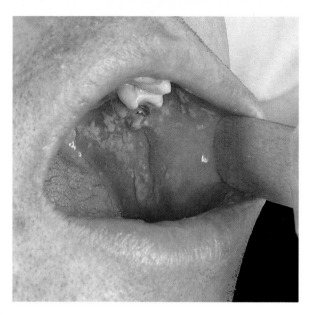

Figure 3.77 Oral candidiasis in a patient taking antibiotics.

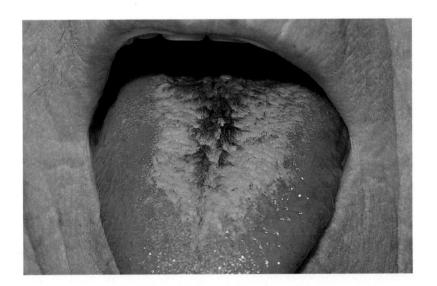

Figure 3.78 Black hairy tongue.

6 Hay KD, Muller HK, Rade PC. D-Penicillamine-induced mucocutaneous lesions with features of pemphigus. *Oral Surg* 1978; **45**: 385–95.
7 Glenert U. Drug stomatitis due to gold therapy. *Oral Surg* 1984; **58**: 52–6.
8 Gall H. Allergien auf zahnärztliche Werkstoffe und Dentalpharmaka. *Hautarzt* 1983; **34**: 326–31.
9 Wiesenfeld D, Ferguson MM, Forsyth A, *et al.* Allergy to dental gold. *Oral Surg* 1984; **57**: 158–60.
10 Krutchik AN, Buzdar AU. Pigmentation of the tongue and mucous membranes associated with cancer chemotherapy. *South Med J* 1979; **72**: 1615–16.
11 Hertz RS, Beckstead PC, Brown WJ. Epithelial melanosis of the gingiva possibly resulting from the use of oral contraceptives. *J Am Dent Assoc* 1980; **100**: 713–14.

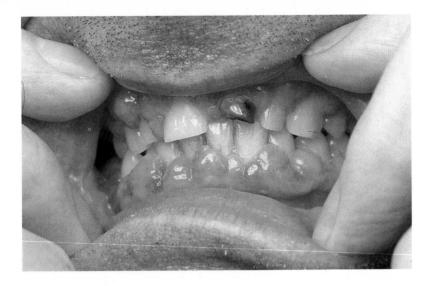

Figure 3.79 Gingival hyperplasia in a patient on combined cyclosporin A and nifedipine therapy. (Courtesy of Dr D.H. McGibbon, St John's Dermatology Centre, London.)

12 Buchner A, Hansen LS. Amalgam pigmentation (amalgam tattoo) of the oral mucosa: a clinicopathologic study of 268 cases. *Oral Surg* 1980; **49**: 139−47.
13 Torack RM. Fungus infections associated with antibiotic and steroid therapy. *Am J Med* 1957; **22**: 872−82.
14 Chervinsky P, Petraco AJ. Incidence of oral candidiasis during therapy with triamcinolone acetonide aerosol. *Ann Allergy* 1979; **43**: 80−3.
15 Hassell TM, Page RC, Narayanan AS, Cooper CG. Diphenylhydantoin (dilantin) gingival hyperplasia: drug induced abnormality of connective tissue. *Proc Natl Acad Sci* 1976; **73**: 2909−12.
16 Benini PL, Crosti C, Sala F, *et al*. Gingival hyperplasia by nifedipine. Report of a case. *Acta Derm Venereol (Stockh)* 1985; **65**: 362−5.
17 Giustiniani S, Robustelli della Cuna F, Marieni M. Hyperplastic gingivitis during diltiazem therapy. *Int J Cardiol* 1987; **15**: 247−9.
18 Frosch PJ, Ruder H, Stiefel A, *et al*. Gingivahyperplasie und Seropapeln unter Cyclosporinbehandlung. *Hautarzt* 1988; **39**: 611−16.

3.34 Oligospermia

This unfortunate effect of certain drugs [1] may come to light only as a result of infertility investigations. Oestrogens, androgens, cyproterone acetate, cytotoxic drugs, including methotrexate given for psoriasis [2], colchicine, most monoamine oxidase inhibitors, ketoconazole, and sulphasalazine have all been incriminated. The synthetic retinoids isotretinoin and etretinate do not seem to affect the numbers of sperm [3,4].

1 Drife JO. Drugs and sperm. *Br Med J* 1982; **284**: 844−5.
2 Sussman A, Leonard JM. Psoriasis, methotrexate, and oligospermia. *Arch Dermatol* 1980; **116**: 215−17.
3 Schill W-B, Wagner A, Nikolowski J, Plewig G. Aromatic retinoid and 13-*cis*-retinoic acid: spermatological investigations. In Orfanos CE, Braun-Falco O, Farber EM, *et al*. (eds) *Retinoids. Advances in Basic Research and Therapy*. Springer Verlag, Berlin, 1981, pp 389−95.
4 Töröck L, Kása M. Spermatological and endocrinological examinations connected with isotretinoin treatment. In Saurat JH (ed.) *Retinoids: New Trends in Research and Therapy*. Karger, Basel, 1985, pp 407−10.

Part 3
Important or
Widely Prescribed Drugs

Chapter 4
Antibacterial Drugs

4.1 β-Lactam antibiotics

Penicillin

Toxic reactions to penicillin are extremely rare and usually only follow massive doses, but can occur with normal doses in patients with renal impairment; encephalopathy may result. By contrast, immunological reactions are common [1–5]; allergy to penicillin has been reported in up to 10% of patients treated [6]. All forms of penicillin, including the semisynthetic penicillins, are cross-allergenic; in general, allergic reactions to semisynthetic compounds are commoner than to natural penicillins. All four types of immunological reaction may occur: urticaria and anaphylactic shock (Type I), haemolytic anaemia or agranulocytosis (Type II), allergic vasculitis or serum sickness-like reaction (Type III) and allergic contact dermatitis [7] (Type IV).

Clinical features

Immediate reactions occur within 1 hour, and take the form of urticaria, laryngeal oedema, bronchospasm, and/or anaphylactic shock. So-called accelerated reactions with the same clinical features develop from 1 to 72 hours later. Reactions occurring more than 72 hours after exposure are termed late reactions; these include maculopapular rashes (Figs 4.1 & 4.2) with scarlatiniform and morbilliform exanthemata, urticaria, serum sickness, erythema multiforme (Fig. 4.3), haemolytic anaemia, thrombocytopenia, and neutropenia. Fever is the commonest reaction. The urticaria has no special features but may persist for months. Attacks of serum sickness usually last about 12 days but, particularly after the depot penicillins, can be much longer. Recurrences sometimes follow the resumption of vigorous use of muscles into which penicillin was injected.

Penicillin antigens

Investigation of the antigenic structures responsible for penicillin allergy first demonstrated a 'major determinant', which is the penicilloyl group formed by spontaneous hydrolysis of penicillin

[137]

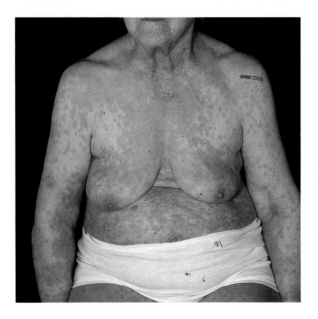

Figure 4.1 Confluent erythema in a patient treated with penicillin, amoxycillin, and flucloxacillin.

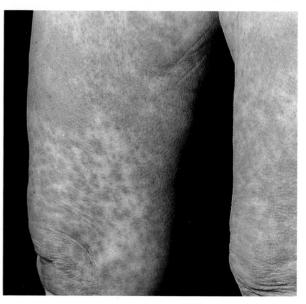

Figure 4.2 Maculopapular purpuric eruption in a patient treated with penicillin, amoxycillin, and flucloxacillin.

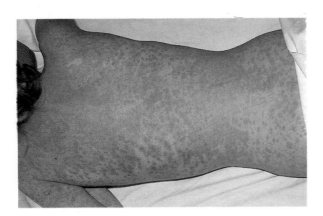

Figure 4.3 Widespread erythema multiforme-like eruption due to penicillin.

(penicilloyl polylysine is used for skin testing); it was subsequently shown that benzyl penicillin is metabolized to produce small amounts of additional antigenic compounds termed 'minor determinants' [3]. Most immediate-type anaphylactic hypersensitivity reactions are mediated by IgE antibodies to minor antigenic determinants, whereas accelerated reactions are usually the result of IgE antibodies directed against the major antigenic determinant [3,4].

Epidemiology

Anaphylactic reactions to penicillin were reported to occur in about 0.015% of treatment courses; fatal reactions occurred in 0.0015–0.002% (i.e. 1 in 50 000–100 000) of treatment courses [8], so that there were several hundred fatalities due to this drug in the US each year [9]. Young and middle aged adults aged 20–49 years are

[138]

at most risk [10]. Atopy does not seem to predispose to a higher frequency of IgE production to, and reactions to, β-lactam antibiotics, but may increase the risk of any reaction being severe [3]. Anaphylaxis is commoner after parenteral administration, and is very rare, but has been recorded, after oral ingestion [10]. Maculopapular reactions occur in about 2% of treatment courses [3]; where there is a history of a prior penicillin reaction, the risk of a subsequent reaction increases to about 10% [11]. A fair proportion (33% in one study) of children may lose their skin test reactivity within a year [12]. In practice, when penicillin is given to children said to be allergic to penicillin, very few experience an adverse reaction [4]. In adults, the rate of disappearance of penicillin-specific IgE is highly variable, from 10 days to indefinite persistence [3]. For a group of penicillin allergic patients, the time lapsed since a previous reaction is inversely related to the risk of a further IgE mediated reaction [11]. In one study, 80−90% of patients were skin-test positive 2 months after an acute allergic reaction, but less than 20% were skin-test positive 10 years later [13]. Nevertheless, patients with a prior history of an IgE-dependent reaction remain at risk of recurrence, even though IgE antibodies become undetectable by skin testing [14]. It should also be appreciated that most serious and fatal allergic reactions to β-lactam antibiotics occur in individuals who have never had a prior allergic reaction; a negative history should therefore not induce a false sense of security [3]. Continuous prophylactic treatment is associated with a very low incidence of reaction [15].

Activation of allergy in a sensitized individual may require only minute amounts of the drug as from contaminated syringes, dental root canal fillings, viral vaccines, contaminated milk or meat products, and contamination of transfused blood [16]. Urticaria and wheezing occurred in the penicillin-sensitive spouse of a man receiving parenteral mezlocillin, and was postulated to have arisen as a result of seminal fluid transmission of penicillin [17].

Other patterns of penicillin reactions

In addition to the reactions detailed above a number of other penicillin-associated conditions have been reported, including erythema multiforme [18], vesicular and bullous eruptions, exfoliative dermatitis [19], vascular purpura or fixed eruptions [1], postinflammatory elastolysis (cutis laxa), which was generalized and eventually fatal in one case [20], and a very few cases of pemphigus vulgaris [21−23], pemphigoid [24] and pustular psoriasis [25]. It has been proposed that penicillin may have a role in chronic 'idiopathic' urticaria [26].

Cloxacillin and flucloxacillin

Cloxacillins cross-react with penicillins but unlike ampicillin do not produce distinctive eruptions. Flucloxacillin rarely elicits primary penicillin hypersensitivity.

1 Beeley L. Allergy to penicillin. *Br Med J* 1984; **288**: 511–12.
2 Erffmeyer JE. Penicillin allergy. *Clin Rev Allergy* 1986; **4**: 171–88.
3 Weiss ME, Adkinson NF. Immediate hypersensitivity reactions to penicillin and related antibiotics. *Clin Allergy* 1989; **18**: 515–40.
4 Anonymous. Penicillin allergy in childhood. *Lancet* 1988; **i**: 420.
5 Weber EA, Knight A. Testing for allergy to antibiotics. *Semin Dermatol* 1989; **8**; 204–12.
6 Van Arsdael PP. The risk of penicillin reactions. *Ann Intern Med* 1968; **69**: 1071.
7 Stejskal VDM, Forsbeck M, Olin R. Side chain-specific lymphocyte responses in workers with occupational allergy induced by penicillins. *Int Arch Allergy Appl Immunol* 1987; **82**: 461–4.
8 Idsøe O, Guthe T, Willcox RR, de Weck AL. Nature and extent of penicillin side reactions, with particular reference to fatalities from anaphylactic shock. *Bull WHO* 1968; **38**: 159–88.
9 Feinberg SM. Allergy from therapeutic products. Incidence, importance, recognition, and prevention. *JAMA* 1961; **178**: 815–18.
10 Simmonds J, Hodges S, Nicol F, Barnett D. Anaphylaxis after oral penicillin. *Br Med J* 1978; **ii**: 1404.
11 Sogn DD. Penicillin allergy. *J Allergy Clin Immunol* 1984; **74**: 589–93.
12 Chandra RK, Joglekar SA, Tomas E. Penicillin allergy: anti-penicillin IgE antibodies and immediate hypersensitivity skin reactions employing major and minor determinants of penicillin. *Arch Dis Child* 1980; **55**: 857–60.
13 Sullivan TJ, Wedner HJ, Shatz GS, *et al.* Skin testing to detect penicillin allergy. *J Allergy Clin Immunol* 1981; **68**: 171–80.
14 Adkinson NF Jr. Risk factors for drug allergy. *J Allergy Clin Immunol* 1984; **74**: 567–72.
15 Wood HF, Simpson R, Feinstein AR, *et al.* Rheumatic fever in children and adolescents. A long-term epidemiologic study of subsequent prophylaxis, streptococcal infections, and clinical sequelae. I. Description of the investigative techniques and the population studied. *Ann Intern Med* 1964; **60** (Suppl. 5): 6–17.
16 Michel J, Sharon R. Non-haemolytic adverse reaction after transfusion of a blood unit containing penicillin. *Br Med J* 1980; **i**: 152–3.
17 Burks JH, Fliegalman R, Sokalski SJ. An unforeseen complication of home parenteral antibiotic therapy. *Arch Intern Med* 1989; **149**: 1603–4.
18 Staretz LR, DeBoom GW. Multiple oral and skin lesions occurring after treatment with penicillin. *J Am Dent Assoc* 1990; **121**: 436–7.
19 Levine BB. Skin rashes with penicillin therapy: current management. *N Engl J Med* 1972; **286**: 42–3.
20 Kerl H, Burg G, Hashimoto K. Fatal, penicillin-induced, generalized, post-inflammatory elastolysis (cutis laxa). *Am J Dermatopathol* 1983; **5**: 267–76.
21 Ruocco V, Rossi A, Pisani M, *et al.* An abortive form of pemphigus vulgaris probably induced by penicillin. *Dermatologica* 1979; **159**: 266–73.
22 Duhra PL, Foulds IS. Penicillin-induced pemphigus vulgaris. *Br J Dermatol* 1988; **118**: 307.
23 Fellner MJ, Mark AS. Penicillin- and ampicillin-induced pemphigus vulgaris. *Int J Dermatol* 1980; **19**: 392–3.
24 Alcalay J, David M, Ingber A, *et al.* Bullous pemphigoid mimicking bullous erythema multiforme: An untoward side effect of penicillins. *J Am Acad Dermatol* 1988; **18**: 345–9.
25 Katz M, Seidenbaum M, Weinrauch L. Penicillin-induced generalized pustular psoriasis. *J Am Acad Dermatol* 1988; **17**: 918–20.
26 Boonk WJ, Van Ketel WG. The role of penicillin in the pathogenesis of chronic urticaria. *Br J Dermatol* 1982; **106**: 183–90.

Ampicillin [1–5]

A morbilliform rash, with onset on the extremities becoming generalized, occurs in 5–10% of patients treated with ampicillin, and usually develops 7–12 days after onset of therapy. This time interval suggests an allergic mechanism, but the rash disappears spontaneously even if ampicillin is continued, and may not develop on re-exposure. Skin tests are generally negative. An urticarial reaction, present in about 1% of patients [2], indicates the presence of Type I IgE-mediated general penicillin allergy. The use of a highly purified preparation has reduced the exanthem rate to 1.4% [3]. Administration of ampicillin when a patient has infectious mononucleosis leads to florid morbilliform and sometimes purpuric eruptions in up to 100% of patients (Figs 4.4 & 4.5) [5,6]. Cutaneous reactions to ampicillin are also increased in cytomegalovirus infection and in chronic lymphatic leukaemia [7,8]. Allopurinol administered concomitantly with ampicillin increases the exanthem rate (to 22%) [9], as does renal insufficiency. Ampicillin has been reported to cause a fixed drug eruption [10], erythema multiforme and Stevens–Johnson syndrome [11], toxic epidermal necrolysis (TEN) [12], Henoch–Schönlein purpura [13], serum sickness [14] and pemphigus vulgaris [15], in individual cases. Administration of ampicillin to a patient with a history of psoriasis resulted in erythroderma on two separate occasions; there was a psoriasiform skin test reaction to intradermal ampicillin but not to a saline control [16]. Re-exposure of patients to ampicillins and other penicillins is contraindicated after urticarial reactions; anaphylactic reactions to ampicillin have been recorded. The risk is far less after morbilliform rashes but is not negligible.

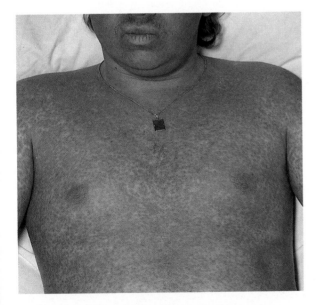

Figure 4.4 Florid morbilliform purpuric eruption in a patient with glandular fever treated with ampicillin.

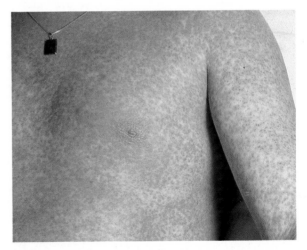

Figure 4.5 Close-up view of eruption in a patient with glandular fever treated with ampicillin.

Methicillin

Methicillin caused reappearance of a recently faded ampicillin rash in a patient with glandular fever [17].

Amoxycillin

Cutaneous eruptions including urticaria, morbilliform, or maculo-papular rashes occur in 1.5−2.1% of treatment courses with amoxycillin [18−20]. Serum sickness has been reported with amoxycillin in children [21]. Amoxycillin has caused a fixed eruption [22], and a curious recurrent localized pustular eruption [23]. This drug has also been implicated in the development of an acute generalized exanthematous pustulosis [24]. Anaphylactic reactions during treatment and rechallenge with amoxycillin have have been reported in three patients with negative skin tests to benzylpenicil-loyl polylysine, and a negative radioallergosorbent (RAST) test with benzylpenicilloyl; in two patients, there were positive skin and RAST tests to amoxycillin [25]. In a further study, 20 of 64 patients diagnosed as having penicillin allergy were found to react to amoxycillin and not to other penicillins [26]. There may be an increased frequency of rash with amoxycillin and clavulanate therapy in human immunodeficiency virus (HIV)-positive patients [27].

1 Almeyda J, Levantine A. Drug reactions XIX. Adverse cutaneous reactions to the penicillins — ampicillin rashes. *Br J Dermatol* 1972; **87**: 293−7.
2 Bass JW, Crowley DM, Steele RW, *et al.* Adverse effects of orally administered ampicillin. *J Pediatr* 1973; **83**: 106−8.
3 Leading Article. Ampicillin rashes. *Br Med J* 1975; **ii**: 708−9.
4 Saurat JH, Ponvert CL, Soubrane CL, *et al.* Sensibilisation à la pénicilline après accident cutané dû à l'ampicilline. *Nouv Presse Méd* 1976: **5**: 25−7.
5 Weiss ME, Adkinson NF. Immediate hypersensitivity reactions to penicillin and related antibiotics. *Clin Allergy* 1988; **18**: 515−40.
6 Pullen H, Wright N, Murdoch J McC. Hypersensitivity reactions to anti-bacterial drugs in infectious mononucleosis. *Lancet* 1967; **ii**: 1176−8.
7 Klemola E. Hypersensitivity reactions to ampicillin in cytomegalovirus mono-nucleosis. *Scand J Infect Dis* 1970; **2**: 29.
8 Cameron SJ, Richmond J. Ampicillin hypersensitivity in lymphatic leukaemia. *Scot Med J* 1972; **16**: 425−7.
9 Jick H, Slone D, Shapiro S, *et al.* Excess of ampicillin rashes associated with allopurinol or hyperuricemia. A report from the Boston Collaborative Drug Surveillance Program, Boston University Medical Center. *N Engl J Med* 1972; **286**: 505−7.
10 Arndt KA, Parrish J. Ampicillin rashes. *Arch Dermatol* 1973; **107**: 74.
11 Gupta HL, Dheman R. Ampicillin induced Stevens−Johnson syndrome. *J Indian Med Assoc* 1979; **72**: 188−9.
12 Tagami H, Tatsuta K, Iwatski K, Yamada M. Delayed hypersensitivity in ampicillin-induced toxic epidermal necrolysis. *Arch Dermatol* 1983; **119**: 910−13.
13 Beeching NJ, Gruer LD, Findlay CD, Geddes AM. A case of Henoch−Schönlein purpura syndrome following oral ampicillin. *J Antimicrob Chemother* 1982; **10**: 479−82.
14 Caldwell JR, Cliff LE. Adverse reactions to antimicrobial agents. *JAMA* 1974; **230**: 77−80.
15 Fellner MJ, Mark AS. Penicillin- and ampicillin-induced pemphigus vulgaris. *Int J Dermatol* 1980; **19**: 392−3.

16 Saito S, Ikezawa Z. Psoriasiform intradermal test reaction to ABPC in a patient with psoriasis and ABPC allergy. *J Dermatol (Tokyo)* 1990; **17**: 677−83.

17 Fields DA. Methicillin rash in infectious mononucleosis. *West J Med* 1981; **133**: 521.

18 Wise PJ, Neu HC. Experience with amoxicillin: an overall summary of clinical trials in the United States. *J Infect Dis* 1974; **129** (Suppl): S266−S267.

19 Levine LR. Quantitative comparison of adverse reactions to cefaclor versus amoxicillin in a surveillance study. *Pediatr Infect Dis* 1985; **4**: 358−61.

20 Bigby M, Jick S, Jick H, Arndt K. Drug-induced cutaneous reactions. A report from the Boston Collaborative Drug Surveillance Program on 15 438 consecutive inpatients, 1975 to 1982. *JAMA* 1986; **256**: 3358−63.

21 Chopra R, Roberts J, Warrington RJ. Severe delayed-onset hypersensitivity reactions to amoxicillin in children. *Can Med Assoc J* 1989; **140**: 921−3.

22 Chowdhury FH. Fixed genital drug eruption. *Practical Med* 1982; **226**: 1450.

23 Shuttleworth D. A localized, recurrent pustular eruption following amoxycillin administration. *Clin Exp Dermatol* 1989; **14**: 367−8.

24 Roujeau J-C, Bioulac-Sage P, Bourseau C, *et al*. Acute generalized exanthematous pustulosis. Analysis of 63 cases. *Arch Dermatol* 1991; **127**: 1333−8.

25 Blanca M, Perez E, Garcia J, *et al*. Anaphylaxis to amoxicillin but good tolerance to benzylpenicillin. *Allergy* 1988; **43**: 508−10.

26 Blanca M, Vega J, Garcia J, *et al*. Allergy to amoxicillin with good tolerance to other penicillins. Study of the incidence of patients allergic to betalactams. *Clin Exp Allergy* 1990; **20**: 475−81.

27 Battegay M, Opravil M, Wütrich B, Lüthy R. Rash with amoxycillin-clavulanate therapy in HIV-infected patients. *Lancet* 1989; **ii**: 1100.

Cephalosporins [1]

Toxic reactions may occur with renal disease. Haemorrhage may result from interference with blood clotting factors. Reactions are more common in penicillin-sensitive patients as a result of cross-sensitivity [2], but primary sensitization is not uncommon [3]. Up to 50% of patients who are skin-test positive to penicillin also have positive skin-test reactions to cephalosporins [4]. However, too few patients with positive skin-test reactions to penicillin have been challenged with cephalosporins, and vice versa, to determine the true incidence of cross-reactivity [5]. Newer cephalosporins are said to demonstrate less cross-reaction with penicillin [6], but they are best avoided in patients with a history of penicillin allergy [5].

Hypersensitivity reactions include various exanthemata, and contact urticaria [7]; cases of anaphylaxis (to cefaclor) [8] and of fatal anaphylactic shock (related to cephalothin) [9] have been reported. Vulvovaginitis and pruritus ani are not uncommon. Exfoliative dermatitis has been attributed to cefoxitin [10]. Disulfiram-like reactions to alcohol have been described with newer members of this group. Pustular reactions have been documented with cephadrine, cephalexin and cephazolin [11−13]. Cephalosporins [14] including cephalexin [15] have been reported to cause TEN, and cephalexin has precipitated pemphigus vulgaris [16]. Cephazolin has caused an unusual fixed drug eruption [17]. A curious photo-recall-like phenomenon followed the use of cephazolin and gentamicin sulphate, in that the eruption was restricted to an area of sunburn sustained 1 month previously [18]. Ceftazidime has been implicated in the development of erythema multiforme [19].

Monobactams

Monobactams (e.g. aztreonam) show weak cross-reactivity with IgE antibodies to penicillin [20,21], but immediate hypersensitivity on first exposure to aztreonam in penicillin-allergic patients has been recorded [22,23]. In general, aztreonam is well tolerated in high-risk patients allergic to other β-lactam antibiotics, but there is a 20% sensitization rate following exposure [24].

Carbapenems

Cross-reactivity and allergic reactions to imipenem occur in patients known to be allergic to penicillin [2,25]. Carbapenems should be avoided in patients with penicillin allergy [5]. Imipenem combined with cilastatin, a non-antibiotic enzyme inhibitor which prevents breakdown of imipenem to nephrotoxic metabolites, may cause phlebitis or pain at the site of infusion [26]. Imipenem has been associated with a pustular eruption [27], and imipenem-cilastatin with palmar–plantar pruritus during infusion in a child with acquired immunodeficiency syndrome (AIDS) [28].

1 Weiss ME, Adkinson NF. Immediate hypersensitivity reactions to penicillin and related antibiotics. *Clin Allergy* 1988; **18**: 515–40.
2 Saxon A, Beall CN, Rohr AS, *et al*. Immediate hypersensitivity reactions to beta-lactam antibiotics. *Ann Intern Med* 1987; **107**: 204–15.
3 Moellering RC Jr, Swartz MN. Drug therapy. The newer cephalosporins. *N Engl J Med* 1976; **294**: 24–8.
4 Sullivan TJ, Wedner HJ, Shatz GS, *et al*. Skin testing to detect penicillin allergy. *J Allergy Clin Immunol* 1981; **68**: 171–80.
5 Weber EA, Knight A. Testing for allergy to antibiotics. *Semin Dermatol* 1989; **8**: 204–12.
6 Korting HC. Zephalosporin-Allergie und Zephalosporin-Penizillin-Kreuzallergie unter besonderer Berücksichtigung für die venerologische Therapie bedeutsamer anaphylaktischer Reaktionen. *Hautarzt* 1984; **35**: 225–9.
7 Tuft L. Contact urticaria from cephalosporins. *Arch Dermatol* 1975; **111**: 1609.
8 Nishioka K, Katayama I, Kobayashi Y, Takijiri C. Anaphylaxis due to cefaclor hypersensitivity. *J Dermatol (Tokyo)* 1986; **13**: 226–7.
9 Spruell FG, Minette LJ, Sturner WQ. Two surgical deaths associated with cephalothin. *JAMA* 1974; **229**: 440–1.
10 Kannangara DW, Smith B, Cohen K. Exfoliative dermatitis during cefoxitin therapy. *Arch Intern Med* 1982; **142**: 1031–2.
11 Kalb R, Grossman ME. Pustular eruption following administration of cephadrine. *Cutis* 1986; **38**: 58–60.
12 Jackson H, Vion B, Levy PM. Generalized eruptive pustular drug rash due to cephalexin. *Dermatologica* 1988; **177**: 292–4.
13 Fayol J, Bernard P, Bonnetblanc JM. Pustular eruption following the administration of cefazolin: A second case report. *J Am Acad Dermatol* 1988; **19**: 571.
14 Nichter LS, Harman DM, Bryant CA, *et al*. Cephalosporin-induced toxic epidermal necrolysis. *J Burn Care Rehabil* 1983; **4**: 358–60.
15 Hogan DJ, Rooney ME. Toxic epidermal necrolysis due to cephalexin. *J Am Acad Dermatol* 1987; **17**: 852.
16 Wolf R, Dechner E, Ophir J, Brenner S. Cephalexin. A nonthiol drug that may induce pemphigus vulgaris. *Int J Dermatol* 1991; **30**: 213–15.
17 Sigal-Nahum M, Konqui A, Gauliet A, Sigal S. Linear fixed drug eruption. *Br J Dermatol* 1988; **118**: 849–51.

18 Flax SH, Uhle P. Photo recall-like phenomenon following the use of cefazolin and gentamicin sulfate. *Cutis* 1990; **46**: 59—61.

19 Pierce TH, Vig SJ, Ingram PM. Ceftazidime in the treatment of lower respiratory tract infection. *J Antimicrob Chemother* 1983; **12** (Suppl A): 21—5.

20 Adkinson NF, Saxon A, Spence MR, Swabb EA. Cross-allergenicity and immunogenicity of aztreonam. *Rev Infect Dis* 1985; **7** (Suppl 4): S613—S621.

21 Saxon A, Hassner A, Swabb EA, *et al.* Lack of cross-reactivity between aztreonam, a monobactam antibiotic, and penicillin-allergic subjects. *J Infect Dis* 1984; **149**: 16.

22 Hantson P, de Coninck B, Horn JL, Mahieu P. Immediate hypersensitivity to aztreonam and imipenem. *Br Med J* 1991; **302**: 294—5.

23 Alvarez JS, Del Castillo JAS, Garcia IS, Ortiz MJA. Immediate hypersensitivity to aztreonam. *Lancet* 1990; **335**: 1094.

24 Moss RB. Sensitization to aztreonam and cross-reactivity with other beta-lactam antibiotics in high-risk patients with cystic fibrosis. *J Allergy Clin Immunol* 1991; **87**: 78—88.

25 Saxon A, Adelman DC, Patel A, *et al.* Imipenem cross-reactivity with penicillin in humans. *J Allergy Clin Immunol* 1988; **82**: 213—17.

26 Anon. Imipenem + cilastatin — a new type of antibiotic. *Drug Ther Bull* 1991; **29**: 43—4.

27 Escallier F, Dalac S, Foucher JL, *et al.* Pustulose exanthématique aiguë généralisée imputabilité a l'imipéneme (Tienam®). *Ann Derm Vénéréol (Paris)* 1989; **116**: 407—9.

28 Machado ARL, Silva CLO, Galvão NAM. Unusual reaction to imipenem—cilastatin in a child with the acquired immunodeficiency syndrome. *J Allergy Clin Immunol* 1991; **87**: 754.

4.2 Tetracyclines

Many of the side-effects are common to all drugs within the group, and cross-sensitivity occurs [1]. Nausea, vomiting and diarrhoea are well-recognized dose-related effects. Oral or vaginal candidiasis may occur as a result of overgrowth of commensals. Resumption of therapy does not necessarily lead to recurrence of the vaginitis [2].

Photosensitivity

All tetracyclines, but especially demethylchlortetracycline, may cause photosensitive eruptions [1,3—9] which clinically resemble exaggerated sunburn, sometimes with blistering. Phototoxicity is thought to be involved in that high serum levels predispose to its occurrence. Reactions to both UV-A and UV-B have been reported. High concentrations of tetracycline are found in sun-damaged skin [3]. Symptoms may persist for months [1]. Photo-onycholysis may develop in finger and (if exposed) toe nails; the thumb (normally less exposed) may be spared [10—13]. Tetracycline therapy is best avoided if there is a prospect of considerable sun exposure. Porphyria cutanea tarda-like changes may develop after chronic sun exposure [9,14]. A photosensitive lichenoid rash has been attributed to demethylchlortetracycline [15].

1 Wright AL, Colver GB. Tetracyclines — how safe are they? *Clin Exp Dermatol* 1988; **13**: 57—61.

2 Hall JH, Lupton ES. Tetracycline therapy for acne: incidence of vaginitis. *Cutis* 1977; **20**: 97—8.

3 Cullen SI, Catalano PM, Helfmann RS. Tetracycline sun sensitivity. *Arch Dermatol* 1966; **93**: 77.

4 Blank H, Cullen SI, Catalano PM. Photosensitivity studies with demethyl-chlortetracycline and doxycycline. *Arch Dermatol* 1968; **97**: 1−2.

5 Frost P, Weinstein GP, Gomez EC. Phototoxic potential of minocycline and doxycycline. *Arch Dermatol* 1972; **105**: 681−3.

6 Ramsay CA. Longwave ultraviolet radiation sensitivity induced by oxytetracycline: a case report. *Clin Exp Dermatol* 1977; **2**: 255−8.

7 Epstein E. High-dose tetracycline therapy. *Arch Dermatol* 1977; **113**: 236.

8 Kaidbey KH, Kligman AM. Identification of systemic phototoxic drugs by human intradermal assay. *J Invest Dermatol* 1978; **70**: 272−4.

9 Hawk JLM. Skin changes resembling hepatic cutaneous porphyria induced by oxytetracycline photosensitization *Clin Exp Dermatol* 1980; **5**: 321−5.

10 Frank SB, Cohen HJ, Minkin W. Photo-onycholysis due to tetracycline hydrochloride and doxycycline. *Arch Dermatol* 1971; **103**: 520−1.

11 Baker H. Photo-onycholysis caused by tetracyclines. *Br Med J* 1977; **ii**: 519−20.

12 Bethell HJN. Photo-onycholysis caused by demethylchlortetracycline. *Br Med J* 1977; **2**: 96.

13 Kestel JL Jr. Photo-onycholysis from minocycline. Side effects of minocycline therapy. *Cutis* 1981; **28**: 53−4.

14 Epstein JH, Tuffanelli DL, Seibert JS, Epstein WL. Porphyria-like cutaneous changes induced by tetracycline hydrochloride photosensitization. *Arch Dermatol* 1976; **112**: 661−6.

15 Jones HE, Lewis CW, Reisner JE. Photosensitive lichenoid eruption associated with demeclocycline. *Arch Dermatol* 1972; **106**: 58−63.

Pigmentation

Methacycline is a rare cause [1]. Long-term minocycline therapy for acne may result in pigmentation; while this is generally held to be a rare event, it may occur in about 3.7% of patients [2−7]. The average time for the development of pigmentary changes was 5 months, and onset of this complication did not seem to be related to cumulative dosage of the drug [6]. Facial hyperpigmentation has been reported in two sisters on long-term minocycline therapy, who were also being treated with Dianette (cyproterone acetate and ethinyloestradiol); it was suggested that pigmentation occurred either as a result of a genetic alteration in the metabolic handling of the drug, or due to accentuation by the concomitant therapy [7]. Other drugs including amitryptyline [3], phenothiazines, and 13-*cis*-retinoic acid have been implicated in the accentuation of minocycline-related hyperpigmentation.

Three types of pigmentation are described with minocycline and may occur in combination or isolation [6]. A focal type with well-demarcated blue−black macules is seen in areas of previous inflammation or scarring, especially in relation to acne scars. Minocycline has been associated with postinflammatory hyperpigmentation in women who have undergone sclerotherapy [8]. We have seen pigmentation related to minocycline therapy for pyoderma gangrenosum (Fig. 4.6). Macular or more diffuse hyperpigmentation may appear distant from acne sites, especially on the extensor surface of the lower legs, forearms and on sun-exposed areas. These two types resolve on cessation of therapy, with a mean

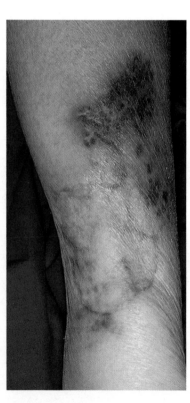

Figure 4.6 Pigmentation around a healed lesion of pyoderma gangrenosum in a patient treated with minocycline. (Courtesy of Dr M.M. Black, St John's Institute of Dermatology, London.)

time to resolution of 12 months [6]. A more persistent diffuse brown−grey change may develop, especially in sun-exposed areas. Pigmentation may also involve nails, bones, teeth, thyroid, aorta and endocardium [9,10]. Histological and electron microscopic studies have demonstrated increased melanin, haemosiderin and either minocycline or a metabolite in the skin [11−13]; pigment may be seen in dermal histiocytes and eccrine myoepithelial cells [12]. Minocycline is metabolized by humans to form a brown−black degradation product [14].

Conjunctival pigmentation may occur with tetracyclines [15,16] and scleral and nail pigmentation with minocycline [17]. Cutaneous osteomas presenting as blue skin nodules, which fluoresce yellow under ultraviolet light, may rarely develop in patients on treatment with tetracycline [18] or minocycline [19] for acne. Yellow discoloration of the nail is an occasional side-effect [20]. Black galactorrhoea occurred in a patient taking both minocycline and phenothiazines [21].

1 Möller H, Rausing A. Methacycline pigmentation: a five-year follow-up. *Acta Derm Venereol (Stockh)* 1980; **60**: 495−501.
2 Basler RSW. Minocycline-related hyperpigmentation. *Arch Dermatol* 1985; **121**: 606−8.
3 Basler RSW, Goetz CS. Synergism of minocycline and amitryptyline in cutaneous hyperpigmentation. *J Am Acad Dermatol* 1985; **12**: 577.
4 Basler RSW. Minocycline-related hyperpigmentation. *Arch Dermatol* 1985; **121**: 606−8.
5 Prigent F, Cavelier-Balloy B, Tollenaere C, Civatte J. Pigmentation cutanée induite par la minocycline: deux cas. *Ann Dermatol Vénéréol (Paris)* 1986; **113**: 227−33.
6 Layton AM, Cunliffe WJ. Minocycline induced pigmentation in the treatment of acne — a review and personal observations. *J Dermatol Treat* 1989; **1**: 9−12.
7 Eedy DJ, Burrows D. Minocycline-induced pigmentation occurring in two sisters. *Clin Exp Dermatol* 1991; **16**: 55−7.
8 Leffell DJ. Minocycline hydrochloride hyperpigmentation complicating treatment of venous ectasia of the extremities. *J Am Acad Dermatol* 1991; **24**: 501−2.
9 Wolfe ID, Reichmister J. Minocycline hyperpigmentation: skin, tooth, nail, and bone involvement. *Cutis* 1984; **33**: 475−8.
10 Butler JM, Marks R, Sutherland R. Cutaneous and cardiac valvular pigmentation with minocycline. *Clin Exp Dermatol* 1985; **10**: 432−7.
11 Sato S, Murphy GF, Bernard JD, *et al*. Ultrastructural and X-ray microanalytical observations on minocycline-related hyperpigmentation of the skin. *J Invest Dermatol* 1981; **77**: 264−71.
12 Argenyi ZB, Finelli L, Bergfeld WF, *et al*. Minocycline-related cutaneous hyperpigmentation as demonstrated by light microscopy, electron microscopy and X-ray energy spectroscopy. *J Cutan Pathol* 1987; **14**: 176−80.
13 Okada N, Moriya K, Nishida K, *et al*. Skin pigmentation associated with minocycline therapy. *Br J Dermatol* 1989; **121**: 247−54.
14 Nelis HJCF, DeLeenheer AP. Metabolism of minocycline in humans. *Drug Metab Dispos* 1982; **10**: 142−6.
15 Brothers DM, Hidayat AA. Conjunctival pigmentation associated with tetracycline medication. *Ophthalmol (Rochester)* 1981; **88**: 1212−15.
16 Messmer E, Font RL, Sheldon G, Murphy D. Pigmented conjunctival cysts following tetracycline/minocycline therapy. Histochemical and electron microscopic observations. *Ophthalmol (Rochester)* 1983; **90**: 1462−8.
17 Angeloni VL, Salasche SJ, Ortiz R. Nail, skin, and scleral pigmentation induced by minocycline. *Cutis* 1988; **42**: 229−33.

18 Walter JF, Macknet KD. Pigmentation of osteoma cutis caused by tetracycline. *Arch Dermatol* 1979; **115**: 1087–8.
19 Moritz DL, Elewski B. Pigmented postacne osteoma cutis in a patient treated with minocycline: Report and review of the literature. *J Am Acad Dermatol* 1991; **24**: 851–3.
20 Hendricks AA. Yellow lunulae with fluorescence after tetracycline therapy. *Arch Dermatol* 1980; **116**: 438–40.
21 Basler RSW, Lynch PJ. Black galactorrhea as a complication of minocycline and phenothiazine therapy. *Arch Dermatol* 1985; **121**: 417–18.

Other cutaneous side-effects

Allergic reactions are far less common than with penicillin. Morbilliform, urticarial, and erythema multiforme-like and bullous eruptions [1,2], exfoliative dermatitis, and erythema nodosum [3] have been reported, as well as a recurrent follicular acneiform eruption in a patient [4]. Gram-negative folliculitis of the face is uncommon but well recognized; *Proteus* may be responsible, and the condition responds to ampicillin [5]. Tetracyclines are a well-known cause of fixed drug eruptions (Fig. 4.7) [6–8], and minocycline [9] and doxycycline [10] have caused Stevens–Johnson syndrome. Toxic epidermal necrolysis has been recorded [11]. It has been suggested that tetracyclines may exacerbate psoriasis [12,13]. An eruption resembling Sweet's syndrome was reproduced on oral challenge with minocycline [14].

1 Shelley WB, Heaton CL. Minocycline sensitivity. *JAMA* 1973; **224**: 125–6.
2 Fawcett IW, Pepys J. Allergy to a tetracycline preparation — a case report. *Clin Allergy* 1976; **6**: 301–4.
3 Bridges AJ, Graziano FM, Calhoun W, Reizner GT. Hyperpigmentation, neutrophilic alveolitis, and erythema nodosum resulting from minocycline. *J Am Acad Dermatol* 1990; **22**: 959–62.

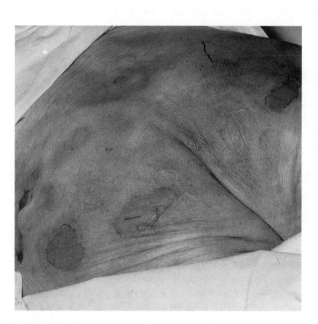

Figure 4.7 Multilocular fixed drug eruption on the buttocks, mimicking toxic epidermal necrolysis, due to doxycycline.

4 Bean SF. Acneiform eruption from tetracycline. *Br J Dermatol* 1971; **85**: 585—6.

5 Leyden JJ, Marples RR, Mills OH Jr, Kligman AM. Gram-negative folliculitis — a complication of antibiotic therapy in acne vulgaris. *Br J Dermatol* 1973; **88**: 533—8

6 Jolly HW, Sherman IJ Jr, Carpenter CL, *et al.* Fixed drug eruptions due to tetracyclines. *Arch Dermatol* 1978; **114**: 1484—5.

7 Fiumara NJ, Yaqub M. Pigmented penile lesions (fixed drug eruptions) associated with tetracycline therapy for sexually transmitted diseases. *Sex Transm Dis* 1980; **8**: 23—5.

8 Chan HL, Wong SN, Lo FL. Tetracycline-induced fixed drug eruptions; influence of dose and structure of tetracyclines. *J Am Acad Dermatol* 1985; **13**: 302—3.

9 Shoji A, Someda Y, Hamada T. Stevens—Johnson syndrome due to minocycline therapy. *Arch Dermatol* 1987; **123**: 18—20.

10 Curley RK, Verbov JL. Stevens—Johnson syndrome due to tetracyclines — a case report (doxycycline) and review of the literature. *Clin Exp Dermatol* 1987; **12**: 124—5.

11 Tatnall FM, Dodd HJ, Sarkany I. Elevated serum amylase in a case of toxic epidermal necrolysis. *Br J Dermatol* 1985; **113**: 629—30.

12 Tsankov M, Botev-Zlatkov M, Lazarova AZ, *et al.* Psoriasis and drugs: Influence of tetracyclines on the course of psoriasis. *J Am Acad Dermatol* 1988; **19**: 629—32.

13 Bergner T, Przybilla B. Psoriasis and tetracyclines. *J Am Acad Dermatol* 1990; **23**: 770.

14 Mensing H, Kowalzick L. Acute febrile neutrophilic dermatosis (Sweet's syndrome) caused by minocycline. *Dermatologica* 1991; **182**: 43—6.

Effects on the fetus and on teeth

There is little evidence that tetracycline is teratogenic [1]. There is an isolated case report of congenital abnormalities in a child whose mother took clomocycline for acne [2]. Yellow discoloration of the teeth due to tetracycline exposure during mineralization of the deciduous or permanent teeth is well known [3—6]. A yellow—brown fluorescent discoloration is formed as a result of a complex with calcium orthophosphate. Tetracyclines should not be given to pregnant women or children under the age of 12 years. Tetracyclines are excreted in breast milk, but chelation with calcium decreases their absorption, so that tooth discoloration is probably prevented [1]. Tetracycline may be deposited up to late adolescence, in calcifying teeth such as the molars, but since these are not normally visible this is not a problem [6]. Minocycline may rarely stain the teeth of adults [7—9].

1 Wright AL, Colver GB. Tetracyclines — how safe are they? *Clin Exp Dermatol* 1988; **13**: 57—61.

2 Corcoran R, Castles JM. Tetracycline for acne vulgaris and possible teratogenesis. *Br Med J* 1977; **ii**: 807—8.

3 Conchie JM, Munroe JD, Anderson DO. The incidence of staining of permanent teeth by the tetracyclines. *Can Med Assoc J* 1970; **103**: 351—6.

4 Grossman ER, Walchek A, Freedman H. Tetracyclines and permanent teeth: the relation between dose and tooth color. *Pediatrics* 1971; **47**: 567—70.

5 Moffitt JM, Cooley RO, Olsen NH, Hefferren JJ. Prediction of tetracycline-induced tooth discolouration. *J Am Dent Assoc* 1974; **88**: 547—52.

6 Grossman ER. Tetracycline and staining of the teeth. *JAMA* 1986; **225**: 2442.

7 Poliak SC, DiGiovanna JJ, Gross EG, *et al.* Minocycline-associated tooth discoloration in young adults. *JAMA* 1985; **254**: 2930—2.

8 Rosen T, Hoffmann TJ. Minocycline-induced discoloration of the permanent teeth. *J Am Acad Dermatol* 1989; **21**: 569.
9 Berger RS, Mandel EN, Hayes TJ, Grimwood RR. Minocycline staining of the oral cavity. *J Am Acad Dermatol* 1989; **21**: 1300−1.

Systemic side-effects

Long-term use of tetracycline for acne may rarely result in benign intracranial hypertension [1,2]. Since retinoids may potentiate this effect, it is safest not to use them in combination with tetracycline therapy for acne. Oesophageal ulceration has been described in a number of patients [3]. With the exception of doxycycline and minocycline, tetracyclines may exacerbate renal failure. Combination therapy with tetracyclines and nephrotoxic drugs such as gentamicin or diuretics should be avoided [4]. Deteriorated tetracyclines have caused a nephropathy accompanied by an exanthematic eruption. Patients should be warned not to use outdated or poorly stored tetracycline, since degraded tetracycline can cause a Fanconi-type syndrome comprising renal tubular acidosis, proteinuria [5,6] and lactic acidosis [7]. A severe, self-limiting eruption associated with acute hepatic failure, fatal in one instance, has been reported in two patients after a few weeks of routine therapy with minocycline for acne [8]. Pulmonary infiltration with eosinophilic or neutrophilic alveolitis has been rarely described in associated with tetracycline or minocycline therapy [9−11]. There have been isolated case reports linking tetracycline with systemic lupus erythematosus [12].

1 Walters BNJ, Gubbay SS. Tetracycline and benign intracranial hypertension: report of five cases. *Br Med J* 1979; **282**: 19−20.
2 Pearson MG, Littlewood SM, Bowden AN. Tetracycline and benign intracranial hypertension. *Br Med J* 1981; **282**: 568−9.
3 Channer KS, Hollanders D. Tetracycline-induced oesophageal ulceration. *Br Med J* 1981; **282**: 1359−60.
4 Wright AL, Colver GB. Tetracyclines − how safe are they? *Clin Exp Dermatol* 1988; **13**: 57−61.
5 Moser RH. Bibliographies on diseases: medical progress. Reactions to tetracyclines. *Clin Pharmacol Ther* 1966; **7**: 117−31.
6 Frimpter GW, Timpanelli AE, Eisenmenger WJ, *et al*. Reversible 'Fanconi syndrome' caused by degraded tetracycline. *JAMA* 1963; **184**: 111−13.
7 Montoliu J, Carrera M, Darnell A, *et al*. Lactic acidosis and Fanconi's syndrome due to degraded tetracycline. *Br Med J* 1981; **281**: 1576−7.
8 Davies MG, Kersey PJW. Acute hepatitis and exfoliative dermatitis associated with minocycline. *Br Med J* 1989; **298**: 1523−4.
9 Ho D, Tashkin DP, Bein ME, Sharma O. Pulmonary infiltrates and eosinophilia associated with tetracycline. *Chest* 1979; **76**: 33−5.
10 Otero M, Goodpasture HG. Pulmonary infiltrates and eosinophilia from minocycline. *Br J Dermatol* 1983; **250**: 2602.
11 Yokoyama A, Mizushima Y, Suzuki H, *et al*. Acute eosinophilic pneumonia induced by minocycline: prominent Kerley B lines as a feature of positive re-challenge test. *Jpn J Med* 1990; **29**: 195−8.
12 Domz CA, Minamara DH, Hozapfel HF. Tetracycline provocation in lupus erythematosus. *Ann Intern Med* 1959; **50**: 1217.

Absorption of tetracyclines is reduced when taken with meals, especially those containing calcium or iron, such as milk, or drugs such as iron or antacids [1]. The decrease in serum levels following a test meal has been reported as follows: oxytetracycline 50% [1], minocycline 13% [1], and doxycycline 20% [2]. Oxytetracycline may have a hypoglycaemic effect on insulin-dependent diabetics [3], and tetracyclines can potentiate the action of warfarin by depressing prothrombin activity, and elevate serum levels of lithium given simultaneously [4].

1 Leyden JJ. Absorption of minocycline HCl and tetracycline hydrochloride. Effect of food, milk and iron. *J Am Acad Dermatol* 1985; **12**: 308–12.
2 Welling PG, Koch PA, Lau CC, Craig WA. Bioavailability of tetracycline and doxycycline in fasted and nonfasted subjects. *Antimicrob Agents Chemother* 1977; **11**: 462–9.
3 Miller JB. Hypoglycaemic effect of oxytetracycline. *Br Med J* 1966; **2**: 1007.
4 McGennis AJ. Lithium carbonate and tetracycline interaction. *Br Med J* 1978; i: 1183.

Tetracyclines and the contraceptive pill

Tetracyclines have been reported to interfere with the action of the contraceptive pill [1,2]. It is standard practice to inform female patients of this and to suggest an additional or alternative method of contraception while on medication. However, there is controversy as to whether there really is a significant risk of interaction [3–5].

1 Bacon JF, Shenfield GM. Pregnancy attributable to interaction between tetracycline and oral contraceptives. *Br Med J* 1980; **280**: 293.
2 Hughes BR, Cunliffe WJ. Interactions between the oral contraceptive pill and antibiotics. *Br J Dermatol* 1990; **122**: 717–18.
3 Fleischer AB Jr, Resnick SD. The effect of antibiotics on the efficacy of oral contraceptives. *Arch Dermatol* 1989; **125**: 1562–4.
4 Orme ML'E, Back DJ. Interactions between oral contraceptive steroids and broad-spectrum antibiotics. *Clin Exp Dermatol* 1986; **11**: 327–31.
5 De Groot AC, Eshuis H, Stricker BHC. Oral contraceptives and antibiotics in acne. *Br J Dermatol* 1991; **124**: 212.

4.3 Sulphonamides

Reactions occur in 1–5% of those exposed, and slow acetylators are at greater risk [1–6]. Reactions are commoner in patients with AIDS [7]. Type I reactions (urticaria and anaphylaxis) are rare but recorded. Phototoxic and photo-allergic eruptions (Fig. 4.8) occur [8,9]. Morbilliform and rubelliform rashes are seen, and erythema multiforme, Stevens–Johnson syndrome and toxic epidermal necrolysis [10–14], erythema nodosum [1], generalized exfoliative dermatitis [1,15,16] and fixed eruptions [17] are all well known. In addition, a lupus-like syndrome and allergic vasculitis [18] are documented. Agranulocytosis or haemolytic anaemia is occasionally precipitated.

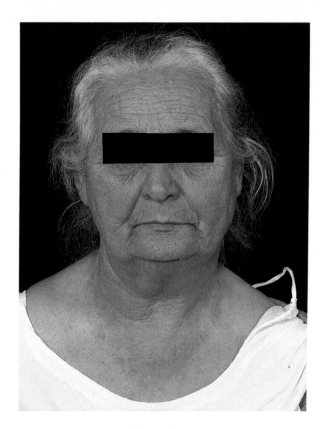

Figure 4.8 Photo-allergic eruption due to trimethoprim–sulphamethoxazole.

1 Koch-Weser J, Sidel VW, Dexter M, *et al*. Adverse reactions to sulfisoxazole, sulfamethoxazole, and nitrofurantoin. Manifestations and specific reaction rates during 2,118 courses of therapy. *Arch Intern Med* 1971; **128**: 399–404.

2 Sehgal UN, Rege VL, Kharangate UN. Fixed drug eruptions caused by medications: a report from India. *Int J Dermatol* 1978; **17**: 78–81.

3 Kauppinen K, Stubb S. Drug eruptions: Causative agents and clinical types. A series of inpatients during a 10-year period. *Acta Derm Venereol (Stockh)* 1984; **64**: 320–4.

4 Bigby M, Jick S, Jick H, Arndt K. Drug-induced cutaneous reactions. A report from Boston Collaborative Drug Surveillance Program on 15 438 consecutive inpatients, 1975 to 1982. *JAMA* 1986; **256**: 3358–63.

5 Anon. Hypersensitivity to sulphonamides — A clue? (Editorial). *Lancet* 1986; **ii**: 958–9.

6 Rieder MJ, Uetrecht J, Shear NH, *et al*. Diagnosis of sulfonamide hypersensitivity reactions by *in-vitro* 'rechallenge' with hydroxylamine metabolites. *Ann Intern Med* 1989; **110**: 286–9.

7 De Raeve L, Song M, Van Maldergem L. Adverse cutaneous drug reactions in AIDS. *Br J Dermatol* 1988; **119**: 521–3.

8 Epstein JH. Photoallergy. A review. *Arch Dermatol* 1972; **106**: 741–8.

9 Hawk JLM. Photosensitizing agents used in the United Kingdom. *Clin Exp Dermatol* 1984; **9**: 300–2.

10 Kauppinen K. Cutaneous reactions to drugs. With special reference to severe mucocutaneous bullous eruptions and sulphonamides. *Acta Derm Venereol (Stockh)* 1972; **52** (Suppl 68): 1–89.

11 Carrol OM, Bryan PA, Robinson RJ. Stevens–Johnson-syndrome associated with long-acting sulfonamides. *JAMA* 1966; **195**: 691–3.

12 Aberer W, Stingl G, Wolff K. Stevens–Johnson-Syndrom und toxische epidermale Nekrolyse nach Sulfonamideinahme. *Hautarzt* 1982; **33**: 484–90.

13 Chan H-L, Stern RS, Arndt KA, *et al*. The incidence of erythema multiforme,

Stevens–Johnson syndrome, and toxic epidermal necrolysis. A population-based study with particular reference to reactions caused by drugs among outpatients. *Arch Dermatol* 1990; **126**: 43–7.

14 Schöpf E, Stühmer A, Rzany B, *et al.* Toxic epidermal necrolysis and Stevens–Johnson syndrome. An epidemiologic study from West Germany. *Arch Dermatol* 1991; **127**: 839–42.
15 Nicolis GD, Helwig EB. Exfoliative dermatitis. A clinicopathologic study of 135 cases. *Arch Dermatol* 1973; **108**: 788–97.
16 Sehgal VN, Srivastava G. Exfoliative dermatitis. A prospective study of 80 patients. *Dermatologica* 1986; **173**: 278–84.
17 Sehgal VN, Gangwani OP. Fixed drug eruption. Current concepts. *Int J Dermatol* 1987; **26**: 67–74.
18 Lehr D. Sulfonamide vasculitis. *J Clin Pharmacol* 1972; **2**: 181–9.

Sulphasalazine

Rashes occur in 1–5% of patients, but desensitization is possible [1]. Of 23 patients treated with sulphasalazine for psoriasis four developed a cutaneous eruption, the nature of which was not specified [2]. Photosensitivity [3] and a fixed eruption [4] have been documented. Toxic epidermal necrolysis, erythroid hypoplasia and agranulocytosis have been reported [5]. Bronchiolitis obliterans and alveolitis are well-recognized complications, and acute hypersensitivity pneumonia is recorded. Lupus erythematosus, including cerebral lupus, may be induced [6]. Reversible oligospermia may occur [7], and reversible hair loss has been attributed to use of this drug in enemata [8]. Many of the above adverse effects are attributable to the carrier molecule, sulphapyridine, which delivers 5-aminosalicylic acid, the component of sulphasalazine active in ulcerative colitis, to its site of action in the colon; patients who are slow acetylators may be especially prone to side-effects [9]. Urticaria, and possibly the renal toxicity, are due to the 5-amino salicylic acid component [10].

Mesalazine (5-aminosalicylic acid)

Fever, erythematous skin eruption and lung involvement, with bilateral interstitial opacities on chest X-ray and restricted pulmonary carbon dioxide diffusion, was reported in a patient with a previous history of a skin eruption following sulphasalazine [11]. This drug may cause renal damage, and has been associated in a case report with fatal bone marrow suppression and thrombocytopenia [12].

Olsalazine

This drug, which consists of a dimer of two molecules of 5-aminosalicylic acid linked by an azo bond, dispenses with the unwanted effects of sulphapyridine. None the less, up to one in five patients experience diarrhoea, rash, nausea and abdominal pain severe enough to stop the drug [10].

Sulphamethoxypyridazine

Obliterative bronchiolitis and alveolitis have been documented in a patient with linear IgA disease of adults [13].

1 Holdsworth CD. Sulphasalazine desensitisation. *Br Med J* 1981; **282**: 110.
2 Gupta AK, Ellis CN, Siegel MT, *et al*. Sulfasalazine improves psoriasis. A double-blind analysis. *Arch Dermatol* 1990; **126**: 487−93.
3 Watkinson G. Sulfasalazine: a review of 40 years' experience. *Drugs* 1986; **32**: 1−11.
4 Kanwar AJ, Singh M, Yunus M, Belhaj MS. Fixed eruption to sulphasalazine. *Dermatologica* 1987; **174**: 104.
5 Maddocks JL, Slater DN. Toxic epidermal necrolysis, agranulocytosis and erythroid hypoplasia associated with sulphasalazine. *J R Soc Med* 1980; **73**: 587−8.
6 Rafferty P, Young AC, Haeny MR. Sulphasalazine-induced cerebral lupus erythematosus. *Postgrad Med J* 1982; **58**: 98−9.
7 Drife JO. Drugs and sperm. *Br Med J* 1982; **84**: 844−5.
8 Kutty PK, Raman KRK, Hawken K, Barrowman JA. Hair loss and 5-aminosalicylic acid enemas. *Ann Intern Med* 1982; **97**: 785−6.
9 Das KM, Eastwood MA, McManus JPA, Sircus W. Adverse reactions during salicylazosulfapyridine therapy and the relation with drug metabolism and acetylator phenotype. *N Engl J Med* 1973; **289**: 491−5.
10 Olsalazine − a further choice in ulcerative colitis. *Drug Ther Bull* 1990; **28**: 57−8.
11 Le Gros V, Saveuse H, Lesur G, Brion N. Lung and skin hypersensitivity to 5-aminosalicylic acid. *Br Med J* 1991; **302**: 970.
12 Daneshmend TK. Mesalazine-associated thrombocytopenia. *Lancet* 1991; **337**: 1297−8.
13 Godfrey KM, Wojnarowska F, Friedland JS. Obliterative bronchiolitis and alveolitis associated with sulphamethoxypyridazine (Lederkyn) therapy for linear IgA disease of adults. *Br J Dermatol* 1990; **123**: 125−31.

Sulphadoxine

This sulphonamide is used in malaria prophylaxis in combination with pyrimethamine. The risk of reactions seems to be very low, but drug fever, toxic epidermal necrolysis and photodermatitis have been recorded [1]. Stevens−Johnson syndrome may occur with Fansidar (pyrimethamine and sulphadoxine) for malaria prophylaxis [1−4] or with sulphadoxine alone [5]. Toxic epidermal necrolysis has occurred with Fansidar in an AIDS patient [6].

1 Koch-Weser J, Hodel C, Leimer R, Styk S. Adverse reactions to pyrimethamine/sulfadoxine. *Lancet* 1982; **ii**: 1459.
2 Hornstein OP, Ruprecht KW. Fansidar-induced Stevens−Johnson syndrome. *N Engl J Med* 1982; **307**: 1529−30.
3 Miller KD, Lobel HO, Satriale RF, *et al*. Severe cutaneous reactions among American travelers using pyrimethamine−sulfadoxine (Fansidar) for malaria prophylaxis. *Am J Trop Med Hyg* 1986; **35**: 451−8.
4 Ortel B, Sivayathorn A, Hönigsmann H. An unusual combination of phototoxicity and Stevens−Johnson syndrome due to antimalarial therapy. *Dermatologica* 1989; **178**: 39−42.
5 Hernborg A. Stevens−Johnson syndrome after mass prophylaxis with sulfadoxine for cholera in Mozambique. *Lancet* 1985; **i**: 1072−3.
6 Raviglione MC, Dinan WA, Pablos-Mendez A, *et al*. Fatal toxic epidermal necrolysis during prophylaxis with pyrimethamine and sulfadoxine in a

human immunodeficiency virus-infected person. *Arch Intern Med* 1988; **148**: 2863−5.

Trimethoprim−sulphamethoxazole (co-trimoxazole)

The general incidence and patterns of reactions to this mixture of sulphamethoxazole and trimethoprim are about the same as for sulphonamides in general; cutaneous reactions are seen in 3.3% of patients [1−4]. Severe cutaneous reactions of all types occur in about 1 per 100000 users of the drug [3,4]. There is a greatly increased incidence of reactions in patients with AIDS [5−12]. In the case shown in Figs 4.9 and 4.10, the drug was deemed to be essential and was continued despite occurrence of the eruption; the latter initially worsened but then resolved spontaneously. Fixed eruptions occur [13−16], and may be due to the sulphonamide or trimethoprim components; a widespread fixed eruption mimicking toxic epidermal necrolysis has been documented in one case [17]. Pustular reactions have been documented [18]. Severe reactions have included erythema multiforme or Stevens−Johnson syndrome [19,20] which has been fatal [20], TEN in AIDS patients [10], cutaneous vasculitis [21], and fatal agranulocytosis [22].

Trimethoprim

Used alone, this substance causes less reaction than sulphonamides; fixed eruption has been proven [23,24].

1 Lawson DH, Jick H. Adverse reactions to co-trimoxazole in hospitalized patients. *Am J Med Sci* 1976; **275**: 53−7.

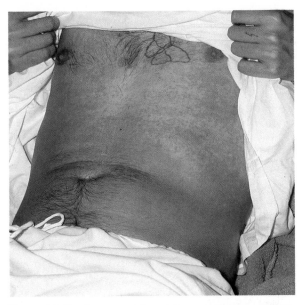

Figure 4.9 Confluent maculopapular eruption in an AIDS patient treated with trimethoprim−sulphamethoxazole.

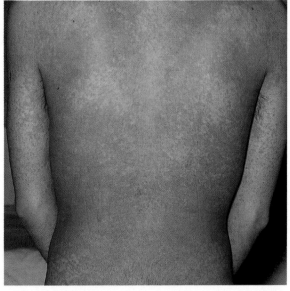

Figure 4.10 Extensive maculopapular eruption in an AIDS patient treated with trimethoprim−sulphamethoxazole.

2 Jick J. Adverse reactions to trimethoprim−sulphamethoxazole in hospitalized patients. *Rev Infect Dis* 1982; **4**: 426−8.

3 Lawson DH, Paice BJ. Adverse reactions to trimethoprim−sulfamethoxasole. *Rev Infect Dis* 1982; **4**: 429−33.

4 Huisman MV, Buller HR, TenCate JW. Co-trimoxasole toxicity. *Lancet* 1984; **ii**: 1152.

5 Jaffe HS, Amman J, Abrams DI, *et al.* Complication of cotrimoxazole in treatment of AIDS associated *Pneumocystis carinii* pneumonia in homosexual men. *Lancet* 1983; **ii**: 1109−11.

6 Mitsuyasu R, Groopman J, Volberding P. Cutaneous reaction to trimethoprim−sulfamethoxazole in patients with AIDS and Kaposi's sarcoma. *N Engl J Med* 1983; **308**: 1535−6.

7 Gordin FM, Simon GL, Wofsy CB, *et al.* Adverse reactions to trimethoprim sulfamethoxazole in patients with the acquired immune deficiency syndrome. *Ann Intern Med* 1984; **100**: 495−9.

8 Cohn DL, Penley KA, Judson FN, *et al.* The acquired immunodeficiency syndrome and a trimethoprim−sulfamethoxazole-adverse reaction. *Ann Intern Med* 1984; **100**: 311.

9 Kovacs JA, Hiemenz JW, Macher AM, *et al. Pneumocystis carinii* pneumonia: a comparison between patients with the acquired immunodeficiency syndrome and patients with other immunodeficiencies. *Ann Intern Med* 1984; **100**: 663−71.

10 De Raeve L, Song M, Van Maldergem L. Adverse cutaneous drug reactions in AIDS. *Br J Dermatol* 1988; **119**: 521−3.

11 Arnold P, Guglielmo J, Hollander H. Severe hypersensitivity reaction upon rechallenge with trimethoprim−sulfamethoxazole in a patient with AIDS. *Drug Intell Clin Pharm* 1988; **22**: 43−4.

12 Coopman SA, Stern RS. Cutaneous drug reactions in human immuno-deficiency virus infection. *Arch Dermatol* 1991; **127**: 714−17.

13 Talbot MD. Fixed genital drug reaction. *Practitioner* 1980; **224**: 823−4.

14 Varsano I, Amir Y. Fixed drug eruption due to cotrimoxasole. *Dermatologica* 1989; **178**: 232.

15 Van Voorhees A, Stenn KS. Histological phases of bactrim-induced fixed drug eruption. The report of one case. *Am J Dermatopathol* 1987; **9**: 528−32.

16 Bharija SC, Belhaj MS. Fixed drug eruption due to cotrimoxazole. *Australas J Dermatol* 1989; **30**: 43−4.

17 Baird BJ, De Villez RL. Widespread bullous fixed drug eruption mimicking toxic epidermal necrolysis. *Int J Dermatol* 1988; **27**: 170−4.

18 MacDonald KJS, Green CM, Kenicer KJA. Pustular dermatosis induced by co-trimoxazole. *Br Med J* 1986; **293**: 1279−80.

19 Azinge NO, Garrick GA. Stevens−Johnson syndrome (erythema multiforme) following ingestion of trimethoprim−sulfamethoxazole on two separate occasions in the same person. A case report. *J Allergy Clin Immunol* 1978; **62**: 125−6.

20 Beck MH, Portnoy B. Severe erythema multiforme complicated by fatal gastrointestinal involvement following co-trimoxasole therapy. *Clin Exp Dermatol* 1979; **4**: 201−4.

21 Wåhlin A, Rosman N. Skin manifestations with vasculitis due to co-trimoxazole. *Lancet* 1976; **ii**: 1415.

22 Lawson DH, Henry DA, Jick H. Fatal agranulocytosis attributed to co-trimoxazole therapy. *Br Med J* 1976; **ii**: 316.

23 Kanwar AJ, Bharija SC, Singh M, Belhaj MS. Fixed drug eruption to trimethoprim. *Dermatologica* 1986; **172**: 230−1.

24 Hughes BR, Holt PJA, Marks R. Trimethoprim associated fixed drug eruption. *Br J Dermatol* 1987; **116**: 241−2.

4.4 Aminoglycosides

Gentamicin, tobramycin, streptomycin and kanamycin cross-react and are all potentially ototoxic and nephrotoxic. Exanthematic eruptions are common with streptomycin, developing in 5% or more of patients. Continued treatment may lead to generalized exfoliative dermatitis with these drugs [1] in a minority, but in a proportion of patients the rash subsides and treatment can be continued. Fever and eosinophilia may be associated with the reactions. Urticaria, maculopapular rashes, drug fever and eosinophilia are well recognized with this group of drugs. Skin necrosis following subcutaneous injection of aminoglycoside antibiotics (gentamicin, sisomycin, and netilmicin) has been reported in elderly females with a history of thrombosis being treated with heparin anticoagulant therapy [2−4]. The reaction has also occurred following intramuscular sisomycin in a patient with defective fibrinolysis and abnormal neutrophil function [5]. A toxic erythema with generalized follicular pustulosis has been documented with streptomycin [6].

1 Karp S, Bakris G, Cooney A, *et al*. Exfoliative dermatitis secondary to tobramycin sulfate. *Cutis* 1991; **47**: 331−2.
2 Taillandier J, Manigaud G, Fixy P, Dumont D. Nécroses cutanées induites par la gentamicine sous-cutanée. *Presse Méd* 1984; **13**: 1574−5.
3 Duterque M, Hubert Asso AM, Corrard A. Lésions nécrotiques par injections sous cutanées de gentamicine et de sisomicine. *Ann Dermatol Vénéréol (Paris)* 1985; **112**: 707−8.
4 Bernard P, Paris M, Cantanzano G, Bonnetblanc JM. Vascularite cutanée localisée induite par la Nétilmicine. *Presse Méd* 1987; **16**: 915−16.
5 Grob JJ, Mege JL, Follano J, *et al*. Skin necrosis after injection of aminosides. Arthus reaction, local toxicity, thrombotic process or pathergy? *Dermatologica* 1990; **181**: 258−62.
6 Kushimoto H, Aoki T. Toxic erythema with generalized follicular pustules caused by streptomycin. *Arch Dermatol* 1981; **117**: 444−5.

4.5 Miscellaneous antibiotics

Chloramphenicol

Although contact dermatitis from topical application is common, hypersensitivity skin reactions to oral therapy are rare. Macular, papular and urticarial eruptions are reported [1]. Pruritus may be prominent. Erythema multiforme and epidermal necrolysis [2] occur rarely. There is a risk of aplastic anaemia [3] and death has exceptionally followed the use of eye drops [4].

1 Unsdek HE, Curtiss WP, Neill EJ. Skin eruption due to chloramphenicol (Chloromycetin®). *Arch Dermatol Syphil* 1951; **64**: 217.
2 Mathé P, Aubert L, Labouche F, *et al*. Syndrome de Lyell. Etiologie médicamenteuse: rôle probable de chloramphénicol. *J Méd Bordeaux* 1965; **42**: 1367−76.
3 Hargraves MM, Mills SD, Heck FJ. Aplastic anemia associated with the administration of chloramphenicol. *JAMA* 1952; **149**: 1293−300.
4 Fraunfelder FT, Bagby GC. Ocular chloramphenicol and aplastic anemia. *N Engl J Med* 1983; **308**: 1536.

Clindamycin and lincomycin

These antibiotics have become particularly associated with a potentially lethal pseudomembranous colitis due to superinfection with *Clostridium difficile* [1–3]. Vancomycin or metronidazole are the treatments of choice for this complication. Hypersensitivity skin reactions are rare with lincomycin but common with clindamycin, occurring in up to 10% of patients. Erythema multiforme and anaphylaxis are very rare [4].

1 Dantzig PI. The safety of long-term clindamycin therapy for acne. *Arch Dermatol* 1976; **112**: 53–4.
2 Tan SG, Cunliffe WJ. The unwanted effects of clindamycin in acne. *Br J Dermatol* 1976; **94**: 313–15.
3 Leading Article. Antibiotic-associated colitis: a progress report. *Br Med J* 1978; i: 669–71.
4 Lochmann O, Kohout P, Vymola F. Anaphylactic shock following the administration of clindamycin. *J Hyg Epiderm Microbiol Immunol* 1977; **21**: 441–7.

Erythromycin

This is one of the most innocuous antibiotics in current use. Cholestasis caused by the estolate ester is the only potentially serious side-effect. Hypersensitivity skin reactions are rare but when they occur skin tests may be positive [1].

1 Van Ketel WG. Immediate and delayed-type allergy to erythromycin. *Contact Dermatitis* 1976; **2**: 363–4.

Fusidic acid

Topical use can lead to contact dermatitis but hypersensitivity reactions to oral or parenteral use are very rare; jaundice has accompanied intravenous use.

Spiramycin

Rashes, usually transient erythema, may occur in up to 1% of cases with use of this macrolide drug. Spiramycin, given for toxoplasmosis in pregnancy, was associated in one case with an erythematous maculopapular pruritic eruption with eosinophilia and raised γ-glutamyl transpeptidase [1]. The drug has caused an allergic vasculitis [2].

1 Ostlere LS, Langtry JAA, Staughton RCD. Allergy to spiramycin during prophylactic treatment of fetal toxoplasmosis. *Br Med J* 1991; **302**: 970.
2 Galland MC, Rodor F, Jouglard J. Spiramycin allergic vasculitis: first report. *Therapie* 1987; **42**: 227–9.

Vancomycin

Allergic skin reactions are not uncommon, occurring in up to 5% of patients. Rapid intravenous infusion of vancomycin can cause a histamine-induced anaphylactoid reaction characterized by flushing, a maculopapular eruption of the neck, face, trunk and extremities, the so-called 'red man syndrome', prolonged hypotension, and in rare cases cardiac arrest [1]. Desensitization has been successfully achieved in a patient with this complication [2]. Vancomycin has been reported to have induced a transient linear IgA bullous dermatosis which recurred on rechallenge [3].

1 Pau AK, Khakoo R. Red-neck syndrome with slow infusion of vancomycin. *N Engl J Med* 1985; **313**: 756−7.
2 Lin RY. Desensitization in the management of vancomycin hypersensitivity. *Arch Intern Med* 1990; **150**: 2197−8.
3 Baden LA, Apovian C, Imber MJ, Dover JS. Vancomycin-induced linear IgA bullous dermatosis. *Arch Dermatol* 1988; **124**: 1186−8.

4.6 Antituberculous drugs

The following drugs are reported to cause contact dermatitis: isoniazid, rifampicin, ethambutol, *p*-aminosalicylic acid, streptomycin, and kanamycin [1]. The incidence of other reactions to individual drugs is difficult to assess because several drugs are usually used in combination.

Ethambutol

Hypersensitivity reactions are very rare. Side-effects are largely confined to visual disturbances, with loss of acuity, colour blindness, and restricted visual fields; these are usually reversible if the drug is stopped promptly. Patients should have ophthalmic assessments prior to and during therapy.

Ethionamide

Eczema, chiefly affecting the forehead, acneiform eruptions, butterfly eruptions on the face, stomatitis, alopecia and purpura have been reported.

Isoniazid

Allergic skin reactions occur in less than 1% of patients. An acneiform eruption, usually occurring in slow inactivators of the drug, is well recognized [2,3]. Urticaria, purpura, and a lupus erythematosus-like syndrome [4,5] have been reported. Rarely, a pellagra-like syndrome has been induced in malnourished patients, due to metabolic antagonism of nicotinic acid with resultant pyridoxine deficiency [2,6]. Exfoliative dermatitis has been reported [7].

Rifampicin

Cutaneous hypersensitivity reactions are very uncommon. There have been isolated reports of bullous erythema multiforme, TEN [8] and pemphigus [9,10]; existing pemphigus may also be exacerbated [11]. Altered liver function, usually transient, and thrombocytopenic purpura may occur. Rifampicin has precipitated porphyria cutanea tarda [12]. It induces liver enzymes and may thus reduce the effectiveness of a number of drugs including oral contraceptives.

Streptomycin

See aminoglycosides above.

Thiacetazone

Severe cutaneous hypersensitivity reactions have been reported, including maculopapular rashes which progress to mucosal involvement with constitutional symptoms, and Stevens—Johnson syndrome [13]. Skin rashes occur in 4−17% of cases [14]. Cutaneous hypersensitivity reactions have been reported in 20% of HIV-seropositive patients, compared with 1% of HIV-seronegative patients who receive the drug as part treatment for tuberculosis; 3 of 93 HIV-positive patients died as a result of toxic epidermal necrolysis [14]. Figurate erythematous eruptions resembling erythema annulare centrifugum may occur [15].

1 Holdiness MR. Contact dermatitis to antituberculous drugs. *Contact Dermatitis* 1986; **15**: 282−8.
2 Cohen LK, George W, Smith R. Isoniazid-induced acne and pellagra. Occurrence in slow acetylators of isoniazid. *Arch Dermatol* 1974; **109**: 377−81.
3 Oliwiecki S, Burton JL. Severe acne due to isoniazid. *Clin Exp Dermatol* 1988; **13**: 283−4.
4 Grunwald M, David M, Feuerman EJ. Appearance of lupus erythematosus in a patient with lichen planus treated by isoniazide. *Dermatologica* 1982; **165**: 172−7.
5 Sim E, Gill EW, Sim RB. Drugs that induce systemic lupus erythematosus inhibit complement C4. *Lancet* 1984; **ii**: 422−4.
6 Schmutz JL, Cuny JF, Trechot P, *et al*. Les érythemes pellagroïdes médicamenteux. Une observations d'érythème pellagroïde secondaire a l'isoniazide. *Ann Dermatol Vénéréol (Paris)* 1987; **114**: 569−76.
7 Rosin MA, King LE Jr. Isoniazid-induced exfoliative dermatitis. *South Med J* 1982; **75**: 81.
8 Okano M, Kitano Y, Igarashi T. Toxic epidermal necrolysis due to rifampicin. *J Am Acad Dermatol* 1987; **17**: 303−4.
9 Gange RW, Rhodes EL, Edwards CO, Powell MEA. Pemphigus induced by rifampicin. *Br J Dermatol* 1976; **95**: 445−8.
10 Lee CW, Lim JH, Kang HJ. Pemphigus foliaceus induced by rifampicin. *Br J Dermatol* 1984; **111**: 619−22.
11 Miyagawa S, Yamanashi Y, Okuchi T, *et al*. Exacerbation of pemphigus by rifampicin. *Br J Dermatol* 1986; **114**: 729−32.
12 Millar JW. Rifampicin-induced porphyria cutanea tarda. *Br J Dis Chest* 1980; **74**: 405−8.
13 Fegan D, Glennon J. Cutaneous sensitivity to thiacetazone. *Lancet* 1991; **337**: 1036.
14 Nunn P, Kibuga D, Gathua S, *et al*. Cutaneous hypersensitivity reactions due to thiacetazone in HIV-1 seropositive patients treated for tuberculosis. *Lancet* 1991; **337**: 627−30.
15 Ramesh V. Eruption resembling erythema annulare centrifugum. *Australas J Dermatol* 1987; **28**: 44.

4.7 Antileprosy drugs

Clofazimine

This drug regularly causes a reversible, dose-dependent brown–orange pigmentation of the skin (Fig. 4.11) [1–3]. Biopsy specimens from two lepromatous leprosy patients on long-term clofazimine therapy revealed ceroid-lipofuscin pigment as well as clofazimine inside macrophage phagolysosomes [3]. Reddish-blue pigmentation occurred in scarred areas of lupus erythematosus in one patient [4]. Xeroderma, pruritus, phototoxicity, acne and non-specific rashes are described [2]. Gastrointestinal symptoms may occur early due to direct irritation of the gut and are quickly reversible; ulcerative enteritis may occur after 9–14 months of treatment. After high-dose prolonged therapy, persistent diarrhoea, abdominal pain and weight loss, associated with deposition of crystalline clofazimine in the small intestinal submucosa and mesenteric lymph nodes, may occur [5,6]. Splenic infarction has been associated with this syndrome [7,8].

1 Thomsen K, Rothenborg HW. Clofazimine in the treatment of pyoderma gangrenosum. *Arch Dermatol* 1979; **115**: 851–2.
2 Yawalker SJ, Vischer W. Lamprene (clofazimine) in leprosy. Basic information. *Lepr Rev* 1979; **50**: 135–44.
3 Job CK, Yoder L, Jacobson RR, Hastings RC. Skin pigmentation from clofazimine therapy in leprosy patients: A reappraisal. *J Am Acad Dermatol* 1990; **23**: 236–41.
4 Kossard S, Doherty E, McColl I, Ryman W. Autofluorescence of clofazimine in discoid lupus erythematosus. *J Am Acad Dermatol* 1987; **17**: 867–71.
5 Harvey RF, Harman RRM, Black C, *et al*. Abdominal pain and malabsorption due to tissue deposition of clofazimine (Lamprene) crystals. *Br J Dermatol* 1977; **97** (Suppl. 15): 19.

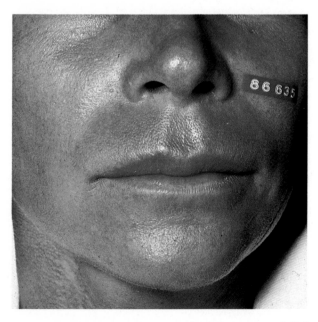

Figure 4.11 Reddish-brown pigmentation due to clofazamine.

6 Venencie PY, Cortez A, Orieux G, *et al.* Clofazimine enteropathy. *J Am Acad Dermatol* 1986; **15**: 290–1.
7 Jopling WAH. Complications of treatment with clofazimine (Lamprene: B.663). *Lepr Rev* 1976; **47**: 1–3.
8 McDougall AC, Horsfall WR, Hede JE, Chaplin AJ. Splenic infarction and tissue accumulation of crystals associated with the use of clofazimine (Lamprene: B.663) in the treatment of pyoderma gangrenosum. *Br J Dermatol* 1980; **102**: 227–30.

Dapsone

Fixed eruptions occur in 3% of West Africans being treated for leprosy [1,2]. Erythema multiforme [1] and exfoliative dermatitis [2] have also been described during leprosy treatment. Another uncommon side-effect is a hypersensitivity reaction within the first month with fever, exfoliative dermatitis, hepatitis, lymphadenopathy and anaemia [3]. A fatal infectious mononucleosis-like syndrome developed in a Burmese boy during induction of treatment for lepromatous leprosy [4].

Haematological side-effects

Red cell life is always shortened, but clinical haemolytic anaemia is uncommon; patients with low red cell glucose-6-phosphate dehydrogenase levels [5], and slow acetylators [6] are at a special risk of developing this complication. Methaemoglobinaemia and Heinz-body formation are seen. Agranulocytosis is rare but well recognized and may occur in the first weeks of therapy [7,8]. For patients receiving the drug for dermatitis herpetiformis, this side-effect occurred at a median dosage of 100 mg daily and a median duration of therapy of 7 weeks [8]. The total risk was one case per 3000 patient years of exposure to the drug; however, agranulocytosis was estimated to occur in 1 in 240 to 1 in 425 new patients receiving dapsone for dermatitis herpetiformis [8]. Agranulocytosis occurred in approximately 1 in 10 000–20 000 US soldiers receiving dapsone for malarial prophylaxis [9]. Elderly patients do not tolerate dapsone well, and sulphapyridine or sulphamethoxypridazine (the latter obtainable on a named patient basis from Lederle Laboratories) is to be preferred for IgA-related diseases.

Other side-effects

Severe but usually reversible hypoalbuminaemia due to failure of albumin production [10,11] or of an atypical nephrotic syndrome, may occur. Rarely, dapsone causes a peripheral neuropathy [12] and optic atrophy [13]; permanent retinal damage has followed overdosage [14]. Occasionally a psychosis may be precipitated [15].

1 Dutta RK. Erythema multiforme bullosum due to dapsone. *Lepr India* 1980; **52**: 306–9.
2 Browne SG. Antileprosy drugs. *Br Med J* 1971; **iv**: 558–9.

3 Tomecki KJ, Catalano CJ. Dapsone hypersensitivity: The sulfone syndrome revisited. *Arch Dermatol* 1981; **117**: 38–9.

4 Frey HM, Gershon AA, Borkowsky W, Bullock WE. Fatal reaction to dapsone during treatment of leprosy. *Ann Intern Med* 1981; **94**: 777–9.

5 Beutler E. Glucose-6-Phosphate dehydrogenase deficiency. *Lancet* 1991; **324**: 169–74.

6 Ellard GA, Gammon PT, Savin LA, Tan RSH. Dapsone acetylation in dermatitis herpetiformis. *Br J Dermatol* 1974; **90**: 441–4.

7 Potter MN, Yates P, Slade R, Kennedy CTC. Agranulocytosis caused by dapsone therapy for granuloma annulare. *J Am Acad Dermatol* 1989; **20**: 87–8.

8 Hörnstein P, Keisu M, Wiholm B-E. The incidence of agranulocytosis during treatment of dermatitis herpetiformis with dapsone as reported in Sweden, 1972 through 1988. *Arch Dermatol* 1990; **126**: 919–22.

9 Ognibene AJ. Agranulocytosis due to dapsone. *Ann Intern Med* 1970; **75**: 521–4.

10 Kingham JG, Swain P, Swarbrick ET, *et al.* Dapsone and severe hypoalbuminaemia: a report of two cases. *Lancet* 1979; **ii**: 662–4.

11 Cowan RE, Wright JT. Dapsone and severe hypoalbuminaemia in dermatitis herpetiformis. *Br J Dermatol* 1981; **104**: 201–4.

12 Ahrens EM, Meckler RJ, Callen JP. Dapsone-induced peripheral neuropathy. *Int J Dermatol* 1986; **25**: 314–16.

13 Homeida M, Babikr A, Daneshmend TK. Dapsone-induced optic atrophy and motor neuropathy. *Br Med J* 1980; **281**: 1180.

14 Kenner DJ, Holt K, Agnello R, Chester GH. Permanent retinal damage following massive dapsone overdose. *Br J Ophthalmol* 1980; **64**: 741–4.

15 Fine J-D, Katz SI, Donahue MJ, Hendricks AA. Psychiatric reaction to dapsone and sulfapyridine. *J Am Acad Dermatol* 1983; **9**: 274–5.

Thalidomide

Teratogenicity (phocomelia), gastric intolerance, drowsiness, neuropsychiatric upset, and sensory peripheral neuropathy developing after several months, have been reported [1]. A dermatitis associated with eosinophilia develops in a few cases of erythema nodosum leprosum treated with thalidomide over several years [2]. Hypersensitivity reactions characterized by fever, tachycardia, and an extensive erythematous macular eruption developed on rechallenge in a number of patients with HIV infection treated with thalidomide for severe aphthous oropharyngeal ulceration [3].

1 Revuz J. Actualité du thalidomide. *Ann Dermatol Vénéréol (Paris)* 1990; **117**: 313–21.

2 Waters MFR. An internally controlled double blind trial of thalidomide in severe erythema nodosum leprosum. *Lepr Rev* 1971; **42**: 26–42.

3 Williams I, Weller IVD, Malin A, *et al.* Thalidomide hypersensitivity in AIDS. *Lancet* 1991; **337**: 436–7.

4.8 Metronidazole and tinidazole

Metronidazole

Pruritus and fixed eruptions [1,2] are rare. A pityriasis rosea-like eruption has been described [3]. A reversible peripheral neuropathy may complicate prolonged therapy.

Tinidazole

A fixed eruption with cross-reactivity with metronidazole has been reported [4,5].

1 Naik RPC, Singh G. Fixed drug eruption due to metronidazole. *Dermatologica* 1977; **155**: 59−60.
2 Shelley WB, Shelley ED. Fixed drug eruption due to metronidazole. *Cutis* 1987; **39**: 393−4.
3 Maize JC, Tomecki KJ. Pityriasis rosea-like drug eruption secondary to metronidazole. *Arch Dermatol* 1977; **113**: 1457−8.
4 Kanwar AJ, Sharma R, Rajagopalan M, Kaur S. Fixed drug eruption due to tinidazole with cross-reactivity with metronidazole. *Dermatologica* 1990; **181**: 277.
5 Mishra D, Mobashir M, Zaheer MS. Fixed drug eruption and cross-reactivity between tinidazole and metronidazole. *Int J Dermatol* 1990; **29**: 740.

4.9 Quinolones

These compounds are related to nalidixic acid [1−5]. Gastrointestinal side-effects occur in up to 6% of patients. Hypersensitivity reactions involving the skin have been reported in 0.5−2% of patients, and in up to 2.4% of patients receiving cinoxacin [1−5]; they most frequently manifest themselves as rash or pruritus. Fever, urticaria, angioedema and anaphylactoid reactions are rare. Anaphylactic or anaphylactoid reactions have been documented with cinoxacin [6], ciprofloxacin [7] and pipemidic acid [8]. Fixed drug eruption due to pipemidic acid is recorded [9]. Norfloxacin has caused a pustular eruption [10]. Ciprofloxacin [11,12], pefloxacin and fleroxacin [13] have been associated with photosensitivity. Pefloxacin and ofloxacin have caused photo-onycholysis [14]. Hypersensitivity leucocytoclastic vasculitis has been reported with both ofloxacin and ciprofloxacin [15,16]. Intravenous administration of ciprofloxacin through small veins at the dorsum of the hands may be associated with local reactions at the site of infusion [17]. Ciprofloxacin has been associated with toxic epidermal necrolysis (TEN) in isolated cases [18].

Nalidixic acid

Cutaneous reactions are common, occurring in up to 5% of patients; various hypersensitivity reactions are seen, including exfoliative dermatitis. Phototoxicity is now well recognized [11,19−22]. A bullous photodermatitis may occur, usually on the hands or feet; chronic scarring and increased skin fragility may mimic porphyria cutanea tarda. Long-wave ultraviolet light is responsible [22]. A lupus-like syndrome has been reported [23], as well as transient alopecia.

1 Christ W, Lehnert T, Ulbrich B. Specific toxicologic aspects of the quinolones. *Rev Infect Dis* 1988; **10** (Suppl 1): S141−S146.
2 Wolfson JS, Hooper DC. Fluoroquinolone antimicrobial agents. *Clin Microbiol Rev* 1989; **2**: 378−424.

3 Hooper DC, Wolfson JS. Fluoroquinolone antimicrobial agents. *N Engl J Med* 1991; **324**: 384−94.

4 Sisca TS, Heel RC, Romankiewicz JA. Cinoxacin: a review of its pharmacological properties and therapeutic efficacy in the treatment of urinary tract infections. *Drugs* 1983; **25**: 544−69.

5 Campoli-Richards DM, Monck JP, Price A, *et al*. Ciprofloxacin. A review of its antibacterial activity, pharmacokinetic properties and therapeutic use. *Drugs* 1988; **35**: 373−447.

6 Stricker BHC, Slagboom G, Demaeseneer R, *et al*. Anaphylactic reactions to cinoxacin. *Br Med J* 1988; **297**: 1434−5.

7 Davis H, McGoodwin E, Reed TG. Anaphylactoid reactions reported after treatment with ciprofloxacin. *Ann Intern Med* 1989; **111**: 1041−3.

8 Gerber D. Anaphylaxis with pipemidic acid. *S Afr Med J* 1985; **67**: 999.

9 Miyagawa S, Yamashina Y, Hirota S, Shirai T. Fixed drug eruption due to pipemidic acid. *J Dermatol (Tokyo)* 1991; **18**: 59−60.

10 Shelley ED, Shelley WB. The subcorneal pustular drug eruption: An example induced by norfloxacin. *Cutis* 1988; **42**: 24−7.

11 Nederost ST, Dijkstra JWE, Handel DW. Drug-induced photosensitivity reaction. *Arch Dermatol* 1989; **125**: 433−4.

12 Ferguson J, Johnson BE. Ciprofloxacine-induced photosensitivity: *in vitro* and *in vivo* studies. *Br J Dermatol* 1990; **123**: 9−20.

13 Bowie WR, Willetts V, Jewesson PJ. Adverse reactions in a dose-ranging study with a new long-acting fluoroquinolone, fleroxacin. *Antimicrob Agents Chemother* 1989; **33**: 1778−82.

14 Baran R, Brun P. Photoonycholysis induced by the fluoroquinolones pefloxacine and ofloxacine. Report on 2 cases. *Dermatologica* 1986; **173**: 185−8.

15 Huminer C, Cohen JD, Majafla R, Dux S. Hypersensitivity vasculitis due to ofloxacin. *Br Med J* 1989; **299**: 303.

16 Choc U, Rothschield BM, Laitman L. Ciprofloxacin-induced vasculitis. *N Engl J Med* 1989; **320**: 257−8.

17 Thorsteinsson SB, Bergan T, Johannesson G, *et al*. Tolerance of ciprofloxacin at injection site, systemic safety and effect on electroencephalogram. *Chemotherapy* 1987; **33**: 448−51.

18 Tham TCK, Allen G, Hayes D, *et al*. Possible association between toxic epidermal necrolysis and ciprofloxacin. *Lancet* 1991; **338**: 522.

19 Baes H. Photosensitivity caused by nalidixic acid. *Dermatologica* 1968; **136**: 61−4.

20 Birkett DA, Garretts M, Stevenson CJ. Phototoxic bullous eruptions due to nalidixic acid. *Br J Dermatol* 1969; **81**: 342−4.

21 Ramsay CA, Obreshkova E. Photosensitivity from nalidixic acid. *Br J Dermatol* 1974; **91**: 523−8.

22 Rosén K, Swanbeck G. Phototoxic reactions from some common drugs provoked by a high-intensity UVA lamp. *Acta Derm Venereol (Stockh)* 1982; **62**: 246−8.

23 Rubinstein A. LE-like disease caused by nalidixic acid. *N Engl J Med* 1979; **301**: 1288.

4.10 Urinary tract antibiotics

Nitrofurantoin

Pruritus, morbilliform rashes and urticaria may be seen occasionally. Erythema multiforme, erythema nodosum [1], exfoliative dermatitis, and a lupus erythematosus-like syndrome [2] are documented. Acute or chronic pulmonary reactions may accompany these skin manifestations, and may lead to pulmonary fibrosis [3]. Polyneuritis is a dose-dependent toxic reaction. Hepatitis, cholestatic jaundice and marrow suppression may occur rarely. Abnormal immunoelectrophoretic patterns may be induced [4].

1 Chisholm JC, Hepner M. Nitrofurantoin induced erythema nodosum. *J Natl Med Assoc* 1981; **73**: 59−61.
2 Selross O, Edgren J. Lupus-like syndrome associated with pulmonary reaction to nitrofurantoin. *Acta Med Scand* 1975; **197**: 125−9.
3 Rantala H, Kirvelä O, Anttolainen I. Nitrofurantoin lung in a child. *Lancet* 1979; **ii**: 799−800.
4 Teppo AM, Haltia K, Wager O. Immunoelectrophoretic 'tailing' of albumin line due to albumin−IgG antibody complexes: a side effect of nitrofurantoin treatment? *Scand J Immunol* 1976; **5**: 249−61.

4.11 Topical antibiotics

The side-effects of topical antibiotics have been reviewed [1]. Allergic contact dermatitis is rare with topical clindamycin, erythromycin and tetracycline, polymyxin B and gentamicin, and mupirocin, but is more frequent with neomycin. The appearance of resistance to gentamicin [2] and mupirocin [1] has been associated with widespread topical use; thus indiscriminate use may render these agents ineffective.

Bacitracin

Anaphylaxis due to bacitracin allergy has followed topical application of this antibiotic [3−5]. The patients had received multiple prior exposures and previous local reactions of pruritus, urticaria, or possible allergic contact dermatitis. Two patients with anaphylactic reactions to Polyfax ointment, containing polymyxin B and bacitracin, have been reported; one had previously documented positive patch tests to Polyfax, and the other had clinical intolerance to the preparation [6]. Intracutaneous injection of bacitracin in sensitive individuals induces histamine release with large wheal and flare reactions [7].

Chloramphenicol

Urticaria and angioedema have been described with topical use [8]. Fatal aplastic anaemia has followed the use of eye drops containing this antibiotic [9].

Sulphonamides

Erythema multiforme and Stevens−Johnson syndrome have been reported from topical preparations [10,11].

1 Hirschmann JV. Topical antibiotics in dermatology. *Arch Dermatol* 1988; **124**: 1691−700.
2 Noble WC. Choice of topical antibiotic: A microbiological viewpoint. *Clin Exp Dermatol* 1981; **6**: 503−7.

3 Roupe G, Strannegård Ö. Anaphylactic shock elicited by topical administration of bacitracin. *Arch Dermatol* 1969; **100**: 450–2.

4 Shechter JF, Wilkinson RD, Del Carpio J. Anaphylaxis following the use of bacitracin ointment: Report of a case and review of the literature. *Arch Dermatol* 1984; **120**: 909–11.

5 Katz BE, Fisher AA. Bacitracin: a unique topical antibiotic sensitiser. *J Am Acad Dermatol* 1987; **17**: 1016–24.

6 Eedy DJ, McMillan JC, Bingham EA. Anaphylactic reactions to topical antibiotic combinations. *Postgrad Med J* 1990; **66**: 858–9.

7 Bjorkner B, Moller H. Bacitracin: a cutaneous allergen and histamine releaser. *Acta Derm Venereol (Stockh)* 1973; **53**: 487–91.

8 Schewach-Millet M, Shpiro D. Urticaria and angioedema due to topically applied chloramphenicol ointment. *Arch Dermatol* 1985; **121**: 587.

9 Fraunfelder FT, Bagby GC. Ocular chloramphenicol and aplastic anemia. *N Engl J Med* 1983; **308**: 1536.

10 Gottschalk HR, Stone OJ. Stevens–Johnson syndrome from ophthalmic sulphonamide. *Arch Dermatol* 1976; **112**: 513–14.

11 Genvert GI, Cohen EJ, Donnenfeld ED, Blecher MH. Erythema multiforme after use of topical sulfacetamide. *Am J Ophthalmol* 1985; **99**: 465–8.

Chapter 5
Antifungal and Antiviral Drugs

5.1 Antifungal drugs

Dermatological aspects of antifungal drugs have been reviewed [1].

1 Lesher JL, Smith JG Jr. Antifungal agents in dermatology. *J Am Acad Dermatol* 1987; **17**: 383−94.

Amphotericin

Skin reactions are rare. The 'grey syndrome', characterized by ashen colour, acral cyanosis and prostration may occur as an immediate reaction to infusion.

Fluconazole

Angioedema has occurred [1]. An anaphylactic reaction occurred in a patient who had previously received ketoconazole and metronidazole, suggesting cross-sensitization [2], and Stevens−Johnson syndrome has been reported in a patient with acquired immunodeficiency syndrome (AIDS) [3].

1 Abbott M, Hughes DL, Patel R, Kinghorn GR. Angio-oedema after fluconazole. *Lancet* 1991; **338**: 633.
2 Neuhaus G, Pavic N, Pletscher M. Anaphylactic reaction after oral fluconazole. *Br Med J* 1991; **302**: 1341.
3 Gussenhoven MJE, Haak A, Peereboom-Wynia JDR, van't Wout JW. Stevens−Johnson syndrome after fluconazole. *Lancet* 1991; **338**: 120.

Flucytosine

Transitory macular and urticarial rashes have been seen. A toxic erythema occurred in a patient [1]. Anaphylaxis has been reported in a patient with AIDS [2]. Bone marrow depression can occur.

1 Thyss A, Viens P, Ticchioni M, *et al*. Toxicodermie au cours d'un traitement par 5 fluorocytosine. *Ann Dermatol Vénéréol (Paris)* 1987; **114**: 1131−2.
2 Kotani S, Hirose S, Niiya K, *et al*. Anaphylaxis to flucytosine in a patient with AIDS. *JAMA* 1988; **260**: 3275−6.

Griseofulvin

Reactions to griseofulvin are uncommon and usually mild; headaches and gastrointestinal disturbances are the most frequent. Morbilliform, erythematous (Fig. 5.1), or rarely haemorrhagic eruptions are occasionally seen [1,2]. Photodermatitis [3,4], with sensitivity to wavelengths above 320 nm, is by no means rare; clinically these are mainly eczematous, although pellagra-like changes may be seen [4]. The reaction is thought to be photo-allergic and photopatch tests are positive in some cases; there may be photo-cross-reactivity with penicillin [4]. Histology may be non-specific; direct immunofluorescence showed immunoglobulin and complement at the dermo-epidermal junction and around papillary blood vessels in one series [4]. Urticaria and a fixed drug eruption [5,6], cold urticaria [7], severe angioedema [8], erythema multiforme [9], serum sickness [10], exfoliative dermatitis [11], and toxic epidermal necrolysis [12,13] are recorded. Exacerbation of lupus erythematosus has been reported [14–18], with fatality in one case [17]. Patients with anti-SSA/Ro and SSB/La antibodies may be at an increased risk of developing a drug eruption [18,19]. Temporary granulocytopenia has been reported, and proteinuria may occur. Griseofulvin may interfere with the action of anticoagulants and the contraceptive pill [20], and should be avoided in pregnancy.

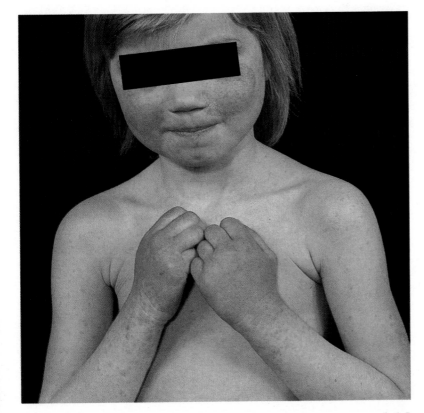

Figure 5.1 Erythematous eruption due to griseofulvin; note dermatophyte infection of the left cheek.

1 Faergemann J, Maibach H. Griseofulvin and ketoconazole in dermatology. *Semin Dermatol* 1983; **2**: 262–9.

2 Von Pöhler H, Michalski H. Allergisches Exanthem nach Griseofulvin. *Dermatol Monatsschr* 1972; **58**: 383–90.

3 Jarratt M. Drug photosensitization. *Int J Dermatol* 1976; **15**: 317–23.

4 Kojima T, Hasegawa T, Ishida H, *et al.* Griseofulvin-induced photodermatitis. Report of six cases. *J Dermatol (Tokyo)* 1988; **15**: 76–82.

5 Feinstein A, Sofer E, Trau H, Schewach-Millet M. Urticaria and fixed drug eruption in a patient treated with griseofulvin. *J Am Acad Dermatol* 1984; **10**: 915–17.

6 Savage J. Fixed drug eruption to griseofulvin. *Br J Dermatol* 1977; **97**: 107–8.

7 Chang T. Cold urticaria and photosensitivity due to griseofulvin. *JAMA* 1965; **193**: 848–50.

8 Goldblatt S. Severe reaction to griseofulvin: sensitivity investigation. *Arch Dermatol* 1961; **83**: 936–7.

9 Rustin NHA, Bunker CB, Dowd P, Robinson TWE. Erythema multiforme due to griseofulvin. *Br J Dermatol* 1989; **120**: 455–8.

10 Prazak G, Ferguson JS, Comer JE, McNeil BS. Treatment of tinea pedis with griseofulvin. *Arch Dermatol* 1960; **81**: 821–6.

11 Reaves LE III. Exfoliative dermatitis occurring in a patient treated with griseofulvin. *J Am Geriat Soc* 1964; **12**: 889–92.

12 Taylor B, Duffill M. Toxic epidermal necrolysis from griseofulvin. *J Am Acad Dermatol* 1988; **19**: 565–7.

13 Mion G, Verdon G, Le Gulluche Y, *et al.* Fatal toxic epidermal necrolysis after griseofulvin. *Lancet* 1989; **ii**: 1331.

14 Alexander S. Lupus erythematosus in two patients after griseofulvin treatment of *Trichophyton rubrum* infection. *Br J Dermatol* 1962; **74**: 72–4.

15 Anderson WA, Torre D. Griseofulvin and lupus erythematosus. *J Med Soc N J* 1966; **63**: 161–2.

16 Watsky MS, Linfield YL. Lupus erythematosus exacerbated by griseofulvin. *Cutis* 1976; **17**: 361–3.

17 Madhok R, Zoma A, Capell H. Fatal exacerbation of systemic lupus erythematosus after treatment with griseofulvin. *Br Med J* 1985; **291**: 249–50.

18 Miyagawa S, Okuchi T, Shiomi Y, Sakamoto K. Subacute cutaneous lupus erythematosus lesions precipitated by griseofulvin. *J Am Acad Dermatol* 1989; **21**: 343–6.

19 Miyagawa S, Sakamoto K. Adverse reactions to griseofulvin in patients with circulating anti-SSA/Ro and SSB/La autoantibodies. *Am J Med* 1989; **87**: 100–2.

20 Coté J. Interaction of griseofulvin and oral contraceptives. *J Am Acad Dermatol* 1990; **22**: 124–5.

Ketoconazole

Pruritus and gastrointestinal upset are the most frequent side-effects [1]. Severe anaphylaxis has been observed in two patients, one of whom had previously reacted to topical miconazole [2]. Other adverse reactions include exfoliative erythroderma [3]. The drug may block testosterone synthesis, causing dose-dependent lowering of serum testosterone and resultant oligospermia, impotence, decreased libido, and gynaecomastia in some men [4–6]. It also blocks the cortisol response to adrenocorticotrophic hormones, and may lead to adrenal insufficiency [6–8]. Hypothyroidism has been documented [9].

The most serious side-effect is idiosyncratic hepatitis, which occurs in about 1 in 10000 patients, and which may lead to fulminant and potentially fatal hepatic necrosis [10–16].

1 Faergemann J, Maibach H. Griseofulvin and ketoconazole in dermatology. *Semin Dermatol* 1983; **2**: 262−9.
2 Van Dijke CPH, Veerman FR, Haverkamp HC. Anaphylactic reactions to ketoconazole. *Br Med J* 1983; **287**: 1673.
3 Rand R, Sober AJ, Olmstead PM. Ketoconazole therapy and exfoliative erthroderma. *Arch Dermatol* 1983; **119**: 97−8.
4 Graybill JR, Drutz DJ. Ketoconazole: a major innovation for treatment of fungal disease. *Ann Intern Med* 1980; **93**: 921−3.
5 Moncada B, Baranda L. Ketoconazole and gynecomastia. *J Am Acad Dermatol* 1982; **7**: 557−8.
6 Pont A, Graybill JR, Craven PC, *et al*. High-dose ketoconazole therapy and adrenal and testicular function in humans. *Arch Intern Med* 1984; **144**: 2150−3.
7 Pont A, Williams P, Loose D, *et al*. Ketoconazole blocks adrenal steroid synthesis. *Ann Intern Med* 1982; **97**: 370−2.
8 Sonino N. The use of ketoconazole as an inhibitor of steroid production. *N Engl J Med* 1987; **317**: 812−18.
9 Kitching NH. Hypothroidism after treatment with ketoconazole. *Br Med J* 1986; **293**: 993−4.
10 Horsburgh CR Jr, Kirkpatrick CJ, Teutsch CB. Ketoconazole and the liver. *Lancet* 1982; **i**: 860.
11 Stern RS. Ketoconazole: Assessing its risks. *J Am Acad Dermatol* 1982; **6**: 544.
12 Rollman O, Lööf L. Hepatic toxicity of ketoconazole. *Br J Dermatol* 1983; **108**: 376−8.
13 Duarte PA, Chow CC, Simmons F, Ruskin J. Fatal hepatitis associated with ketoconazole therapy. *Arch Intern Med* 1984; **144**: 1069−70.
14 Lewis J, Zimmerman HJ, Benson GD, Ishak KG. Hepatic injury associated with ketoconazole therapy: Analysis of 33 cases. *Gastroenterology* 1984; **86**: 503−13.
15 Lake-Bakaar G, Scheuer PJ, Sherlock S. Hepatic reactions associated with ketoconazole in the United Kingdom. *Br Med J* 1987; **294**: 419−22.
16 Knight TE, Shikuma CY, Knight J. Ketoconazole-induced fulminant hepatitis necessitating liver transplantation. *J Am Acad Dermatol* 1991; **25**: 398−400.

Nystatin

A fixed drug eruption has been reported [1], as has Stevens−Johnson syndrome in an isolated case [2].

1 Pareek SS. Nystatin-induced fixed eruption. *Br J Dermatol* 1980; **103**: 679−80.
2 Garty B-Z. Stevens−Johnson syndrome associated with nystatin treatment. *Arch Dermatol* 1991; **127**: 741−2.

5.2 Antiviral drugs

Acyclovir

In general, there are very few side-effects [1]. Intravenous use may cause inflammation and phlebitis. A nephropathy may develop with intravenous use, especially in patients with renal failure, due to renal precipitation of the drug; the dose should be reduced in patients with impaired renal function. An encephalopathy may occur. Peripheral oedema has been reported very rarely [2,3].

1 Arndt KA. Adverse reactions to acyclovir: topical, oral, and intravenous. *J Am Acad Dermatol* 1988; **18**: 188−90.

2 Hisler BM, Daneshvar SA, Aronson PJ, Hashimoto K. Peripheral edema and oral acyclovir. *J Am Acad Dermatol* 1988; **18**: 1142−3.
3 Medina S, Torrelo A, España A, Ledo A. Edema and oral acyclovir. *Int J Dermatol* 1991; **30**: 305−6.

Azidothymidine (zidovudine)

This drug, used in the management of AIDS, may cause gastrointestinal upset and marrow suppression (with serious anaemia in 32% and leucopenia in 37%), myalgia, headache and insomnia [1−4]. Such side-effects have been reported in health care workers treated with zidovudine for attempted prophylaxis of human immunodeficiency virus (HIV) infection following accidental needlestick injury [5,6]. Zidovudine-related thrombocytopenia resulted in ecchymoses around Kaposi's sarcoma lesions in a patient with AIDS, simulating rapid intracutaneous spread of neoplasm [7]. Vaginal tumours have been documented in rodents. Diffuse pigmentation, as well as isolated hyperpigmented spots on the palms, soles and fingers, pigmentation of the fingernails and buccal mucosa, have been described [8−13]. Postural hypotension has been recorded [14]. Hypertrichosis of the eyelids has occurred [15]. A possible link with neutrophilic eccrine hidradenitis has been postulated in HIV-infected patients [16].

1 Gill PS, Rarick M, Brynes RK, *et al*. Azidothymidine associated with bone marrow failure in AIDS. *Ann Intern Med* 1987; **107**: 502−5.
2 Richman DD, Fiscal MA, Grieco MH, *et al*. The toxicity of azidothymidine (AZT) in the treatment of patients with AIDS or AIDS-related complex: a double blind, placebo-controlled trial. *N Engl J Med* 1987; **317**: 192−7.
3 Gelmon K, Montaner JS, Fanning M, *et al*. Nature, time course and dose dependence of zidovudine-related side-effects: results from the Multicenter Canadian Azidothymidine Trial. *AIDS* 1989; **3**: 555−61.
4 Moore RD, Creagh-Kirk T, Keruly J, *et al*. Long-term safety and efficacy of zidovudine in patients with advanced human immunodeficiency virus infection. *Arch Intern Med* 1991; **151**: 981−6.
5 Centers for Disease Control. Public health service statement on management of occupational exposure to human immunodeficiency virus, including considerations regarding zidovudine post-exposure use. *MMWR* 1990; **39**: 1−14.
6 Jeffries DJ. Zidovudine after occupational exposure to HIV. Hospitals should be able to give it within an hour. *Br Med J* 1991; **302**: 1349−51.
7 Barnett JH, Gilson E. Zidovudine-related thrombocytopenia simulating rapid growth of Kaposi's sarcoma. *Arch Dermatol* 1991; **127**: 1068−9.
8 Azon-Masoliver A, Mallolas J, Gatell J, Castel T. Zidovudine-induced nail pigmentation. *Arch Dermatol* 1988; **124**: 1570−1.
9 Fisher CA, McPoland PR. Azidothymidine-induced nail pigmentation. *Cutis* 1989; **43**: 552−4.
10 Bendick C, Rasokat H, Steigleder GK. Azidothymidine-induced hyperpigmentation of skin and nails. *Arch Dermatol* 1989; **125**: 1285−6.
11 Greenberg RG, Berger TG. Nail and mucocutaneous hyperpigmentation with azidothymidine therapy. *J Am Acad Dermatol* 1990; **22**: 327−30.
12 Grau-Massanes M, Millan F, Febrer MI, *et al*. Pigmented nail bands and mucocutaneous pigmentation in HIV-positive patients treated with zidovudine. *J Am Acad Dermatol* 1990; **22**: 687−8.
13 Tadini G, D'Orso M, Cusini M, *et al*. Oral mucosa pigmentation: A new side-effect of azidothymidine therapy in patients with acquired immunodeficiency syndrome. *Arch Dermatol* 1991; **127**: 267−8.

14 Loke RHT, Murray-Lyon IM, Carter GD. Postural hypotension related to zidovudine in a patient infected with HIV. *Br Med J* 1990; **300**: 163–4.

15 Klutman NE, Hinthorn DR. Excessive growth of eyelashes in a patient with AIDS being treated with zidovudine. *N Engl J Med* 1991; **324**: 1896.

16 Smith KJ, Skelton HG III, James WD, *et al*. Neutrophilic eccrine hidradenitis in HIV-infected patients. *J Am Acad Dermatol* 1990; **23**: 945–7.

Foscarnet

A generalized cutaneous rash has been reported with use of this drug in AIDS [1].

1 Green ST, Nathwani D, Goldberg DJ, *et al*. Generalised cutaneous rash associated with foscarnet usage in AIDS. *J Infect* 1990; **21**: 227–8.

Dideoxycytidine

A maculopapular reaction with oral ulceration developed in 70% of patients treated with this new anti-AIDS agent, but resolved spontaneously in those who continued on therapy [1].

1 McNeely MC, Yarchoan R, Broder S, Lawley TJ. Dermatologic complications associated with administration of 2′,3′-dideoxycytidine in patients with human immunodeficiency virus infection. *J Am Acad Dermatol* 1989; **21**: 1213–17.

Idoxuridine

Severe alopecia and loss of nails followed parenteral use [1].

1 Nolan DC, Carruthers MM, Lerner AM. *Herpesvirus hominis* encephalitis in Michigan: report of thirteen cases, including six treated with idoxuridine. *N Engl J Med* 1970; **282**: 10–13.

Chapter 6
Antimalarial and Antihelminthic Drugs

6.1 Antimalarials

The reactions to antimalarial agents have been reviewed recently [1,2].

1 Ribrioux A. Antipaludéens de synthese et peau. *Ann Dermatol Vénéréol (Paris)* 1990; **117**: 975–90.
2 Ochsendorf FR, Runne U. Chloroquin und Hydroxychloroquin: Nebenwirkungsprofil wichtiger Therapeutika. *Hautarzt* 1991; **42**: 140–6.

Chloroquine and hydroxychloroquine

Pruritus is common in Africans on acute or prolonged treatment, but rare in Europeans [1–4]. Pigmentary changes develop in about 25% of patients receiving any of the antimalarials for more than 4 months [5–8]; chloroquine binds to melanin [8]. Blackish-purple patches on the shins are often seen, and brown–grey pigmentation may appear in light-exposed skin [7]. The nail beds may be pigmented diffusely or in transverse bands, and the hard palate is diffusely pigmented. By contrast, red–blonde (but not dark) hair may be bleached [9].

Photosensitivity may be seen [10]; in addition, certain types of porphyria may be provoked [11]. Effects on psoriasis are unpredictable, but precipitation of severe psoriasis has long been recognized [12–17], including erythroderma [17]. However, 88% of a series of 50 psoriatics who were treated with standard doses of chloroquine noted no change in their psoriasis [18]. Lichenoid eruptions are uncommon, and erythema annulare centrifugum is rare [19]. Toxic epidermal necrolysis with oral involvement has been documented. A pustular eruption with hydroxychloroquine has been reported [20]. Toxic psychosis has been described with hydroxychloroquine [21]. All antimalarials are potentially teratogenic.

Chloroquine and hydroxychloroquine may cause serious ophthalmic side-effects [22,23]. Corneal deposits occur in 95% of patients on long-term therapy, but of these 95% are asymptomatic [24]. A potentially irreversible retinopathy leading to blindness may develop in 0.45–2% of cases [25,26]. The retinal changes may progress after the drug is stopped. Use of less than 250 mg (or 4 mg/kg) daily of chloroquine, with pretreatment and 6-monthly ophthalmological assessment, using an Amsler grid, is recommended. Malarial prophylaxis with two tablets weekly is said not to carry an appreciable risk.

1 Osifo NG. Chloroquine induced pruritus among patients with malaria. *Arch Dermatol* 1984; **120**: 80−2.

2 Ekpechi OI, Okoro AN. A pattern of pruritus to chloroquine. *Arch Dermatol* 1964; **89**: 631−2.

3 Spencer HC, Poulter NR, Lury JD, Poulter CJ. Chloroquine-associated pruritus in a European. *Br Med J* 1982; **285**: 1703−4.

4 Salako LA. Toxicity and side-effects of antimalarials in Africa: a critical review. *Bull WHO* 1984; **62** (Suppl): 63−8.

5 Dall JLC, Keane JA. Disturbances of pigmentation with chloroquine. *Br Med J* 1959; **i**: 1387−9.

6 Tuffanelli D, Abraham RK, Dubois EJ. Pigmentation from antimalarial therapy; its possible relationship to the ocular lesions. *Arch Dermatol* 1963; **88**: 419−26.

7 Levy H. Chloroquine-induced pigmentation. Case reports. *S Afr Med J* 1982; **2**: 735−7.

8 Sams WM, Epstein JH. The affinity of melanin for chloroquine. *J Invest Dermatol* 1965; **45**: 482−8.

9 Dupré A, Ortonne J-P, Viraben R, Arfeux F. Choroquine-induced hypopigmentation of hair and freckles. Association with congenital renal failure. *Arch Dermatol* 1985; **121**: 1164−6.

10 Van Weelden H, Bolling HH, Baart de la Faille H, Van Der Leun JC. Photosensitivity caused by chloroquine. *Arch Dermatol* 1982; **118**: 290.

11 Davis MJ, Vander Ploeg DE. Acute porphyria and coproporphyrinuria following chloroquine therapy: a report of two cases. *Arch Dermatol* 1957; **75**: 796−800.

12 O'Quinn SE, Kennedy CB, Naylor LZ. Psoriasis, ultraviolet light and chloroquine. *Arch Dermatol* 1964; **90**: 211−16.

13 Baker H. The influence of chloroquine and related drugs on psoriasis and keratoderma blenorrhagicum. *Br J Dermatol* 1966; **78**: 161−6.

14 Abel EA, Dicicco LM, Orenberg EK, *et al.* Drugs in exacerbation of psoriasis. *J Am Acad Dermatol* 1986; **15**: 1007−22.

15 Nicolas J-F, Mauduit G, Haond J, *et al.* Psoriasis grave induit par la chloroquine (nivaquine). *Ann Dermatol Vénéréol (Paris)* 1988; **115**: 289−93.

16 Luzar MJ. Hydroxychloroquine in psoriatic arthropathy: Exacerbation of psoriatic skin lesions. *J Rheumatol* 1982; **9**: 462−4.

17 Slagel GA, James WD. Plaquenil-induced erythroderma. *J Am Acad Dermatol* 1985; **12**: 857−62.

18 Katugampola G, Katugampola S. Chloroquine and psoriasis. *Int J Dermatol* 1990; **29**: 153−4.

19 Ashurst PJ. Erythema annulare centrifugum. Due to hydroxychloroquine sulfate and chloroquine sulfate. *Arch Dermatol* 1967; **95**: 37−9.

20 Lotem M, Ingber A, Segal R, Sandbank M. Generalized pustular drug rash induced by hydroxychloroquine. *Acta Derm Venereol (Stockh)* 1990; **70**: 250−1.

21 Ward WQ, Walter-Ryan WG, Shehi GM. Toxic psychosis: A complication of antimalarial therapy. *J Am Acad Dermatol* 1985; **12**: 863−5.

22 Olansky AJ. Antimalarials and ophthalmologic safety. *J Am Acad Dermatol* 1982; **6**: 19−23.

23 Portnoy JZ, Callen JP. Ophthalmologic aspects of chloroquine and hydroxychloroquine safety. *Int J Dermatol* 1983; **22**: 273−8.

24 Easterbrook M. Ocular side effects and safety of antimalarial agents. *Am J Med* 1988; **85**; 23−9.

25 Marks JS. Choroquine retinopathy: is there a safe daily dose? *Ann Rheum Dis* 1982; **41**: 52−8.

26 Easterbrook M. Dose relationships in patients with early chloroquine retinopathy. *J Rheumatol* 1987; **14**: 472−5.

Mefloquine

Dizziness, nausea, erythema, and neurological disturbance are documented, and a case report of Stevens–Johnson syndrome has been recorded [1].

1 Van Den Ende E, Van Gompel A, Colebunders R, Van Den Ende J. Mefloquine-induced Stevens–Johnson syndrome. *Lancet* 1991; **337**: 683.

Mepacrine (atabrine, quinacrine)

This drug constantly causes yellow staining of the skin which may involve the conjunctiva and may mimic jaundice [1]. Lichenoid eruptions are well known. Large numbers of military personnel given mepacrine for malaria prophylaxis in World War II developed a tropical lichenoid dermatitis, which was quickly followed by anhidrosis, cutaneous atrophy, alopecia, nail changes, altered pigmentation and keratoderma [2,3]. A few patients developed localized bluish-black hyperpigmentation confined to the palate, face, pretibial area and nail beds after prolonged administration of more than a year. Years later, lichenoid nodules, scaly red plaques, atrophic lesions on the soles, erosions and leucoplakia of the tongue and fungating warty growths appeared [3,4]. Progression to squamous cell carcinoma, especially on the palm, has occurred. Ocular toxicity is much less than with chloroquine.

1 Leigh JM, Kennedy CTC, Ramsey JD, Henderson WJ. Mepacrine pigmentation in systemic lupus erythematosus. *Br J Dermatol* 1979; **101**: 147–53.
2 Bauer F. Late sequelae of atabrine dermatitis: a new premalignant entity. *Aust J Dermatol* 1978; **19**: 9–12.
3 Bauer F. Quinacrine hydrochloride drug eruption (tropical lichenoid dermatitis). Its early and late sequelae and its malignant potential. A review. *J Am Acad Dermatol* 1981; **4**: 239–48.
4 Callaway JL. Late sequelae of quinacrine dermatitis, a new premalignant entity. *J Am Acad Dermatol* 1979; **1**: 456.

Pyrimethamine

This folate antagonist can cause agranulocytosis even in very low dosage, especially when combined with dapsone [1]. A lichenoid eruption has been reported [2], as has photosensitivity. The reported rate for all serious reactions to pyrimethamine–sulphadoxine (Fansidar) was 1 in 2100 prescriptions, and for cutaneous reactions including Stevens–Johnson syndrome was 1 in 4900, with a fatality rate of 1 in 11 100 [3]. Similar rates for severe reactions to pyrimethamine–dapsone (Maloprim) were 1 in 9100 prescriptions, and for blood dyscrasias 1 in 20 000, with a fatality rate of 1 in 75 000. Epidermal necrolysis, angioedema, bullous disorders and serious hepatic disorders also occurred. Since few serious reactions have been recorded with chloroquine and proguanil, it has been recommended that use of compound antimalarials should be restricted [3].

1 Friman G, Nyström-Rosander C, Jonsell G, *et al.* Agranulocytosis associated with malaria prophylaxis with Maloprim. *Br Med J* 1983; **286**: 1244–5.
2 Cutler TP. Lichen planus caused by pyrimethamine. *Clin Exp Dermatol* 1980; **5**: 253–6.
3 Phillips-Howard PA, West LJ. Serious adverse drug reactions to pyrimethamine–sulphadoxine, pyrimethamine–dapsone and to amodiaquine in Britain. *J R Soc Med* 1990; **83**: 82–5.

Quinine

Purpura may or may not be thrombocytopenic [1,2]. Erythematous, urticarial, photo-allergic [3–5], bullous and fixed eruptions are recorded. Lichenoid eruptions are rare. If contact allergic sensitivity is already present, eczematous reactions may occur, as in 'systemic contact-type eczema' [6]. Splinter haemorrhages, and a maculopapular and a photosensitive papulonecrotic eruption, due to a lymphocytic vasculitis, has been recorded in one case [7].

1 Belkin GA. Cocktail purpura. An unusual case of quinine sensitivity. *Ann Intern Med* 1967; **66**: 583–6.
2 Helmly RB, Bergin JJ, Shulman NR. Quinine-induced purpura: observation on antibody titers. *Arch Intern Med* 1967; **20**: 59–62.
3 Ljunggren B, Sjövall P. Systemic quinine photosensitivity. *Arch Dermatol* 1986; **122**: 909–11.
4 Ferguson J, Addo HA, Johnson BE, *et al.* Quinine induced photosensitivity: clinical and experimental studies. *Br J Dermatol* 1987; **117**: 631–40.
5 Diffey BL, Farr PM, Adams SJ. The action spectrum in quinine photosensitivity. *Br J Dermatol* 1988; **118**: 679–85.
6 Calnan CD, Caron GA. Quinine sensitivity. *Br Med J* 1961; **ii**: 1750–2.
7 Harland CC, Millard LG. Another quirk of quinine. *Br Med J* 1991; **302**: 295.

6.2 Antihelminthics

Amocarzine (CGP 6140)

This macro- and micro-filaricidal drug used for the therapy of onchocerciasis may be associated with dizziness and pruritus with or without a rash [1].

1 Poltera AA, Zea-Flores G, Guderian R, *et al.* Onchocercacidal effects of amocarzine (CGP 6140) in Latin America. *Lancet* 1991; **337**: 583–4.

Benzimidazole compounds

These are used both for the therapy of intestinal helminthiasis and also for hydatid disease; fever, gastrointestinal upset, reversible neutropenia, and transient abnormalities in liver function are reported. Telogen effluvium has been documented with both albendazole [1,2] and mebendazole.

1 Karawifa MA, Yasawi MI, Mohamed AE. Hair loss as a complication of albendazole therapy. *Saudi Med J* 1988; **9**: 530.
2 Garcia-Muret MP, Sitjas D, Tuneu L, de Moragas JM. Telogen effluvium associated with albendazole therapy. *Int J Dermatol* 1990; **29**: 669–70.

Ivermectin

Fever, rash, pruritus, local swelling and tender regional lymphadenopathy are documented [1]. The incidence of moderate adverse
reactions including pruritus, localized rash and fever was 4% in a
study of patients with onchocerciasis from Ecuador [2], and increased
itching and/or rash occurred in 8% of cases in another study [3].
Patients with reactive onchodermatitis (*sowda*) may have severe
pruritus and limb swelling with ivermectin [4].

1 Bryan RT, Stokes SL, Spencer HC. Expatriates treated with ivermectin. *Lancet*
  1991; **337**: 304.
2 Guderian RH, Beck BJ, Proano S Jr, Mackenzie CD. Onchocerciasis in Ecuador,
  1980–86: epidemiological evaluation of the disease in the Esmerldas province.
  Eur J Epidemiol 1989; **5**: 294–302.
3 Whitworth JAG, Maude GH, Luty AJF. Expatriates treated with ivermectin.
  Lancet 1991; **337**: 625–6.
4 Guderian RH, Anselmi M, Sempertegui R, Cooper PJ. Adverse reactions to
  ivermectin in reactive onchodermatitis. *Lancet* 1991; **337**: 188.

Levamisole

Prolonged use at high dosage as an immunostimulant is associated
with type I reactions with itching, pruritus and urticaria. Lichenoid
[1] and non-specific [2] rashes, leucocytoclastic vasculitis with a
reticular livedo pattern due to circulating immune complexes [3],
and cutaneous necrotizing vasculitis [4] have been reported.

1 Kirby JD, Black MM, McGibbon D. Levamisole-induced lichenoid eruptions. *J
  R Soc Med* 1980; **73**: 208–11.
2 Parkinson DR, Cano PO, Jerry LM, *et al*. Complications of cancer immunotherapy with levamisole. *Lancet* 1977; **ii**: 1129–32.
3 Macfarlane DG, Bacon PA. Levamisole-induced vasculitis due to circulating
  immune complexes. *Br Med J* 1978; **i**: 407–8.
4 Scheinberg MA, Bezera JBG, Almeida LA, Silveira LA. Cutaneous necrotising
  vasculitis induced by levamisole. *Br Med J* 1978; **i**: 408.

Niridazole

Urticaria and a pellagra-like dermatitis have been described.

Piperazine

Occupational dermatitis has been caused [1]. Previous contact sensitization induced by ethylenediamine has led to severe cross-
reactions on subsequent oral administration of piperazine, including
generalized exfoliative dermatitis [2].

1 Calnan CD. Occupational piperazine dermatitis. *Contact Dermatitis* 1975; **1**:
  126.
2 Burry JN. Ethylenediamine sensitivity with a systemic reaction to piperazine
  treatment. *Contact Dermatitis* 1978; **4**: 380.

Tetrachlorethylene

This drug has caused toxic epidermal necrolysis.

Thiabendazole

An unusual body odour is well known after the administration of this drug. Skin reactions, consisting of urticaria or maculopapular rashes, are infrequent and usually mild and transient. Erythema multiforme [1] and toxic epidermal necrolysis [2] has been reported.

1 Humphreys F, Cox NH. Thiabendazole-induced erythema multiforme with lesions around melanocytic naevi. *Br J Dermatol* 1988; **118**: 855−6.
2 Robinson HM, Samorodin CS. Thiabendazole-induced toxic epidermal necrolysis. *Arch Dermatol* 1976; **112**: 1757−60.

6.3 Drugs for *Pneumocystis*

Pentamidine

This drug is increasingly being used in the treatment and prophylaxis of *Pneumocystis carinii* pneumonia in patients with acquired immunodeficiency syndrome (AIDS). Urticaria, or maculopapular eruption proceeding to erythroderma, has been reported with nebulized therapy [1,2]. Toxic epidermal necrolysis may occur with systemic therapy [3,4].

1 Leen CLS, Mandal BK. Rash due to nebulized pentamidine. *Lancet* 1988; **ii**: 1250−1.
2 Berger TG, Tappero JW, Leoung GS, Jacobson MA. Aerosolized pentamidine and cutaneous eruptions. *Ann Intern Med* 1989; **110**: 1035−6.
3 Wang JJ, Freeman AI, Gaeta JF, Sinks LF. Unusual complications of pentamidine in the treatment of *Pneumocystis carinii* pneumonia. *J Pediatr* 1970; **77**: 311−14.
4 Walzer PD, Perl DP, Krogstadt DJ, *et al. Pneumocystis carinii* pneumonia in the United States: Epidemiologic, diagnostic and clinical features. *Ann Intern Med* 1974; **80**: 83−93.

Chapter 7
Non-steroidal Anti-inflammatory Agents

7.1 Acetylsalicylic acid and related compounds

Aspirin

Reactions to aspirin [1–4] occur in 0.3% of normal subjects [2,4]; these are usually sporadic, but occasionally more than one family member may be affected, and an HLA linkage has been reported [5]. Urticaria or angioedema (Fig. 7.1) is the commonest reaction [1]. Patients suffering from chronic idiopathic urticaria are often made worse by aspirin [6,7]; this probably has a non-allergic basis. Patients with chronic urticaria or angioedema have a risk of up to 30% of developing a flare in the condition following administration of aspirin or a non-steroidal anti-inflammatory agent [3]. The reaction is dose dependent and is greater when the urticaria is in an active phase. Aspirin may render the skin of such patients more reactive to histamine [5]. The syndrome of nasal polyposis, bronchial asthma and aspirin intolerance is well known [4,8]; up to 40% of patients with nasal polyps, and 4% of patients with asthma, may develop bronchoconstriction on exposure to aspirin, but only 2% develop urticaria [4]. Anaphylactoid responses may occur [3]; these may involve abnormalities of platelet function [9]. Cross-sensitivity between aspirin and tartrazine is thought to be rare [3]. Oral desensitization is feasible if essential, and may be maintained by daily aspirin intake [3]. Other reported reactions include purpura (Fig. 7.2), scarlatiniform erythema, erythema multiforme, fixed eruption, and a lichenoid eruption (which recurred on challenge) [10], but all are rare [1]. Neonatal petechiae may result from aspirin therapy of the mother [11]. Aspirin has provoked generalized pustular psoriasis [12]. Oral ulceration may follow prolonged chewing of aspirin [13], and at the site of an insoluble aspirin tablet placed at the side of an aching tooth. Nephropathy, marrow depression and gastric haemorrhage are well-recognized hazards. The elderly are at an increased risk of developing such complications [14]. The drug may interfere with renal clearance, e.g. of methotrexate. Aspirin is safe to administer to patients with glucose-6-phosphate deficiency [15].

1 Baker H, Moore-Robinson M. Drug reactions. IX. Cutaneous responses to aspirin and its derivatives. *Br J Dermatol* 1970; **82**: 319–21.

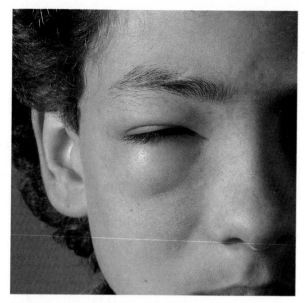 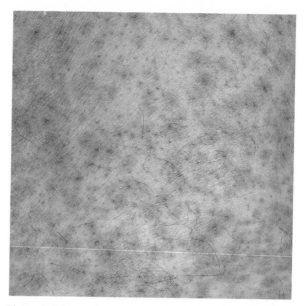

Figure 7.1 Angioedema due to acetylsalicylic acid.

Figure 7.2 Purpuric eruption due to acetylsalicylic acid.

2 Settipane RA, Constantine HP, Settipane GA. Aspirin intolerance and recurrent urticaria in normal adults and children. Epidemiology and review. *Allergy* 1980; **35**: 149−54.

3 Stevenson DD. Diagnosis, prevention and treatment of adverse reactions to aspirin and nonsteroidal anti-inflammatory drugs. *J Allergy Clin Immunol* 1984; **74**: 617−22.

4 Morassut P, Yang W, Karsh J. Aspirin intolerance. *Semin Arthritis Rheum* 1989; **19**: 22−30.

5 Mullarkey MF, Thomas PS, Hansen JA, *et al.* Association of aspirin-sensitive asthma with HLA-DQw2. *Am Rev Respir Dis* 1986; **133**: 261−3.

6 Champion RH, Roberts SOB, Carpenter RG, Roger JH. Urticaria and angiooedema. A review of 554 patients. *Br J Dermatol* 1969; **81**: 588−97.

7 Doeglas HMG. Reactions to aspirin and food additives in patients with chronic urticaria, including the physical urticarias. *Br J Dermatol* 1975; **93**: 135−44.

8 Samter M, Beers RF. Intolerance to aspirin. Clinical studies and consideration of its pathogenesis. *Ann Intern Med* 1968; **68**: 975−83.

9 Wüthrich B. Azetylsalizylsäure-Pseudoallergie: eine Anomalie der Thrombozyten-Funktion? *Hautarzt* 1988; **39**: 631−4.

10 Bharija SC, Belhaj MS. Acetylsalicylic acid may induce a lichenoid eruption. *Dermatologica* 1988; **177**: 19.

11 Stuart MJ, Gross SJ, Elrad H, Graeber JE. Effects of acetylsalicylic-acid ingestion on maternal and neonatal hemostasis. *N Engl J Med* 1982; **307**: 909−12.

12 Shelley WB. Birch pollen and aspirin psoriasis. *JAMA* 1964; **189**: 985−8.

13 Claman NH. Mouth ulcers associated with prolonged chewing of gum containing aspirin. *JAMA* 1967; **202**: 651−2.

14 Karsh J. Adverse reactions and interactions with aspirin. Considerations in the treatment of the elderly patient. *Drug Saf* 1990; **5**: 317−27.

15 Beutler E. Glucose-6-phosphate dehydrogenase deficiency. *Lancet* 1991; **324**: 169−74.

Diflunisal

Various cutaneous reactions have been reported in up to 5% of patients, including pruritus, urticaria, exanthems, Stevens−Johnson

[181]

syndrome, erythroderma [1], and a lichenoid photoreactive rash [2]. A non-pigmenting fixed drug eruption has been documented [3].

1 Chan L, Winearls C, Oliver D, *et al.* Acute interstitial nephritis and erythroderma associated with diflunisal. *Br Med J* 1980; **280**: 84−5.
2 Street ML, Winkelmann RK. Lichenoid photoreactive epidermal necrosis with diflunisal. *J Am Acad Dermatol* 1989; **20**: 850−1.
3 Roetzheim RG, Herold AH, Van Durme DJ. Nonpigmenting fixed drug eruption caused by diflunisal. *J Am Acad Dermatol* 1991; **24**: 1021−2.

Paracetamol

Allergic reactions are very rare, especially considering that it has been estimated that more than 1.4 billion tablets are sold per annum in the UK [1,2]. Urticaria [3], anaphylaxis, a widespread maculo-papular eruption, fixed eruption [2,4,5], and exfoliative dermatitis [6] have been seen.

1 Stricker BHC, Meyboom RHB, Lindquist M. Acute hypersensitivity reactions to paracetamol. *Br Med J* 1985; **291**: 938−9.
2 Meyrick Thomas RH, Munro DD. Fixed drug eruption due to paracetamol. *Br J Dermatol* 1986; **115**: 357−9.
3 Cole FOA. Urticaria from paracetamol. *Clin Exp Dermatol* 1985; **10**: 404.
4 Valsecchi R. Fixed drug eruption to paracetamol. *Dermatologica* 1989; **179**: 51−8.
5 Duhra P, Porter DI. Paracetamol-induced fixed drug eruption with positive immunofluorescence findings. *Clin Exp Dermatol* 1990; **15**: 293−5.
6 Girdhar A, Bagga AK, Girdhar BF. Exfoliative dermatitis due to paracetamol. *Ind J Dermatol Venereol Lepr* 1984; **50**: 162−3.

Phenacetin (acetaminophen)

Fixed drug eruption [1,2] and a bullous pemphigoid-like eruption [3] have been documented.

1 Guin JD, Haynie LS, Jackson D, Baker GF. Wandering fixed drug eruption: A mucocutaneous reaction to acetaminophen. *J Am Acad Dermatol* 1987; **3**: 399−402.
2 Guin JD, Baker GF. Chronic fixed drug eruption caused by acetaminophen. *Cutis* 1988; **41**: 106−8.
3 Kashihara M, Danno K, Miyachi Y, *et al.* Bullous pemphigoid-like lesions induced by phenacetin. Report of a case and an immunopathologic study. *Arch Dermatol* 1984; **120**: 1196−9.

Salicylamide

Use of teething jellies containing this substance has resulted in severe urticaria in infants [1].

1 Bentley-Phillips B. Infantile urticaria caused by salicylamide teething powder. *Br J Dermatol* 1968; **80**: 341.

7.2 Other non-steroidal anti-inflammatory agents

Dermatological aspects of the non-steroidal anti-inflammatory drugs (NSAIDs) have been extensively reviewed [1−8]. All of these drugs inhibit the enzyme cyclooxygenase, and decrease the production of prostaglandins and thromboxanes [8]. NSAIDs represent about 5% of all prescriptions in the UK [7] and US [4]; nearly 1 in 7 Americans were treated with an NSAID in 1984, and in 1986 100 million prescriptions for these drugs were written in the US [9]. NSAIDs accounted for 25% of all suspected adverse drug reactions reported to the UK Committee on Safety of Medicines in 1986 [7,10]. Reactions to NSAIDs occur in about 1 in 50000 administrations; NSAIDs should be avoided in patients known to be intolerant of aspirin [11]. Benoxaprofen, piroxicam, meclofenamate sodium, sulindac, and zomepirac sodium had the highest reaction rates relative to the number of new prescriptions in the US [3,4]. Benoxaprofen and zomepirac sodium (which caused anaphylactoid reactions) have subsequently been withdrawn. By contrast, naproxen, fenoprofen, ibuprofen, and indomethacin all had low rates of reaction; ibuprofen is available as a non-prescription drug in the US.

All of the NSAIDs, but particularly phenylbutazone, piroxicam, fenbufen, sulindac (and benoxaprofen before it was withdrawn), may cause Stevens–Johnson syndrome or toxic epidermal necrolysis (TEN) [8]. Tolmetin is associated with anaphylactoid reactions. Most of the NSAIDs causing photosensitivity are phenylpropionic acid derivatives: benoxaprofen (now withdrawn), carprofen, ketoprofen, tiaprofenic acid, naproxen, and nabumetone [12–17]. NSAIDs which cause photosensitivity absorb ultraviolet radiation at longer than 310 nm, resulting in the generation of singlet oxygen molecules which damage cell membranes [12]. The cutaneous photosensitivity appears to be elicited by a phototoxic mechanism [12–14,17]. The phototoxic reactions with NSAIDs are immediate, consisting of itching, burning, erythema, and at higher fluences whealing; this contrasts with the delayed reactions associated with psoralens and tetracyclines, which produce abnormal delayed erythema or exaggerated sunburn. Propionic acid derivatives may also precipitate photo-urticaria by mast cell degranulation [16]. Piroxicam, an enolic acid derivative structurally unrelated to phenylpropionic acid, is the most frequently cited non-phenylpropionic acid NSAID to cause photosensitivity [13,14,18]; phototoxicity to the parent drug has not been elicited in volunteers or experimental animals, although a phototoxic metabolite has been identified *in vitro*. Indomethacin, sulindac [19], meclofenamate sodium, and phenylbutazone have all been associated with photosensitivity [4]. NSAIDs may cause pseudoporphyria changes [20].

Drug exanthemata and urticaria occur in 0.2–9% of patients treated with NSAIDs [4,8]. Drug exanthemata develop in 1.2% of patients on phenylbutazone, and 0.3% of patients on indomethacin [8]; they are most frequently associated with diflunisal, sulindac, meclofenamate sodium, piroxicam, and phenylbutazone. All of the NSAIDs, but particularly aspirin and tolmetin, may cause urticaria and anaphylactoid reactions, especially in a patient with a history of aspirin-induced urticaria. NSAIDs should therefore be avoided in patients with aspirin 'hypersensitivity' [8]. Oral lichenoid lesions have also been recorded with NSAIDs [21]. Psoriasis has been reported anecdotally to be exacerbated by indomethacin and meclofenamate sodium, but there is no definitive evidence that NSAIDs consistently exacerbate psoriasis [7]. Pyrazolone NSAIDs are the only group which cause fixed drug eruptions at all commonly. While all NSAIDs may precipitate exfoliative erythroderma, this is commonest with phenylbutazone [8].

Apart from the cutaneous complications, NSAIDs may cause a variety of adverse effects [9], including gastrointestinal bleeding, intestinal perforations, and acute deterioration in renal function with interstitial nephritis [22]; the elderly and patients with impaired renal function or receiving concomitant diuretic therapy are most at risk. Aplastic anaemia is a recognized complication, and has occurred in the same individual with two different NSAIDs (sulindac and fenbufen) [23]. Hepatic syndromes, pneumonitis and neurological problems such as headache, aseptic meningitis and dizziness are recorded [9]. Niflumic acid and diclofenac both precipitated a dermatomyositis-like syndrome in a patient [24]. The potential for adverse interactions between NSAIDs and other drugs is considerable [9].

1 Almeyda J, Baker H. Drug reactions XII. Cutaneous reactions to anti-rheumatic drugs. *Br J Dermatol* 1970; **83**: 707−11.
2 Bailin PL, Matkaluk RM. Cutaneous reactions to rheumatological drugs. *Clin Rheum Dis* 1982; **8**: 493−516.
3 Stern RS, Bigby M. An expanded profile of cutaneous reactions to nonsteroid anti-inflammatory drugs. Reports to a specialty-based system for spontaneous reporting of adverse reactions to drugs. *JAMA* 1984; **252**: 1433−7.
4 Bigby M, Stern R. Cutaneous reactions to non-steroidal anti-inflammatory drugs. A review. *J Am Acad Dermatol* 1985; **12**: 866−76.
5 O'Brien WM, Bagby GF. Rare reactions to nonsteroidal anti-inflammatory drugs. *J Rheumatol* 1985; **12**: 13−20.
6 Roujeau JC. Clinical aspects of skin reactions to NSAIDs. *Scand J Rheumatol* 1987; **65** (Suppl): 131−4.
7 Greaves MW. Pharmacology and significance of nonsteroidal anti-inflammatory drugs in the treatment of skin diseases. *J Am Acad Dermatol* 1987; **16**: 751−64.
8 Bigby M. Nonsteroidal anti-inflammatory drug reactions. *Semin Dermatol* 1989; **8**: 182−6.
9 Brooks PM, Day RO. Nonsteroidal antiinflammatory drugs − differences and similarities. *N Engl J Med* 1991; **324**: 1716−25.
10 Committee on Safety of Medicines. Nonsteroidal anti-inflammatory drugs and serious gastrointestinal adverse reaction − 1. *Br Med J* 1986; **292**: 614.
11 Morassut P, Yang W, Karsh J. Aspirin intolerance. *Semin Arthritis Rheum* 1989; **19**: 22−30.
12 Ljunggren B. Propionic acid-derived nonsteroidal anti-inflammatory drugs are phototoxic *in vitro*. *Photodermatol* 1985; **2**: 3−9.
13 Stern RS. Phototoxic reactions to piroxicam and other nonsteroidal antiinflammatory agents. *N Engl J Med* 1983; **309**: 186−7.
14 Diffey BL, Daymond TJ, Fairgreaves H. Phototoxic reactions to piroxicam, naproxen and tiaprofenic acid. *Br J Rheumatol* 1983; **22**: 239−42.
15 Przybilla B, Ring J, Schwab U, *et al*. Photosensibilisierende Eigenschaften nichtsteroidaler Antirheumatika im Photopatch-Test. *Hautarzt* 1987; **38**: 18−25.

16 Kaidbey KH, Mitchell FN. Photosensitizing potential of certain nonsteroidal anti-inflammatory agents. *Arch Dermatol* 1989; **125**: 783−6.

17 Kochevar IE. Phototoxicity of nonsteroidal inflammatory drugs. Coincidence or specific mechanism? *Arch Dermatol* 1989; **125**: 824−6.

18 Serrano G, Bonillo J, Aliaga AET, *et al*. Piroxicam-induced photosensitivity and contact sensitivity to thiosalicylic acid. *J Am Acad Dermatol* 1990; **23**: 479−83.

19 Jeanmougin M, Manciet J-R, Duterque M, *et al*. Photosensibilisation au sulindac. *Ann Dermatol Vénéréol (Paris)* 1987; **114**: 1400−1.

20 Taylor BJ, Duffill MB. Pseudoporphyria from nonsteroidal anti-inflammatory drugs. *N Z Med J* 1987; **100**: 322−3.

21 Hamburger J, Potts AJC. Non-steroidal anti-inflammatory drugs and oral lichenoid reactions. *Br Med J* 1983; **287**; 1258.

22 Clive DM, Stoff JS. Renal syndromes associated with nonsteroidal anti-inflammatory drugs. *N Engl J Med* 1984; **310**: 563−72.

23 Andrews R, Russell N. Aplastic anaemia associated with a non-steroidal anti-inflammatory drug: relapse after exposure to another such drug. *Br Med J* 1990; **301**: 38.

24 Grob JJ, Collet AM, Bonerandi JJ. Dermatomyositis-like syndrome induced by nonsteroidal anti-inflammatory agents. *Dermatologica* 1989; **178**: 58−9.

Proprionic acid derivatives

Benoxaprofen

This drug was withdrawn in 1982 because of multiple side-effects including fatal cholestatic jaundice [1−4]. Over 60% of treated patients developed adverse effects [1], with photosensitivity occurring in 30%, often accompanied by photo-onycholysis [1,2,4−6]. It is discussed here partly because it has been claimed that benoxaprofen-induced photosensitivity may be persistent [6,7], and partly as an illustration of the potential side-effects of this group of drugs. However, it has been proposed that chronic episodic light reactivity following previous benoxaprofen therapy results from systemic administration of other photoactive drugs including NSAIDs [8]. Milia, especially on sun-exposed areas [9] and eruptive tumours on exposed skin [10] were documented. Other cutaneous complications included urticaria, pruritus, hypertrichosis, reversal of male-pattern baldness and accelerated hair and nail growth [11], erythema multiforme [12] and toxic epidermal necrolysis (TEN) [13].

1 Halsey JP, Cardoe N. Benoxaprofen: Side effect profile in 300 patients. *Br Med J* 1982; **284**: 1365−8.

2 Hindson C, Daymond T, Diffey B, Lawlor F. Side effects of benoxaprofen. *Br Med J* 1982: **284**: 1368−9.

3 Taggart HM, Alderdice JM. Fatal cholestatic jaundice in elderly patients taking benoxaprofen. *Br Med J* 1982; **284**: 1372.

4 Allen BR. Comment: benoxaprofen and the skin. *Br J Dermatol* 1983; **109**: 361−4.

5 Ferguson J, Addo HA, McGill PE, *et al*. A study of benoxaprofen-induced photosensitivity. *Br J Dermatol* 1982; **107**: 429−41.

6 Sneddon IB. Persistent phototoxicity after benoxaprofen. *Br J Dermatol* 1986; **115**: 515−16.

7 Ramakrishnan S, Macleod P, Tyrrel CJ. Acute radiation skin reaction and persistent photosensitivity after benoxaprofen. *Lancet* 1988; **ii**: 913.

8 Frain-Bell W. A study of persistent photosensitivity as a sequel of the prior

administration of the drug benoxaprofen. *Br J Dermatol* 1989; **121**: 551−62.

9 Stuart DRM. Milia due to benoxaprofen. *Br J Dermatol* 1982; **106**: 613.

10 Findlay GH, Hull PR. Eruptive tumours on sun-exposed skin after benoxaprofen. *Lancet* 1982; **ii**: 95.

11 Fenton DA, English JS, Wilkinson JD. Reversal of male-pattern baldness, hypertrichosis, and accelerated hair and nail growth in patients receiving benoxaprofen. *Br Med J* 1982; **284**: 1228−9.

12 Taylor AEM, Goff D, Hindson TC. Association between Stevens−Johnson syndrome and benoxaprofen. *Br Med J* 1981; **282**: 1433.

13 Fenton DA, English JS. Toxic epidermal necrolysis, leucopenia and thrombocytopenic purpura − a further complication of benoxaprofen therapy. *Clin Exp Dermatol* 1982; **7**: 277−80.

Carprofen

This drug also causes photosensitivity [1].

1 Merot Y, Harms M, Saurat JH. Photosensibilisation au caprofén (imadyl), un nouvel anti-inflammatoire non stéroidien. *Dermatologica* 1983; **166**: 301−7.

Fenbufen

Morbilliform and erythematous rashes, erythema multiforme [1], Stevens−Johnson syndrome, and allergic vasculitis have been recorded rarely. Fenbufen has caused exfoliative dermatitis, haemolytic anaemia and hepatitis [2], and was the drug implicated most commonly in adverse reactions reported to the Committee on Safety of Medicines in 1986 and 1987. A florid erythematous rash with pulmonary eosinophilia has been described in four cases [3].

1 Peacock A, Ledingham J. Fenbufen-induced erythema multiforme. *Br Med J* 1981; **283**: 582.

2 Muthiah MM. Severe hypersensitivity reaction to fenbufen. *Br Med J* 1988; **297**: 1614.

3 Burton GH. Rash and pulmonary eosinophilia associated with fenbufen. *Br Med J* 1990; **300**: 82−3.

Fenoprofen

This drug has caused pruritus, urticaria, vesicobullous eruption, thrombocytopenic purpura, and toxic epidermal necrolysis [1].

1 Stotts JS, Fang ML, Dannaker CJ, Steinman HK. Fenoprofen-induced toxic epidermal necrolysis. *J Am Acad Dermatol* 1988; **18**: 755−7.

Ibuprofen

Pruritus is the only common cutaneous reaction. When used in rheumatoid arthritis, rashes are rare, but patients with systemic lupus erythematosus (SLE) are liable to develop a generalized rash with fever and abdominal symptoms [1]. Angioedema/urticaria [2], fixed eruptions, vesicobullous rashes, erythema multiforme, vasculitis, and alopecia occur [3]. Psoriasis has been reported to be exacerbated [4]. This drug is available over the counter in the UK.

[186]

1 Shoenfeld Y, Livni E, Shaklai M, Pinkhas J. Sensitization to ibuprofen in SLE. *JAMA* 1980; **244**: 547−8.
2 Shelley ED, Shelley WB. Ibuprofen urticaria. *J Am Acad Dermatol* 1987; **17**: 1057−8.
3 Meyer HC. Alopecia associated with ibuprofen. *JAMA* 1979; **242**: 142.
4 Ben-Chetrit E, Rubinow A. Exacerbation of psoriasis by ibuprofen. *Cutis* 1986; **38**: 45.

Ketoprofen

Topical application has caused photo-allergic contact dermatitis [1] and systemic ketoprofen has caused pseudoporphyria.

1 Alomar A. Ketoprofen photodermatitis. *Contact Dermatitis* 1985; **12**: 112−13.

Naproxen

The incidence of side-effects is low given the widespread and long-term use of naproxen. Rashes occur in about 5% of patients; pruritus is the commonest symptom. Naproxen is associated with a photo-sensitivity dermatitis [1] and pseudoporphyria [2−6]; most naproxen photo-urticarial reactions are evoked by the UV-A band. Urticaria/angioedema, purpura, hyperhidrosis, acneiform problems in women [7], vasculitis [8,9], vesicobullous and fixed drug eruptions [10], erythema multiforme, a pustular reaction [11] and lichen planus-like reaction [12] have all been reported.

1 Shelley WB, Elpern DJ, Shelley ED. Naproxen photosensitization demonstrated by challenge. *Cutis* 1986; **38**: 169−70.
2 Farr PM, Diffey BL. Pseudoporphyria due to naproxen. *Lancet* 1985; **i**: 1166−7.
3 Judd LE, Henderson DW, Hill DC. Naproxen-induced pseudoporphyria: A clinical and ultrastructural study. *Arch Dermatol* 1986; **122**: 451−4.
4 Mayou S, Black MM. Pseudoporphyria due to naproxen. *Br J Dermatol* 1986; **114**: 519−20.
5 Burns DA. Naproxen pseudoporphyria in a patient with vitiligo. *Clin Exp Dermatol* 1987; **12**: 296−7.
6 Levy ML, Barron KS, Eichenfield A, Honig PJ. Naproxen-induced pseudoporphyria: a distinctive photodermatitis. *J Pediatr* 1990; **117**: 660−4.
7 Hamman CO. Severe primary dysmenorrhea treated with naproxen. A prospective, double-blind crossover investigation. *Prostaglandins* 1980; **19**: 651−7.
8 Grennan DM, Jolly J, Holloway LJ, Palmer DG. Vasculitis in a patient receiving naproxen. *N Z Med J* 1979; **89**: 48−9.
9 Singhal PC, Faulkner M, Venkatesham J, Molho L. Hypersensitivity angiitis associated with naproxen. *Ann Allergy* 1989; **63**: 107−9.
10 Habbema L, Bruynzeel DP. Fixed drug eruption due to naproxen. *Dermatologica* 1987; **174**: 184−5.
11 Grattan CEH. Generalized pustular drug rash due to naproxen. *Dermatologica* 1989; **179**: 57−8.
12 Heymann WR, Lerman JS, Luftschein S. Naproxen-induced lichen planus. *J Am Acad Dermatol* 1984; **10**: 299−301.

Tiaprofenic acid

This drug may cause photosensitivity [1].

1 Neumann RA, Knobler RM, Lindemayr H. Tiaprofenic acid induced photo-sensitivity. *Contact Dermatitis* 1989; **20**: 270−3.

Phenylacetic acids

Diclofenac

A variety of cutaneous adverse effects [1,2], including pruritus, urticaria, various exanthemata, papulovesicular eruptions [3], vasculitis [4], a bullous eruption associated with linear basement membrane deposition of IgA [5], and fatal erythema multiforme [1], have been recorded.

1 Ciucci AG. A review of spontaneously reported adverse drug reactions with diclofenac sodium (voltarol). *Rheum Rehab* 1979; **Suppl 2**: 116−21.
2 O'Brien WM. Adverse reactions to nonsteroidal antiinflammatory drugs. Diclofenac compared with other nonsteroidal antiinflammatory drugs. *Am J Med* 1986; **80**: 70−80.
3 Seigneuric C, Nougué J, Plantavid M. Erythème polymorphe avec atteinte muqueuse: responsabilité du diclofénac? *Ann Dermatol Vénéréol (Paris)* 1982; **109**: 287.
4 Bonafé J-L, Mazières B, Bouteiller G. Trisymptôme de Gougerot induit par les anti-inflammatoires. Rôle du diclofénac? *Ann Dermatol Vénéréol (Paris)* 1982; **109**: 283−4.
5 Gabrielson TØ, Staerfelt F, Thune PO. Drug induced bullous dermatosis with linear IgA deposits along the basement membrane. *Acta Derm Venereol (Stockh)* 1981; **61**: 439−41.

Oxicams

Piroxicam

This drug may cause adverse cutaneous reactions in 2−3% of patients [1,2]. More than two-thirds of affected patients have photosensitivity; lesions may be vesicobullous or eczematous, and occur within 3 days of starting therapy in 50% of cases [3−10]. Photosensitivity may result from phototoxic metabolites [7]. Photocontact dermatitis developed in three patients after the application of a gel containing 0.5% proxicam. Patch tests were positive to thiomersal and thiosalicylic acid and photopatch tests with piroxicam were positive. Patch tests in patients with systemic photosensitivity to piroxicam were also positive for thiomersal and thiosalicylic acid. Contact allergic sensitivity to the latter is a marker for patients with a high risk of developing photosensitivity reactions to piroxicam [10].

Other eruptions include maculopapular [11] or lichenoid rashes, urticaria, alopecia, erythema multiforme (Fig. 7.3) [12], and vasculitis [13]. Classical fixed drug eruption [14,15] and a non-pigmenting fixed drug reaction [16] have also been reported. Piroxicam was thought to have triggered subacute lupus erythematosus in a patient with Sjögren's and seronegative arthritis [17]. Isolated case reports

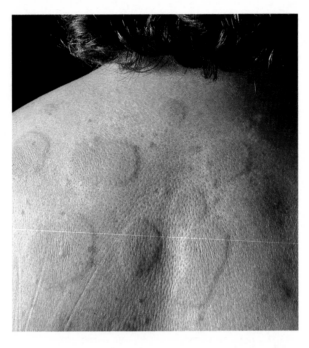

Figure 7.3 Erythema multiforme-like eruption due to piroxicam.

of fatal pemphigus vulgaris [18] and fatal toxic epidermal necrolysis (TEN) [19] have appeared. Blood dyscrasias have been reported.

1 Pitts N. Efficacy and safety of piroxicam. *Am J Med* 1982; **72** (Suppl 2A): 77−87.
2 Gerber D. Adverse reactions of piroxicam. *Drug Intell Clin Pharm* 1987; **21**: 707−10.
3 Stern RS. Phototoxic reactions to piroxicam and other nonsteroidal anti-inflammatory agents. *N Engl J Med* 1983; **309**: 186−7.
4 Diffey BL, Daymond TJ, Fairgreaves H. Phototoxic reactions to piroxicam, naproxen and tiaprofenic acid. *Br J Rheumatol* 1983; **22**: 239−42.
5 Serrano G, Bonillo J, Aliaga A, *et al*. Piroxicam-induced photosensitivity. *J Am Acad Dermatol* 1984; **11**: 113−20.
6 McKerrow KJ, Greig DE. Piroxicam-induced photosensitive dermatitis. *J Am Acad Dermatol* 1986; **15**: 1237−41.
7 Kochevar IE, Morison WL, Lamm JL, *et al*. Possible mechanism of piroxicam-induced photosensitivity. *Arch Dermatol* 1986; **122**: 1283−7.
8 Kaidbey KH, Mitchell FN. Photosensitizing potential of certain nonsteroidal anti-inflammatory agents. *Arch Dermatol* 1989; **125**: 783−6.
9 Kochevar IE. Phototoxicity of nonsteroidal inflammatory drugs. Coincidence or specific mechanism? *Arch Dermatol* 1989; **125**: 824−6.
10 Serrano G, Bonillo J, Aliaga AET, *et al*. Piroxicam-induced photosensitivity and contact sensitivity to thiosalicylic acid. *J Am Acad Dermatol* 1990; **23**: 479−83.
11 Faure M, Goujon C, Perrot H, *et al*. Accidents cutanés provoqués par le piroxicam. A propos de trois observations. *Ann Dermatol Vénéréol (Paris)* 1982; **109**: 255−8.
12 Bertail M-A, Cavelier B, Civatte J. Réaction au piroxicam (Feldène®). A type d'ectoderme érosive pluri-orificielle. *Ann Dermatol Vénéréol (Paris)* 1982 **109**: 261−2.
13 Goebel KN, Mueller-Brodman W. Reversible overt nephropathy with Henoch−Schönlein purpura due to piroxicam. *Br Med J* 1982; **284**: 311−12.
14 Stubb S, Reitamo S. Fixed drug eruption caused by piroxicam. *J Am Acad Dermatol* 1990; **22**: 1111−12.
15 de la Hoz B, Soria C, Fraj J, *et al*. Fixed drug eruption due to piroxicam. *Int J Dermatol* 1990; **29**: 672−3.

16 Valsecchi R, Cainelli T. Nonpigmenting fixed drug reaction to piroxicam. *J Am Acad Dermatol* 1989; **21**: 1300.
17 Roura M, Lopez-Gil F, Umbert P. Systemic lupus erythematosus exacerbated by piroxicam. *Dermatologica* 1991; **182**: 56–8.
18 Martin RL, McSweeny GW, Schneider J. Fatal pemphigus vulgaris in a patient taking piroxicam. *N Engl J Med* 1983; **309**: 795–6.
19 Roujeau JC, Revuz I, Touraine R, *et al*. Syndrome de Lyell au cours d'un traitement par un nouvel antiinflammatoire. *Nouv Presse Méd* 1981; **10**: 3407–8.

Anthranilic acids

Meclofenamate sodium

Rashes occur in up to 9% of patients. More than two-thirds of reactions have been exanthematous, with prominent pruritus; vasculitic, purpuric or petechial reactions are also noted, as well as occasional urticaria, fixed drug eruption, erythema multiforme [1], exfoliative erythroderma and a vesicobullous reaction. It has been reported to exacerbate psoriasis [2].

1 Harrington T, Davis D. Erythema multiforme induced by meclofenamate sodium. *J Rheumatol* 1983; **10**: 169–70.
2 Meyerhoff JO. Exacerbation of psoriasis with meclofenamate. *N Engl J Med* 1983; **309**: 496.

Mefenamic acid

Urticaria, a morbilliform eruption, fixed drug eruption [1,2] and generalized exfoliative dermatitis are documented.

1 Wilson DL, Otter A. Fixed drug eruption associated with mefenamic acid. *Br Med J* 1986; **293**: 1243.
2 Watson A, Watt G. Fixed drug eruption to mefenamic acid. *Australas J Dermatol* 1986; **27**: 6–7.

Heterocyclic acetic acids

Indomethacin

Allergic reactions are very uncommon but pruritus, urticaria, purpura and morbilliform eruptions are documented. Stomatitis [1] and thrombocytopenia occur rarely, as well as a generalized exfoliative dermatitis and TEN [2]. Vasculitis has been documented [3]. There have been rare reports of exacerbation of psoriasis [4,5]; however, indomethacin in a standard dose of 75 mg daily had no significant harmful effect on psoriasis in a series of patients treated with the Ingram regime of coal tar bath, sub-erythemal ultraviolet B phototherapy, and dithranol in Lassar's paste [6]. Exacerbation of dermatitis herpetiformis has been recorded [7].

1 Guggenheimer J, Ismail YH. Oral ulcerations associated with indomethacin therapy: report of three cases. *J Am Dent Assoc* 1975; **90**: 632–4.

2 O'Sullivan M, Hanly JG, Molloy M. A case of toxic epidermal necrolysis secondary to indomethacin. *Br J Rheumatol* 1983; **22**: 47−9.
3 Marsh FP, Almeyda JR, Levy IS. Non-thrombocytopenic purpura and acute glomerulonephritis after indomethacin therapy. *Ann Rheum Dis* 1971; **30**: 501−5.
4 Katayama H, Kawada A. Exacerbation of psoriasis induced by indomethacin. *J Dermatol (Tokyo)* 1981; **8**: 323−7.
5 Powles AV, Griffiths CEM, Seifert MH, Fry L. Exacerbation of psoriasis by indomethacin. *Br J Dermatol* 1987; **117**: 799−800.
6 Sheehan-Dare RA, Goodfield MJD, Rowell NR. The effect of oral indomethacin on psoriasis treated with the Ingram regime. *Br J Dermatol* 1991; **125**: 253−5.
7 Griffiths CEM, Leonard JN, Fry L. Dermatitis herpetiformis exacerbated by indomethacin. *Br J Dermatol* 1985; **112**: 443−5.

Sulindac

Rashes occur in up to 9% of patients. The drug has caused anaphylaxis [1] and anaphylactoid reactions [2], photosensitivity [3], facial and oral erythema, a pernio-like reaction [4] and fixed drug eruption [5]. Stevens−Johnson syndrome [6−8], TEN [6,9], serum sickness, and exfoliative erythroderma are documented. Blood dyscrasias, toxic hepatitis, pancreatitis, and aseptic meningitis in patients with SLE are recorded.

1 Smith F, Lindberg P. Life-threatening hypersensitivity to sulindac. *JAMA* 1980; **244**: 269−70.
2 Hyson CP, Kazakoff MA. A severe multisystem reaction to sunlindac. *Arch Intern Med* 1991; **151**: 387−8.
3 Jeanmougin M, Manciet J-R, Duterque M, *et al*. Photosensibilization au sulindac. *Ann Dermatol Vénéréol (Paris)* 1987; **114**: 1400−1.
4 Reinertsen J. Unusual pernio-like reaction to sulindac. *Arthritis Rheum* 1981; **24**: 1215.
5 Aram HA. Fixed drug eruption due to sulindac. *Int J Dermatol* 1984; **23**: 421.
6 Levitt L, Pearson RW. Sulindac-induced Stevens−Johnson toxic epidermal necrolysis syndrome. *JAMA* 1980; **243**: 1262−3.
7 Husain Z, Runge LA, Jabbs JM, Hyla JA. Sulindac-induced Stevens−Johnson syndrome: Report of 3 cases. *J Rheumatol* 1981; **8**: 176−9.
8 Maguire FW. Stevens−Johnson syndrome due to sulindac: a case report and review of the literature. *Del Med J* 1981; **53**: 193−7.
9 Chevrant Breton J, Pibouin M, Allain H, *et al*. Syndrome de Lyell: à propos d'uncas. *Thérapie* 1985; **40**: 67.

Tolmetin

Anaphylactoid reactions are well recognized [1]. Toxic epidermal necrolysis has been recorded.

1 Rossi A, Knapp D. Tolmetin-induced anaphylactoid reactions. *N Engl J Med* 1982; **307**: 499−500.

Pyrazolones

Amidopyrine (aminophenazone)

This is the most dangerous of all analgesics and has caused hundreds of deaths due to blood dyscrasias. It has been withdrawn from western Europe and North America but is still available in certain parts of the world. Toxic epidermal necrolysis, exfoliative dermatitis and erythema multiforme are all well known.

Azapropazone

Photosensitivity is recognized [1]. A multifocal bullous fixed drug eruption resembling erythema multiforme has been reported [2]. A bullous eruption on the face and extremities, with histological features suggestive of pemphigoid but negative immunofluorescence was reported [3]. The drug is contraindicated in patients receiving warfarin, as the latter medication is potentiated [4].

1 Olsson S, Biriell C, Boman G. Photosensitivity during treatment with azapropazone. *Br Med J* 1985; **291**: 939.
2 Sowden JM, Smith AG. Multifocal fixed drug eruption mimicking erythema multiforme. *Clin Exp Dermatol* 1990; **15**: 387–8.
3 Barker DJ, Cotterill JA. Skin eruptions due to azapropazone. *Lancet* 1977; **i**: 90.
4 Win N, Mitchell DC. Azapropazone and warfarin. *Br Med J* 1991; **302**: 969–70.

Phenylbutazone and oxyphenbutazone

Reactions have been frequent and often fatal [1,2]. Therefore, in the UK oxyphenbutazone has been withdrawn and phenylbutazone is restricted to hospital usage for ankylosing spondylitis. Pruritus, morbilliform eruptions, urticaria, and buccal ulceration are the commonest; erythema multiforme, fixed eruptions (especially with oxyphenbutazone), generalized exfoliative dermatitis, and toxic epidermal necrolysis [3] are all well-documented hazards. Drug exanthemata or erythroderma may occur in up to 4% of treated patients with phenylbutazone. Occasional reports of exacerbation of psoriasis have occurred [4]. Rarer reactions have included generalized lymphadenopathy, a Sjögren-like syndrome, nonthrombocytopenic purpura, allergic vasculitis [5] and polyarteritis nodosa. Provocation of temporal arteritis has been reported. A haemorrhagic bullous eruption of the hands was observed in three patients [6]. Cutaneous necrosis has been seen after intramuscular injection. Phenylbutazone causes fluid retention, gastrointestinal bleeding, and bone marrow depression [2]; the hazards of the latter are greatly increased if the dose exceeds 200 mg daily.

1 Van Joost T, Asghar SS, Cormane RH. Skin reactions caused by phenlybutazone. Immunologic studies. *Arch Dermatol* 1974; **110**: 929–33.
2 Inman WHW. Study of fatal bone marrow depression with special reference to phenylbutazone and oxyphenbutazone. *Br Med J* 1977; **i**: 1500–5.
3 Montgomery PR. Toxic epidermal necrolysis due to phenylbutazone. *Br J Dermatol* 1970; **83**: 220.
4 Reshad H, Hargreaves GK, Vickers CFH. Generalized pustular psoriasis precipitated by phenylbutazone and oxyphenbutazone. *Br J Dermatol* 1983; **109**: 111–13.
5 Von Paschoud J-M. Vasculitis allergica cutis durch phenylbutazon. *Dermatologica* 1966; **133**: 76–86.

6 Millard LG. A haemorrhagic bullous eruption of the hands caused by phenyl-butazone: a report of 3 cases. *Acta Derm Venereol (Stockh)* 1977; **57**: 83–6.

7.3 Miscellaneous anti-inflammatory agents

Benzydamine

Photo-allergy has been described to both topical and systemic administration of this drug [1].

1 Frosch PJ, Weickel R. Photokontaktallergie durch Benzydamin (Tantum). *Hautarzt* 1989; **40**: 771–3.

Allopurinol

Dermatological complications occur in up to 10% of cases [1–6]. Acute sensitivity reactions are well known, including scarlatiniform erythema, morbilliform rashes, urticaria or generalized exfoliative dermatitis, which may be associated with fever, eosinophilia, hepatic abnormalities and a nephropathy [2,3,5]. Alopecia [7], ichthyosis [7], vasculitis, Stevens–Johnson syndrome (Fig. 7.4) and toxic epidermal necrolysis (Fig. 7.5) [8,9] have been reported. Allopurinol potentiates the risk of a reaction to ampicillin [10]. Eruptions are commoner in the setting of impaired renal function [11] and with

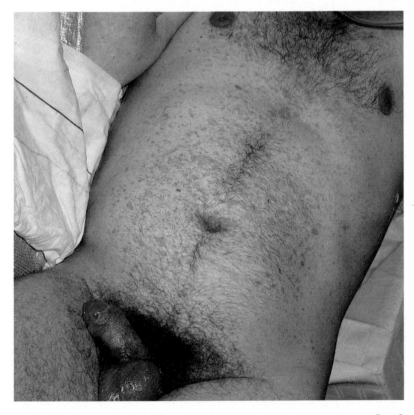

Figure 7.4 Stevens–Johnson syndrome with genital involvement due to allopurinol.

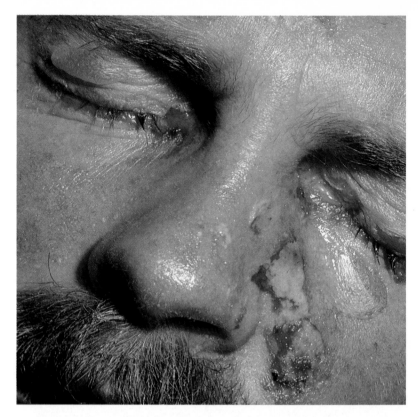

Figure 7.5 Toxic epidermal necrolysis in a patient treated with allopurinol.

concomitant thiazide therapy [12], and may first appear up to 3 weeks after the drug has been discontinued [13].

1 Rundles RW, Metz EM, Silberman HR. Allopurinol in the treatment of gout. *Ann Intern Med* 1966; **64**: 229–58.
2 Mills RM Jr. Severe hypersensitivity reactions associated with allopurinol. *JAMA* 1972; **216**: 799–802.
3 Lupton GP. The allopurinol hypersensitivity syndrome. *J Am Acad Dermatol* 1979; **1**: 365–74.
4 McInnes GT, Lawson DH, Jick H. Acute adverse reactions attributed to allopurinol in hospitalised patients. *Ann Rheum Dis* 1981; **40**: 245–9.
5 Singer JZ, Wallace SL. The allopurinol hypersensitivity syndrome. Unnecessary morbidity and mortality. *Arthritis Rheum* 1986; **29**: 82–7.
6 Foucault V, Pibouin M, Lehry D, *et al.* Accidents médicamenteux sévères et allopurinol. *Ann Dermatol Vénéréol (Paris)* 1988; **115**: 1169–72.
7 Auerbach R, Orentreich N. Alopecia and ichthyosis secondary to allopurinol. *Arch Dermatol* 1968; **98**: 104.
8 Bennett TO, Sugar J, Sahgal S. Ocular manifestations of toxic epidermal necrolysis associated with allopurinol use. *Arch Ophthalmol* 1977; **95**: 1362–4.
9 Dan M, Jedwab M, Peled M, *et al.* Allopurinol-induced toxic epidermal necrolysis. *Int J Dermatol* 1984; **23**: 142–4.
10 Jick H, Slone D, Shapiro S, *et al.* Excess of ampicillin rashes associated with allopurinol or hyperuricemia. A report from the Boston Collaborative Drug Surveillance Program, Boston University Medical Center. *N Engl J Med* 1972; **286**: 505–7.
11 Handke KR, Noone RM, Stone WJ. Severe allopurinol toxicity. Description and guidelines for prevention in patients with renal insufficiency. *Am J Med* 1984; **76**: 47–56.

12 Handke KR. Evaluation of a thiazide allopurinol drug interaction. *Am J Med Sci* 1986; **292**: 213–16.

13 Bigby M, Jick S, Jick H, Arndt K. Drug-induced cutaneous reactions. A report from the Boston Collaborative Drug Surveillance Program on 15 438 consecutive inpatients, 1975 to 1982. *JAMA* 1986; **256**: 3358–63.

Chapter 8
Drugs Acting on the
Central Nervous System

8.1 Antidepressants

Tricyclics and related compounds

Sedative, cardiovascular, anticholinergic, and gastrointestinal side-effects are well known [1,2]. Agranulocytosis may occur occasionally. Cutaneous reactions are rare [1], but include maculopapular rashes, photosensitivity (protriptyline and imipramine), urticaria, pruritus, hyperhidrosis, vasculitis or acne (maprotiline), and Lyell's syndrome (amoxaprine).

1 Gupta MA, Gupta AK, Haberman HF. Psychotropic drugs in dermatology. A review and guidelines for use. *J Am Acad Dermatol* 1986; **14**: 633–45.
2 Gupta MA, Gupta AK, Ellis CN. Antidepressant drugs in dermatology. An update. *Arch Dermatol* 1987; **123**: 647–52.

Amineptine

Severe acne [1] and rosacea [2] have been reported.

1 Thioly-Bensoussan D, Edelson Y, Cardinne A, Grupper C. Acné monstrueuse iatrogène provoquée par le Survector®: première observation mondiale à propos de deux cas. *Nouv Dermatol* 1987; **6**: 535–7.
2 Jeanmougin M, Civatte J, Cavelier-Balloy B. Toxiderme rosaceiforme a l'amineptine (Survector). *Ann Dermatol Vénéréol (Paris)* 1988; **115**: 1185–6.

Amitriptyline

A bullous reaction in a patient with overdosage of amitriptyline and chlorazepate dipotassium has been reported [1]. Alopecia is documented.

1 Herschtal D, Robinson MJ. Blisters of the skin in coma induced by amitriptyline and chlorazepate dipotassium. Report of a case with underlying sweat gland necrosis. *Arch Dermatol* 1979; **115**: 499.

Clomipramine

A photo-allergic eruption has been documented [1].

[196]

1 Ljunggren B, Bojs G. A case of photosensitivity and contact allergy to systemic tricyclic drugs, with unusual features. *Contact Dermatitis* 1991; **24**: 259−65.

Imipramine

This drug has caused urticarial or exanthematic eruptions occasionally [1] and agranulocytosis has occurred. Oedema of the feet is seen in older people. Glossitis and stomatitis are rare, as are transient erythema of the face, photosensitivity and exfoliative dermatitis. Slate-grey pigmentation of exposed skin may develop; golden-yellow granules, which ultrastructurally are electron dense inclusion bodies in phagocytes, fibroblasts and dendrocytes, are seen in the papillary dermis [2]. Cutaneous vasculitis is well documented.

1 Almeyda J. Drug reactions XIII. Cutaneous reactions to imipramine and chlordiazepoxide. *Br J Dermatol* 1971; **84**: 298−9.
2 Hashimoto K, Joselow SA, Tye MJ. Imipramine hyperpigmentation: A slate-gray discoloration caused by long-term imipramine administration. *J Am Acad Dermatol* 1991; **25**: 357−61.

Maprotiline

Acne [1] and vasculitis [2] are recorded.

1 Ponte CD. Maprotiline-induced acne. *Am J Psychiatry* 1982; **139**: 141.
2 Oakley AM, Hodge L. Cutaneous vasculitis from maprotiline. *Aust N Z J Med* 1985; **15**: 256−7.

Mianserin

Erythema multiforme has recently been reported [1].

1 Quraishy E. Erythema multiforme during treatment with mianserin. *Br J Dermatol* 1981; **104**: 481.

Trazodone

This drug has caused leuconychia [1], erythema multiforme [2], and vasculitis [3], and has been implicated in causing a psoriasiform eruption.

1 Longstreth GF, Hershman J. Trazodone-induced hepatotoxicity and leukonychia. *J Am Acad Dermatol* 1985; **13**: 149−50.
2 Ford HE, Jenike MA. Erythema multiforme associated with trazadone therapy. *J Clin Psychiatry* 1985; **46**: 294−5.
3 Mann SC, Walker MM, Messenger GG, *et al*. Leukocytoclastic vasculitis secondary to trazodone treatment. *J Am Acad Dermatol* 1984; **10**: 669−70.

Monoamine-oxidase inhibitors

Iproniazid

Vasculitis and peripheral neuritis are documented.

Phenelzine

Hypersensitivity skin reactions are rare.

Lithium

Skin reactions [1—5] are relatively uncommon. Pustular and psoriasiform lesions induced by this drug have received particular attention. The pustular propensities of lithium have been attributed to lysosomal enzyme release and increased neutrophil chemotaxis [2]. Tetracycline should be avoided in treating these pustular eruptions as it may precipitate serious lithium toxicity. The acneiform 'erysipelas' eruption consists of monomorphic pustules on an erythematous base, tends to affect mainly the arms and legs, is not associated with comedones or cystic lesions, and may be very persistent. Various patterns of folliculitis may occur. Lithium can aggravate pre-existing psoriasis, making it more difficult to control [6—9], and may precipitate a palmoplantar pustular reaction [10] or even generalized pustular psoriasis [11]. Psychiatrists should avoid the use of lithium in psoriatics if possible. Darier's disease may also be exacerbated [12].

Additional reactions described include morbilliform rashes, erythema multiforme [13], a dermatitis herpetiformis-like rash [14], linear IgA bullous dermatosis [15], and a generalized exfoliative eruption [16]. A lupus erythematosus-like syndrome [17] with increased prevalence of antinuclear antibodies [18], toe nail dystrophy [19] and hair loss [20,21] have been reported. None of these effects is related to excessive blood levels of lithium or other evidence of toxicity.

1 Callaway CL, Hendrie HC, Luby ED. Cutaneous conditions observed in patients during treatment with lithium. *Am J Psychiatry* 1968; **124**: 1124—5.
2 Heng MCY. Cutaneous manifestations of lithium toxicity. *Br J Dermatol* 1982; **106**: 107—9.
3 Deandrea D, Walker N, Mehlmauer M, White K. Dermatological reactions to lithium: A review. *J Clin Psychopharmacol* 1982; **2**: 199—204.
4 Sarantidis D, Waters B. A review and controlled study of cutaneous conditions associated with lithium carbonate. *Br J Psychiatry* 1983; **143**: 42—50.
5 Albrecht G. Unerwünschte Wirkungen von Lithium an der Haut. *Hautarzt* 1985; **36**: 77—82.
6 Lazarus GS, Gilgor RS. Psoriasis, polymorphonuclear leukocytes, and lithium carbonate. An important clue. *Arch Dermatol* 1979; **115**: 1183—4.
7 Skoven I, Thormann J. Lithium compound treatment and psoriasis. *Arch Dermatol* 1979; **115**: 1185—7.
8 Abel EA, Dicicco LM, Orenberg EK, *et al*. Drugs in exacerbation of psoriasis. *J Am Acad Dermatol* 1986; **15**: 1007—22.
9 Sasaki T, Saito S, Aihara M, *et al*. Exacerbation of psoriasis during lithium treatment. *J Dermatol (Tokyo)* 1989; **16**: 59—63.
10 White SW. Palmoplantar pustular psoriasis provoked by lithium therapy. *J Am Acad Dermatol* 1982; **7**: 660—2.
11 Lowe NJ, Ridgway HB. Generalized pustular psoriasis precipitated by lithium. *Arch Dermatol* 1978; **114**: 1788—9.
12 Milton GP, Peck GL, Ru J-J, *et al*. Exacerbation of Darier's disease by lithium carbonate. *J Am Acad Dermatol* 1990; **23**: 926—8.

13 Balldin J, Berggren U, Heijer A, Mobacken H. Erythema multiforme caused by lithium. *J Am Acad Dermatol* 1991; **24**: 1015–16.

14 Meinhold JM, West DP, Gurwich E, *et al.* Cutaneous reaction to lithium carbonate: a case report. *J Clin Psychiatry* 1980; **41**: 395–6.

15 McWhirter JD, Hashimoto K, Fayne S, *et al.* Linear IgA bullous dermatosis related to lithium carbonate. *Arch Dermatol* 1987; **123**: 1120–2.

16 Kuhnley EJ, Granoff AL. Exfoliative dermatitis during lithium treatment. *Am J Psychiatry* 1979; **136**: 1340–1.

17 Shukla VR, Borison RL. Lithium and lupuslike syndrome. *JAMA* 1982; **248**: 921–2.

18 Presley AP, Kahn A, Williamson N. Antinuclear antibodies in patients on lithium carbonate. *Br Med J* 1976; **ii**: 280–1.

19 Hooper JF. Lithium carbonate and toenails. *Am J Psychiatry* 1981; **138**: 1519.

20 Dawber R, Mortimer P. Hair loss during lithium treatment. *Br J Dermatol* 1982; **107**: 124–5.

21 Orwin A. Hair loss following lithium therapy. *Br J Dermatol* 1983; **108**: 503–4.

8.2 Hypnotics, sedatives and anxiolytics

Barbiturates

A toxic bullous eruption may appear at pressure points in comatose patients after overdosage [1–4]. In one series, 7.8% of patients admitted with drug-induced coma had such bullae [3]. The bullae are few, large (Fig. 8.1) and may lead to ulceration [2]. Necrotic lesions are seen in 4% of patients recovering from, and in 40% of fatalities related to, a barbiturate-induced coma [4]. Allergic reactions are very uncommon and may be scarlatiniform or morbilliform. Exfoliative dermatitis has proved fatal [5], as has erythema multiforme. Urticaria and serum sickness are very rare as is purpuric capillaritis. Fixed eruptions are well known [6] and particularly occur on the glans penis. Toxic epidermal necrolysis, lupus-like syndrome, purpura, and photosensitivity are recorded [7].

1 Beveridge GW, Lawson AAH. Occurrence of bullous lesions in acute barbiturate intoxication. *Br Med J* 1965; **i**: 835–7.

2 Gröschel D, Gerstein AR, Rosenbaum JM. Skin lesions as a diagnostic aid in barbiturate poisoning. *N Engl J Med* 1970; **283**: 409–10.

3 Pinkus NB. Skin eruptions in drug-induced coma. *Med J Aust* 1971; **2**: 886–8.

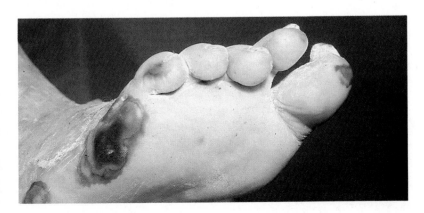

Figure 8.1 Necrotic bullae at pressure points in a patient who took an overdose of barbiturate.

4 Almeyda J, Levantine A. Drug reactions XVII. Cutaneous reactions to barbiturates, chloralhydrate and its derivatives. *Br J Dermatol* 1972; **86**: 313–16.
5 Sneddon IB, Leishman AWD. Severe and fatal phenobarbitone eruptions. *Br Med J* 1952; **i**: 1276–8.
6 Korkij W, Soltani K. Fixed drug eruption. A brief review. *Arch Dermatol* 1984; **120**: 520–4.
7 Gupta MA, Gupta AK, Haberman HF. Psychotropic drugs in dermatology. A review and guidelines for use. *J Am Acad Dermatol* 1986; **14**: 633–45.

Benzodiazepines

Allergic reactions are very rare [1].

Alprazolam

Photosensitivity has been recorded with this newer benzodiazepine [2].

Chlordiazepoxide

Morbilliform erythema, urticaria [3], fixed eruption [4], photo-allergic eczema [5] and exacerbation of porphyria have been recorded. Erythema multiforme and chronic pigmented purpuric eruption occur rarely [6].

Lormetazepam

A fixed drug eruption has been reported [7].

Diazepam and nitrazepam

Bullae similar to those seen after barbiturates may occur in comatose patients after overdosage [8,9]. Thrombophlebitis may follow intravenous injection of diazepam [10]. Hyperpigmentation in previously dermabraded scars has been attributed to diazepam [11]. An eruption comprising oedema, moon face, and generalized erythema, with erosions of cheeks, axillae and the genitocrural area was attributed to nitrazepam; a provocation test was positive [12].

Temazepam

An extensive fixed drug reaction has been reported [13]. Extravasation following attempted femoral vein injection of a suspension of the contents of capsules in tap water, by an addict, resulted in extensive necrosis of genital and pubic skin [14].

1 Edwards JG. Adverse effects of antianxiety drugs. *Drugs* 1981; **22**: 495–514.
2 Kanwar AJ, Gupta R, Das Mehta S, Kaur S. Photosensitivity to alprazolam. *Dermatologica* 1990; **181**: 75.
3 Almeyda J. Drug reactions XIII. Cutaneous reactions to imipramine and chlordiazepoxide. *Br J Dermatol* 1971; **84**: 298–9.

4 Blair HM III. Fixed drug eruption from chlordiazepoxide: report of a case. *Arch Dermatol* 1974; **109**: 914.

5 Luton EF, Finchum RN. Photosensitivity reaction to chlordiazepoxide. *Arch Dermatol* 1965; **91**: 362−3.

6 Nishioka K, Katayama I, Masuzawa M, *et al*. Drug-induced chronic pigmented purpura. *J Dermatol (Tokyo)* 1989; **16**: 220−2.

7 Jafferany M, Haroon TS. Fixed drug eruption with lormetazepam (Noctamid). *Dermatologica* 1988; **177**: 386.

8 Ridley CM. Bullous lesions in nitrazepam-overdosage. *Br Med J* 1971; **iii**: 28.

9 Varma AJ, Fisher BK, Sarin MK. Diazepam-induced coma with bullae and eccrine sweat gland necrosis. *Arch Intern Med* 1977; **137**: 1207−10.

10 Langdon DE, Harlan JR, Bailey RL. Thrombophlebitis with diazepam used intravenously. *JAMA* 1973; **223**: 184−5.

11 Fereira JA, The role of diazepam in skin hyperpigmentation. *Aesthetic Plast Surg* 1980; **4**: 343−8.

12 Shoji A, Kitajima J, Hamada T. Drug eruption caused by nitrazepam in a patient with severe pustular psoriasis successfully treated with methotrexate and etretinate. *J Dermatol (Tokyo)* 1987; **14**: 274−8.

13 Archer CB, English JSC. Extensive fixed drug eruption induced by temazepam. *Clin Exp Dermatol* 1988; **13**: 336−8.

14 Meshikhes AN, Duthie JS. Untitled report. *Br Med J* 1991; **303**: 478.

Miscellaneous drugs

Carbromal

This drug, now rarely used, commonly produced a characteristic capillaritis with punctate purpura and haemosiderin giving a golden-brown discoloration of the skin, especially on the legs [1].

Chloral hydrate

Hypersensitivity reactions are very rare. Chloral is now virtually given only in tablet form as dichloralphenazone, in which the phenazone may cause a fixed eruption [2].

Ethchlorvynol

Overdose has caused bullous lesions [3].

Glutethimide

Dermographism with subsequent erythema, and vesicles which lasted several days, were reported in one comatose patient [4], and bullae in another patient [5] following overdosage. Fixed eruptions are recorded [6].

Meprobamate

Anorexia, drowsiness, dizziness, flushing and gastrointestinal symptoms may occur, especially with high doses. Fixed eruptions may occur [7]. The most characteristic cutaneous reaction, preceded by itching, malaise and fever, is an erythema, starting in the limb flexures which rapidly gives way to a fierce non-thrombocytopenic purpura [8]. A widespread toxic erythema was associated with an anaphylactoid reaction, in a patient in whom patch testing proved useful in diagnosis [9].

1 Peterson WC Jr, Manick KP. Purpuric eruptions associated with use of carbromal and meprobamate. *Arch Dermatol* 1967; **95**: 40−2.
2 McCulloch H, Zeligman I. Fixed drug eruption and epididymitis due to antipyrine. *Arch Dermatol Syphilol* 1951; **64**: 198−9.
3 Brodin MD, Redmond WJ. Bullous eruptions due to Ethchlorvynol. *J Cutan Pathol* 1980; **7**: 326−9.
4 Leavell UW Jr, Coyer JR, Taylor RJ. Dermographism and erythematous lines in glutethimide overdose. *Arch Dermatol* 1972; **106**: 724−5.
5 Burdon JGW, Cade JF. 'Barbiturate burns' caused by glutethimide. *Med J Aust* 1979; **1**: 101−2.
6 Fisher M, Lerman JS. Fixed eruption due to glutethimide. *Arch Dermatol* 1971; **104**: 87−9.
7 Gore HC Jr. Fixed drug eruption cross reaction of meprobamate and carisoprodol. *Arch Dermatol* 1965; **91**: 627.
8 Levan NE. Meprobamate reaction. *Arch Dermatol* 1957; **75**: 437−8.
9 Felix RH, Comaish JS. The value of patch and other skin tests in drug eruptions. *Lancet* 1974; **i**: 1017−19.

8.3 Antipsychotics

The most important clinical side-effects include those on the central nervous and cardiovascular systems and the ocular effects [1,2]. Drugs with high potency such as haloperidol and pimozide, tend to have fewer cardiovascular and anticholinergic effects and are less sedating, but have more neurological effects. Long-term use of antipsychotic agents results in tardive dyskinesia.

Phenothiazines

The side-effects of this group of drugs have been reviewed [1−4].

Chlorpromazine

This drug is still widely used, but many related compounds are now available. Pigmentation of the skin in light-exposed areas after chronic usage may be a problem, especially in women and Negroes [5−11]. Rarely, a purplish or slate-grey pigmentation develops [6]. There may be brown discoloration of cornea and lens [5] and bulbar conjunctiva [7]. Chlorpromazine has an affinity for melanin *in vitro* [8]. Electron microscopy shows many melanosome complexes within lysosomes of dermal macrophages, and electron dense 'chlorpromazine bodies' in macrophages, endothelial cells, and Schwann cells [9,10]; energy-dispersive X-ray microanalysis has revealed the abundant presence of sulphur in these granules, found in the chlorpromazine molecule [10]. Similar pigmentary deposits are found in internal organs [11] and in blood neutrophils and monocytes.

Chlorpromazine has caused lichenoid eruptions [12], exfoliative dermatitis, erythema multiforme, a lupus-like illness [13] with positive antinuclear factor [14] and the lupus anticoagulant [15], and Henoch−Schönlein vasculitis [16]. Phototoxicity is well known [17−19] and phenothiazine-derived antihistamines may cause photosensitivity in atopics and subsequent development of actinic reticuloid [19]. Photocontact urticaria has been documented [20]. Cholestatic jaundice is an important hazard.

Fluspirilene

Subcutaneous nodules may develop at injection sites after long-term high doses of this depot preparation [21].

Thiothixene

A sensitivity reaction has been recorded [22].

Trifluoperazine

A fixed eruption has been recorded [23].

Loxapine

Dermatitis, pruritus and seborrhoea have been recorded, and photosensitivity eruptions may occur occasionally [24].

Levomepromazin

An erythema annulare centrifugum-like pseudolymphomatous eruption has been reported [25].

1 Simpson GM, Pi EH, Sramek JJ Jr. Adverse effects of antipsychotic agents. *Drugs* 1981; **21**: 138−51.
2 Gupta MA, Gupta AK, Haberman HF. Psychotropic drugs in dermatology. A review and guidelines for use. *J Am Acad Dermatol* 1986; **14**: 633−45.
3 Hägermark Ö, Wennersten G, Almeyda J: Drug reactions XIV. Cutaneous side effects of phenothiazines. *Br J Dermatol* 1971; **84**: 605−7.
4 Bond WS, Yee GC. Ocular and cutaneous effects of chronic phenothiazine therapy. *Am J Hosp Pharm* 1980; **37**: 74−8.
5 Greiner AC, Berry K. Skin pigmentation and corneal and lens opacities with prolonged chlorpromazine therapy. *Can Med Assoc J* 1964; **90**: 663−5.
6 Hays GB, Lyle CB Jr, Wheeler CE Jr. Slate-grey color in patients receiving chlorpromazine. *Arch Dermatol* 1964; **90**: 471−6.
7 Satanove A. Pigmentation due to phenothiazines in high and prolonged dosage. *JAMA* 1965; **191**: 263−8.
8 Blois MS Jr. On chlorpromazine binding *in vivo*. *J Invest Dermatol* 1965; **45**: 475−81.
9 Hashimoto K, Wiener W, Albert J, Nelson RG. An electron microscopic study of chlorpromazine pigmentation. *J Invest Dermatol* 1966; **47**: 296−306.
10 Benning TL, McCormack KM, Ingram P, *et al*. Microprobe analysis of chlorpromazine pigmentation. *Arch Dermatol* 1988; **124**: 1541−4.
11 Greiner AC, Nicolson GA. Pigment deposition in viscera associated with

prolonged chlorpromazine therapy. *Can Med Assoc J* 1964; **90**: 627–35.

12 Matsuo I, Ozawa A, Niizuma K, Ohkido M. Lichenoid dermatitis due to chlorpromazine phototoxicity. *Dermatologica* 1979; **159**: 46–9.

13 Pavlidakey GP, Hashimoto K, Heller GL, Daneshvar S. Chlorpromazine-induced lupuslike disease: Case report and review of the literature. *J Am Acad Dermatol* 1985; **13**: 109–115.

14 Zarrabi MH, Zucker S, Miller F, *et al.* Immunologic and coagulation disorders in chlorpromazine-treated patients. *Ann Intern Med* 1979; **91**: 194–9.

15 Canoso RT, Sise HS. Chlorpromazine-induced lupus anticoagulant and associated immunologic abnormalities. *Am J Hematol* 1982; **13**: 121–9.

16 Aram H. Henoch–Schönlein purpura associated induced by chlorpromazine. *J Am Acad Dermatol* 1987; **17**: 139–40.

17 Johnson BE. Cellular mechanisms of chlorpromazine photosensitivity. *Proc R Soc Med* 1974; **67**: 871–3.

18 Ljunggren B. Phenothiazine phototoxicity: toxic chlorpromazine photoproducts. *J Invest Dermatol* 1977; **69**: 383–6.

19 Amblard P, Beani J-C, Reymond J-L. Photo-allergie rémanente aux phénothiazines chez l'atopique. *Ann Dermatol Vénéréol (Paris)* 1982; **109**: 225–8.

20 Lovell CR, Cronin E, Rhodes EL. Photocontact urticaria from chlorpromazine. *Contact Dermatitis* 1986; **14**: 290–1.

21 UK Committee of Safety of Medicines. *Current Problems* 1981; No. 7.

22 Matsuoka LY. Thiothixene drug sensitivity. *J Am Acad Dermatol* 1982; **7**: 405–6.

23 Kanwar AJ, Singh M, El-Sheriff AK, Belhaj MS. Fixed eruption due to trifluoperazine hydrochloride. *Br J Dermatol* 1987; **117**: 798–9.

24 Anonymous. Cloxapine and loxapine for schizophrenia. *Drug Ther Bull* 1991; **29**: 41–2.

25 Blazejak T, Hölzle E. Phenothiazin-induziertes Pseudolymphom. *Hautarzt* 1990; **41**: 161–3.

8.4 Drugs for alcoholism

Cyanamide

This inhibitor of alcohol dehydrogenase, used in the treatment of alcoholism, has been implicated in the development of a lichen planus-like eruption with oesophageal involvement [1].

1 Torrelo A, Soria C, Rocamora A, *et al.* Lichen planus-like eruption with esophageal involvement as a result of cyanamide. *J Am Acad Dermatol* 1990; **23**: 1168–9.

Disulfiram

This drug causes vasomotor flushing, morbilliform rash, and urticaria, as well as eczema in patients sensitized to rubber; it cross-reacts with rubber [1–3]. A toxic pustular eruption is recorded [4].

1 Webb PK, Gibbs SC, Mathias CT, *et al.* Disulfiram hypersensitivity and rubber contact dermatitis. *JAMA* 1979; **241**: 2061.

2 Fischer AA. Dermatologic aspects of disulfiram use. *Cutis* 1982; **30**: 461–524.

3 Minet A, Frankart M, Eggers S, *et al.* Réactions allergiques aux implants de disulfirame. *Ann Dermatol Vénéréol (Paris)* 1989; **116**: 543–45.

4 Larbre B, Larbre JP, Nicolas JF, *et al.* Toxicodermie pustuleuse au disulfirame. A propos d'un cas. *Ann Dermatol Vénéréol (Paris)* 1990; **117**: 721–22.

8.5 Anticonvulsants

There may be cross-reactivity in terms of clinical reactions to the aromatic anticonvulsants (phenytoin, phenobarbital, carbamazepine); arene oxide metabolites may be involved in the pathogenesis of these eruptions [1]. Sodium valproate may be substituted safely.

1 Shear N, Spielberg S. Anticonvulsant hypersensitivity syndrome. *In vitro* assessment of risk. *J Clin Invest* 1989; **82**: 1826–32.

Carbamazepine

Eruptions occur in about 3% of patients and include erythematous (Figs 8.2 & 8.3), morbilliform, urticarial or purpuric (Fig. 8.4) rashes [1–4]. Toxic epidermal necrolysis and exfoliative dermatitis are

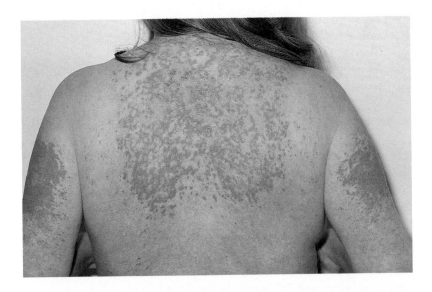

Figure 8.2 Erythematous eruption due to carbamazepine.

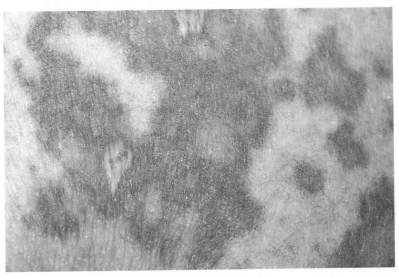

Figure 8.3 Close-up view of carbamazepine eruption demonstrating pustulation within erythematous area.

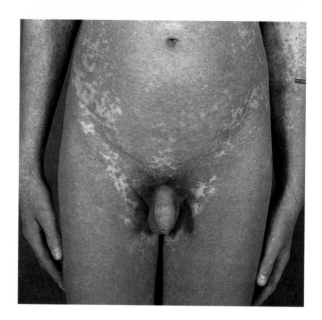

Figure 8.4 Purpuric erythroderma caused by carbamazepine.

well recognized [2,3,5]. Eczema and photosensitivity [6], a lupus erythematosus-like syndrome, dermatomyositis and erythema multiforme [7], as well as a pustular [8,9] and a lichenoid reaction [2,10] are very rare. Lesions with clinical and histological features suggestive of mycosis fungoides have been reported [11,12]. Patch testing has been advocated for the diagnosis of carbamazepine eruptions [13,14], but has resulted in re-induction of exfoliative dermatitis [15]. Desensitization has been achieved by oral induction of tolerance in a patient in whom there was no suitable alternative therapy [16]. Other adverse effects include nausea, vomiting, ataxia, vertigo and drowsiness. Abnormal liver function [17] and bone marrow suppression with occasional deaths due to aplastic anaemia have been recorded [2]. Development of a rash may act as an early warning of marrow toxicity. Carbamazepine therapy during pregnancy carries a 1% risk of development of spina bifida in the offspring [18].

1 Harman PRM. Carbamazepine (Tegretol) drug eruptions. *Br J Dermatol* 1967; **79**: 500−1.
2 Roberts DL, Marks R. Skin reactions to carbamazepine. *Arch Dermatol* 1981; **117**: 273−5.
3 Breathnach SM, McGibbon DH, Ive FA, *et al.* Carbamazepine ('Tegretol') and toxic epidermal necrolysis: report of three cases with histopathological observations. *Clin Exp Dermatol* 1982; **7**: 585−91.
4 Chadwick D, Shan M, Foy P, *et al.* Serum anticonvulsant concentrations and the risk of drug-induced skin eruptions. *J Neurol Neurosurg Psychiatry* 1984; **47**: 642−4.
5 Reed MD, Bertino JA, Blumer JL. Carbamazepine-associated exfoliative dermatitis. *Clin Pharmacol* 1982; **1**: 78−9.
6 Terui T, Tagami H. Eczematous drug eruption from carbamazepine: coexistence of contact and photocontact sensitivity. *Contact Dermatitis* 1989; **20**: 260−4.

7 Simpson JR. 'Collagen disease' due to carbamazepine (Tegretol). *Br Med J* 1966; **ii**: 1434.
8 Staughton RCD, Harper JI, Rowland Payne CME, *et al*. Toxic pustuloderma: a new entity? *J R Soc Med* 1984; **77**: 6–8.
9 Commens CA, Fischer GO. Toxic pustuloderma following carbamazepine therapy. *Arch Dermatol* 1988; **124**: 178–9.
10 Atkin SL, McKenzie TMM, Stevenson CJ. Carbamazepine-induced lichenoid eruption. *Clin Exp Dermatol* 1990; **15**: 382–3.
11 Welykyj S, Gradini R, Nakao J, Massa M. Carbamazepine-induced eruption histologically mimicking mycosis fungoides. *J Cutan Pathol* 1990; **17**: 111–16.
12 Rijlaarsdam U, Scheffer E, Meijer CJLM, *et al*. Mycosis fungoides-like lesions associated with phenytoin and carbamazepine therapy. *J Am Acad Dermatol* 1991; **24**: 216–20.
13 Houwerzijl J, De Gast GC, Nater JP, *et al*. Lymphocyte-stimulation tests and patch tests in carbamazepine hypersensitivity. *Clin Exp Immunol* 1977; **29**: 272–7.
14 Silva R, Machado A, Brandao M, Gonçalo S. Patch test diagnosis in carbamazepine erythroderma. *Contact Dermatitis* 1986; **15**: 254–5.
15 Vaillant L, Camenen I, Lorette G. Patch testing with carbamazepine: reinduction of an exfoliative dermatitis. *Arch Dermatol* 1989; **125**: 299.
16 Eames P. Adverse reaction to carbamazepine managed by desensitization. *Lancet* 1989; **i**: 509–10.
17 Ramsey ID. Carbamazepine induced jaundice. *Br Med J* 1967; **4**: 155.
18 Rosa FW. Spina bifida in infants of women treated with carbamazepine during pregnancy. *N Engl J Med* 1991; **324**: 674–7.

Diphenylhydantoin (phenytoin)

Cutaneous manifestations related to phenytoin have been reviewed [1,2]. About 5% of children develop a mild transient maculopapular rash within 3 weeks of starting treatment. This is more likely to occur if high loading doses are given initially [3,4]. In other series, between 8.5% [5] and 19% [6] of patients receiving phenytoin developed exanthematic rashes [7].

A phenytoin-induced hypersensitivity state, with generalized lymphadenopathy, hepatosplenomegaly, fever, arthralgia, and eosinophilia, occurs in about 1% of patients, and may be accompanied by hepatitis, nephritis, pneumonitis, and haematological abnormalities [8–10]. Skin involvement may lead to a suspicion of lymphoma, the phenytoin-induced pseudolymphoma syndrome [11–16]. Cutaneous lesions may be restricted to a few erythematous plaques [15], or cutaneous nodules [12], or consist of a generalized erythematous maculopapular rash [11], generalized exfoliative dermatitis [13,17], or toxic epidermal necrolysis (TEN) [18]. Generalized pustulation has been recorded as a manifestation of the anticonvulsant hypersensitivity syndrome [19]. Universal depigmentation has resulted from TEN [20]. Cutaneous histopathology in the pseudolymphoma syndrome is often indistinguishable from that of mycosis fungoides, with infiltrating cells having cerebriform nuclei and Pautrier microabscesses [14,16]. The rash resolves after cessation of the drug. However, there is a three-fold risk of true lymphoma on long-term therapy [21,22], and T-cell lymphoma has been reported in an adult [23].

Long-term treatment causes fibroblast proliferation, and may

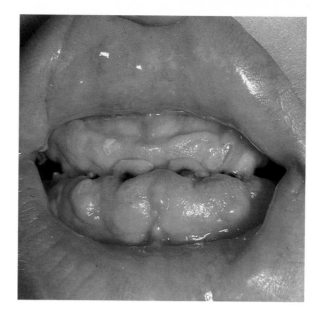

Figure 8.5 Marked gingival hyperplasia caused by long-term phenytoin.

result in dose-dependent gingival hyperplasia (Fig. 8.5) [24,25] or coarsening of the features [26]; hypertrophic retro-auricular folds were reported in an isolated case [27]. Hypertrichosis may be seen. Other reactions have included fixed eruptions [28], including a widespread fixed drug eruption mimicking TEN [29], erythema multiforme [1,3], TEN with cholestasis [30], cutaneous vasculitis [31], a lupus-like syndrome [32], and eosinophilic fasciitis [33]. Delayed bluish discoloration, erythema and oedema, sometimes with bullae, has occurred distal to the site of intravenous injection [34].

Treatment during pregnancy may lead to a characteristic 'fetal syndrome', with general underdevelopment and hypoplasia of phalanges and nails [35] and neonatal acne [36]. Recent controlled observations suggest that acne is neither caused nor worsened by hydantoins [37], despite reports to the contrary [38].

1 Silverman AK, Fairley J, Wong RC. Cutaneous and immunologic reactions to phenytoin. *J Am Acad Dermatol* 1988; **18**: 721–41.
2 Levantine A, Almeyda J. Drug reactions XX. Cutaneous reactions to anticonvulsants. *Br J Dermatol* 1972; **87**: 646–9.
3 Pollack MA, Burk PG, Nathanson G. Mucocutaneous eruptions due to anti epileptic drug therapy in children. *Ann Neurol* 1979; **5**: 262–7.
4 Wilson JT, Höjer B, Tomson G, *et al.* High incidence of a concentration-dependent skin reaction in children treated with phenytoin. *Br Med J* 1978; **i**: 1583–6.
5 Leppik IE, Lapora A, Loewenson R. Seasonal incidence of phenytoin allergy unrelated to plasma levels. *Arch Neurol* 1985; **42**: 120–2.
6 Rapp RP, Norton JA, Young B, Tibbs PA. Cutaneous reactions in head-injured patients receiving phenytoin for seizure prophylaxis. *Neurosurgery* 1983; **13**: 272–5.
7 Robinson HM, Stone JH. Exanthem due to diphenylhydantoin therapy. *Arch Dermatol* 1970; **101**: 462–5.
8 Stanley J, Fallon-Pellici V. Phenytoin hypersensitivity reaction. *Arch Dermatol* 1978; **114**: 1350–3.

9 Brown M, Schubert T. Phenytoin hypersensitivity hepatitis and mono-nucleosis syndrome. *J Clin Gastroenterol* 1986; **8**: 469−77.

10 Shear N, Spielberg S. Anticonvulsant hypersensitivity syndrome. *In vitro* assessment of risk. *J Clin Invest* 1989; **82**: 1826−32.

11 Charlesworth EN. Phenytoin-induced pseudolymphoma syndrome. An immunologic study. *Arch Dermatol* 1977; **113**: 477−80.

12 Adams JD. Localized cutaneous pseudolymphoma associated with phenytoin therapy: A case report. *Australas J Dermatol* 1981; **22**: 28−9.

13 Rosenthal CJ, Noguera CA, Coppola A, Kapelner SN. Pseudolymphoma with mycosis fungoides manifestations, hyperresponsiveness to diphenylhydantoin, and lymphocyte disregulation. *Cancer* 1982; **49**: 2305−14.

14 Kardaun SH, Scheffer E, Vermeer BJ. Drug-induced pseudolymphomatous skin reactions. *Br J Dermatol* 1988; **118**: 545−52.

15 Wolf R, Kahane E, Sandbank M. Mycosis fungoides-like lesions associated with phenytoin therapy. *Arch Dermatol* 1985; **121**: 1181−2.

16 Rijlaarsdam U, Scheffer E, Meijer CJLM, *et al*. Mycosis fungoides-like lesions associated with phenytoin and carbamazepine therapy. *J Am Acad Dermatol* 1991; **24**: 216−20.

17 Danno K, Kume M, Ohta M, *et al*. Erythroderma with generalized lymphadenopathy induced by phenytoin. *J Dermatol (Tokyo)* 1989; **16**: 392−6.

18 Sherertz EF, Jegasothy BV, Lazarus GS. Phenytoin hypersensitivity reaction presenting with toxic epidermal necrolysis and severe hepatitis: report of a patient treated with corticosteroid 'pulse therapy'. *J Am Acad Dermatol* 1985; **12**: 178−81.

19 Kleier RS, Breneman DL, Boiko S. Generalized pustulation as a manifestation of the anticonvulsant hypersensitivity syndrome. *Arch Dermatol* 1991; **127**: 1361−4.

20 Smith DA, Burgdorf WHC. Universal cutaneous depigmentation following phenytoin-induced toxic epidermal necrolysis. *J Am Acad Dermatol* 1984; **10**: 106−9.

21 Tashima CK, De Los Santos R. Lymphoma and anticonvulsant therapy. *JAMA* 1974; **228**: 287−8.

22 Bichel J. Hydantoin derivatives and malignancies of the haemopoietic system. *Acta Med Scand* 1975; **198**: 327−8.

23 Isobe T, Horimatsu T, Fujita T, *et al*. Adult T cell lymphoma following diphenylhydantoin therapy. *Acta Haematol Jpn* 1980; **43**: 711−14.

24 Angelopoulos AP, Goaz PW. Incidence of diphenylhydantoin gingival hyperplasia. *Oral Surg* 1972; **34**: 898−906.

25 Hassell TM, Page RC, Narayanan AS, Cooper CG. Diphenylhydantoin (Dilantin) gingival hyperplasia: drug induced abnormality of connective tissue. *Proc Natl Acad Sci* 1976; **73**: 2909−12.

26 Lefebvre EB, Haining RG, Labbé RF. Coarse facies, calvarial thickening and hyperphosphatasia associated with long-term anticonvulsant therapy. *N Engl J Med* 1972; **286**: 1301−2.

27 Trunnell TN, Waisman M. Hypertrophic retroauricular folds attributable to diphenylhydantoin. *Cutis* 1982; **30**: 207−9.

28 Sweet RD. Fixed skin eruption due to phenytoin sodium. *Lancet* 1950; **i**: 68.

29 Baird BJ, De Villez RL. Widespread bullous fixed drug eruption mimicking toxic epidermal necrolysis. *Int J Dermatol* 1988; **27**: 170−4.

30 Spechler SJ, Sperber H, Doos WG, Koff RS. Cholestasis and toxic epidermal necrolysis associated with phenytoin sodium ingestion: the role of bile duct injury. *Ann Intern Med* 1981; **95**: 455−6.

31 Yermakov VM, Hitti IF, Sutton AL. Necrotizing vasculitis associated with diphenylhydantoin: two fatal cases. *Hum Pathol* 1983; **14**: 182−4.

32 Gleichman H. Systemic lupus erythematosus triggered by diphenylhydantoin. *Arthritis Rheum* 1982; **25**: 1387−8.

33 Buchanan RR, Gordon DA, Muckle TJ, *et al*. The eosinophilic fasciitis syndrome after phenytoin (Dilantin) therapy. *J Rheumatol* 1980; **7**: 733−6.

34 Kilarski DJ, Buchanan C, Von Behren L. Soft tissue damage associated with intravenous phenytoin. *N Engl J Med* 1984; **311**: 1186−7.

35 Nagy R. Fetal hydantoin syndrome. *Arch Dermatol* 1981; **117**: 593−5.

36 Stankler L, Campbell AGM. Neonatal acne vulgaris: A possible feature of the fetal hydantoin syndrome. *Br J Dermatol* 1980; **103**: 453–5.
37 Greenwood R, Fenwick PBC, Cunliffe WJ. Acne and anticonvulsants. *Br Med J* 1983; **287**: 1669–70.
38 Jenkins RB, Ratner AC. Diphenylhydantoin and acne. *N Engl J Med* 1972; **287**: 148.

Sodium valproate

Occasional transient rashes and stomatitis are documented. Temporary hair loss may be followed by increasing curliness of the regrowing hair [1]. Alteration in hair colour has been noted [2]. One case of generalized morphea [3], and two of cutaneous leucocytoclastic vasculitis recurring on challenge [4], have been reported. An extrapyramidal syndrome may be induced [5], and the drug may be teratogenic [6].

1 Jeavons PM, Clark JE, Harding GFA. Valproate and curly hair. *Lancet* 1977; **i**: 359.
2 Herranz JL, Arteaga R, Armijo JA. Change in hair colour induced by valproic acid. *Dev Med Child Neurol* 1981; **23**: 386–7.
3 Goihman-Yahr M, Leal H, Essenfeld-Yahr E. Generalized morphea: a side effect of valproate sodium? *Arch Dermatol* 1980; **116**: 621.
4 Kamper AM, Valentijn RM, Stricker BHC, Purcell PM. Cutaneous vasculitis induced by sodium valproate. *Lancet* 1991; **337**: 497–8.
5 Lautin A, Stanley M, Angrist B, Gershon S. Extrapyramidal syndrome with sodium valproate. *Br Med J* 1979; **ii**: 1035–6.
6 Gomez MR. Possible teratogenicity of valproic acid. *J Paediatr* 1981; **98**: 508–9.

Trimethadione

Serious hypersensitivity reactions may occur, including erythema multiforme, urticaria and generalized exfoliative dermatitis.

8.6 Opioid analgesics and amphetamine

Cutaneous side-effects common to drug abuse following parenteral injection include [1]: infections, abscesses (Fig. 8.6), septic phlebitis, subcutaneous and deep dermal cellulitis, tetanus, widespread urticaria, cutaneous manifestations of primary and secondary syphilis, and endocarditis. Starch and talc granulomas, lymphangitis and lymphadenitis in draining lymph nodes, pigmentary abnormalities including hyperpigmentation over the injected veins, accidental 'soot' tattoos where needles were sterilized over an open flame, scarring, ulceration, necrotizing angiitis and leucocytoclastic vasculitis may supervene.

1 Rosen VJ. Cutaneous manifestations of drug abuse by parenteral injections. *Am J Dermatopathol* 1985; **7**: 79–83.

Buprenorphine

An addict accidentally injected a suspension of crushed tablets into

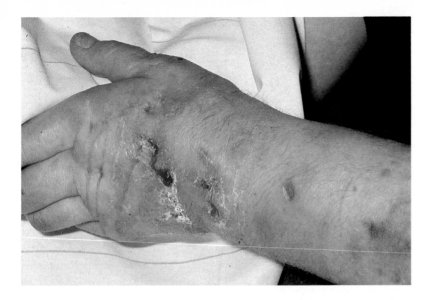

Figure 8.6 Multiple abscesses in a drug addict.

the superficial pudendal artery instead of the femoral vein, and developed pain, oedema and mottling of the penis [1].

1 Naylor AR, Gordon M, Jenkins AMcL. Untitled report. *Br Med J* 1991; **303**: 478.

Codeine

This drug has been associated with pruritus, urticaria (usually due to non-immunological release of histamine) [1,2], macular and maculopapular eruptions, scarlatiniform rashes [1,3], angioneurotic oedema, fixed eruption, a bullous eruption, erythema multiforme, and erythema nodosum.

1 Hunskaar S, Dragsund S. Scarlatiniform rash and urticaria due to codeine. *Ann Allergy* 1985; **54**: 240–1.
2 De Groot AC, Conemans J. Allergic urticarial rash from oral codeine. *Contact Dermatitis* 1986; **14**: 209–14.
3 Voohost R, Sparreboom S. Four cases of recurrent pseudo-scarlet fever caused by phenanthrene alkaloids with a 6-hydroxy group (codeine and morphine). *Ann Allergy* 1980; **44**: 116–20.

Heroin

Use of the dorsal vein of the penis for administration of the drug has produced ulceration [1]. Systemic infections, such as candidiasis, may supervene [2]. Leucocytoclastic vasculitis and necrotizing angiitis has been reported in drug abusers [3–5]. Pigmentation of the tongue may occur as a form of fixed drug eruption in heroin addicts [6]. A possible association with development of pemphigus erythematosus has been suggested [7].

1 White WB, Barrett S. Penile ulcer in heroin abuse: a case report. *Cutis* 1982; **29**: 62–3.

[211]

2 Bielsa I, Miro JM, Herrero C, *et al*. Systemic candidiasis in heroin abusers. *Int J Dermatol* 1987; **26**: 314–19.
3 Citron BP, Halpern M, McCarron M, *et al*. Necrotizing angiitis associated with drug abuse. *N Engl J Med* 1970; **283**: 1003–11.
4 Lignelli GJ, Bucheit WA. Angiitis in drug abusers. *N Engl J Med* 1971; **284**: 112–13.
5 Gendelman H, Linzer M, Barland P, *et al*. Leucocytoclastic vasculitis in an intravenous heroin abuser. *N Y State J Med* 1983; **83**: 984–6.
6 Westerhof W, Wolters EC, Brookbakker JTW, *et al*. Pigmented lesions of the tongue in heroin addicts — fixed drug eruption. *Br J Dermatol* 1983; **109**: 605–10.
7 Fellner MJ, Winiger J. Pemphigus erythematosus and heroin addiction. *Int J Dermatol* 1978; **17**: 308–11.

Morphine

Morphine is a potent histamine releaser and may cause pruritus and urticaria [1]. Profuse sweating is a common effect. Morphine provokes facial flushing blocked by naloxone [2].

1 McLelland J. The mechanism of morphine-induced urticaria. *Arch Dermatol* 1986; **122**: 138–9.
2 Cohen RA, Coffman JD. Naloxone reversal of morphine-induced peripheral vasodilatation. *Clin Pharmacol Ther* 1980; **28**: 541–4.

Pentazocine

Woody induration and subcutaneous tissues at injection sites, perhaps with central ulceration and peripheral pigmentation, and a granulomatous histology, is well recognized [1–7]. Pigmentation, ulceration and a chronic panniculitis have supervened after many years of use. Phlebitis, cellulitis, fibrous myopathy [8] and limb contractures can complicate these changes. Generalized eruptions are rare [9]. Toxic epidermal necrolysis has been reported [10].

1 Parks DL, Perry HO, Muller SA. Cutaneous complications of pentazocine injections. *Arch Dermatol* 1971; **104**: 231–5.
2 Schlicher JE, Zuehlke RL, Lynch PJ. Local changes at the site of pentazocine injection. *Arch Dermatol* 1971; **104**: 90–1.
3 Swanson DW, Weddige RL, Morse RM. Hospitalised pentazocine abusers. *Mayo Clinic Proc* 1973; **48**: 85–93.
4 Schiff BL, Kern AB. Unusual cutaneous manifestations of pentazocine addiction. *JAMA* 1977; **238**: 1542–3.
5 Padilla RS, Becker LE, Hoffman H, Long G. Cutaneous and venous complications of pentazocine abuse. *Arch Dermatol* 1979; **115**: 975–7.
6 Palestine RF, Millns JL, Spigel GT, *et al*. Skin manifestations of pentazocine abuse. *J Am Acad Dermatol* 1980; **2**: 47–55.
7 Mann RJ, Gostelow BE, Meacock DJ, Kennedy CTC. Pentazocine ulcers. *J R Soc Med* 1982; **75**: 903–5.
8 Johnson KR, Hsueh WA, Glusman SM, Arnett FC. Fibrous myopathy: A rheumatic complication of drug abuse. *Arthritis Rheum* 1976; **19**: 923–6.
9 Pedragosa R, Vidal J, Fuentes R, Huguet P. Tricotropism by pentazocine. *Arch Dermatol* 1987; **123**: 297–8.
10 Hunter JAA, Davison AM. Toxic epidermal necrolysis associated with pentazocine therapy and severe reversible renal failure. *Br J Dermatol* 1973; **88**: 287–90.

Methylamphetamine

A link with necrotizing angiitis has been recorded when this drug is used alone or with heroin or *d*-lysergic acid diethylamide [1].

1 Citron BP, Halpern M, McCarron M, *et al*. Necrotizing angiitis associated with drug abuse. *N Engl J Med* 1970; **283**: 1003−11.

8.7 Anti-Parkinsonian drugs

Amantadine

Reversible livedo reticularis has occurred in a high percentage of patients receiving amantadine, a tricyclic amine used in the treatment of Parkinson's disease and influenza A [1,2].

Bromocriptine

Transient livedo reticularis [3], erythromelalgia [4], acrocyanosis with Raynaud's phenomenon [5,6], morphea [7] and swelling of the legs with a sclerodermatous histology [8] have been reported rarely, as has alopecia [9] and psychosis.

Carbidopa

Scleroderma-like reactions have occurred when this drug has been given in conjunction with tryptophan [10,11].

Levodopa

There have been several isolated reports of the occurrence of malignant melanoma [12−14], in certain instances involving multiple primaries, but the association may be by chance alone.

1 Shealy CN, Weeth JB, Mercier D. Livedo reticularis in patients with parkinsonism receiving amantadine. *JAMA* 1970; **212**: 1522−3.
2 Vollum DI, Parkes JD, Doyle D. Livedo reticularis during amantadine treatment. *Br Med J* 1971; **ii**: 627−8.
3 Calne DB, Plotkin C, Neophytides A, *et al*. Long-term treatment of Parkinsonism with bromocriptine. *Lancet* 1978; **i**: 735−7.
4 Eisler T, Hall RP, Kalavar KAR, Calne DB. Erythromelalgia-like eruption in Parkinsonian patients treated with bromocriptine. *Neurology* 1981; **37**: 1368−70.
5 Duvoisin RC. Digital vasospasm with bromocryptine. *Lancet* 1976; **ii**: 204.
6 Pearce I, Pearce JMS. Bromocriptine in Parkinsonism. *Br Med J* 1978; **i**: 1402−4.
7 Leshin B, Piette WW, Caplin RM. Morphea after bromocriptine therapy. *Int J Dermatol* 1989; **28**: 177−9.
8 Dupont E, Olivarius B, Strong MJ. Bromocriptine-induced collagenosis-like symptomatology in Parkinson's disease. *Lancet* 1982; **i**: 850−1.
9 Blum I, Leiba S. Increased hair loss as a side effect of bromocriptine treatment. *N Engl J Med* 1980; **303**: 1418.
10 Sternberg EM, Van Woert MH, Young SN, *et al*. Development of a sclero-

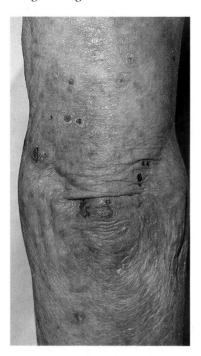

Figure 8.7 Lichenoid eruption due to cinnarazine.

derma-like illness during therapy with L-5-hydroxytryptophan and carbidopa. *N Engl J Med* 1980; **303**: 782−7.

11 Chamson A, Périer C, Frey J. Syndrome sclérodermiforme et poïkilodermique observé au cours d'un traitement par carbidopa et 5-hydroxytryptophanne. Culture de fibroblastes avec analyse biochimique du métabolisme du collagene. *Ann Dermatol Vénéréol (Paris)* 1986; **113**: 71.

12 Sober AJ, Wick MM. Levodopa therapy and malignant melanoma. *JAMA* 1978; **240**: 554−5.

13 Bernstein JE, Medenica M, Soltani K, *et al.* Levodopa administration and multiple primary cutaneous melanomas. *Arch Dermatol* 1980; **116**: 1041−4.

14 Rosin MA, Braun M III. Malignant melanoma and levodopa. *Cutis* 1984; **33**: 572−4.

8.8 Antivertigo drugs and cerebrovascular dilators

Cinnarazine

This drug [1], and its derivative flunarizine [2], have been implicated in the precipitation of lichenoid eruptions (Fig. 8.7). In the case of cinnarazine, clinical and immunofluorescence features of lichen planus were combined with the presence of a circulating anti-basement membrane zone IgG antibody [2]. Other side-effects include drowsiness, depression, and parkinsonism.

1 Miyagawa W, Ohi H, Muramatsu T, *et al.* Lichen planus pemphigoides-like lesions induced by cinnarizine. *Br J Dermatol* 1985; **112**: 607−13.

2 Suys E, De Coninck A, De Pauw I, Roseeuw D. Lichen planus induced by flunarizine. *Dermatologica* 1990; **181**: 71−2.

Chapter 9
Drugs Acting on the Cardiovascular and Respiratory Systems

9.1 Cardiac antiarrhythmic drugs

Amiodarone

This iodinated antiarrhythmic drug causes photosensitivity in 30–50% of patients [1–7]. Symptoms develop within 2 hours of sun exposure as a burning sensation followed by erythema; the action spectrum is UV-A extending to a degree into visible light wavebands above 400 nm [5]. Light sensitivity may persist for up to 4 months after the drug is stopped [1,2]. Blue or grey pigmentation of the face (Fig. 9.1) and other sun-exposed areas, resembling that in argyria, is a much less common late effect, occurring in 2–5% of cases; non-sun-exposed areas may also be involved [4,7–16]. It is induced by a phototoxic reaction involving both UV-B and UV-A [4,7], and is related to both duration and dosage of the drug [15]. Amiodarone-pigmented skin contains the drug and its metabolites in higher concentrations than non-pigmented skin [4]. Iodine-rich amiodarone and its metabolites have been detected bound to lipofuscin within secondary lysosomes in perivascular dermal macrophages [7,12–14]. Electron dense granules and myelin-like bodies are also found in peripheral blood leucocytes [16]. The cutaneous pigmentation slowly fades after discontinuation of therapy, but may persist for months to years [12].

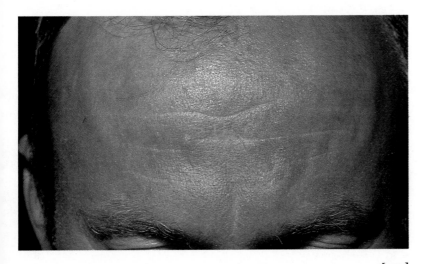

Figure 9.1 Blue–grey discoloration of exposed areas due to amiodarone. (Courtesy of Professor K. Wolff, Vienna.)

Iododerma has occurred with long-term therapy. Vasculitis is recorded [17]. A fatal case of toxic epidermal necrolysis has been reported [18]. The most severe adverse side-effect seen with amiodarone is pulmonary fibrosis, which occurs in 5–10% of exposed patients, and which has a 10% mortality rate. Other problems have been cardiac dysrhythmias, thyroid dysfunction, peripheral neuropathy and reversible corneal deposits [19].

1 Marcus FI, Fontaine GH, Frank R, Grosgogeat Y. Clinical pharmacology and therapeutic applications of the antiarrhythmic agent amiodarone. *Am Heart J* 1981; **101**: 480–93.

2 Chalmers RJ, Muston HL, Srinivas V, Bennett DH. High incidence of amiodarone-induced photosensitivity in North-west England. *Br Med J* 1982; **285**: 341.

3 Walter JF, Bradner H, Curtis GP. Amiodarone photosensitivity. *Arch Dermatol* 1984; **120**: 1591–4.

4 Zachary CB, Slater DN, Holt DW, *et al.* The pathogenesis of amiodarone-induced pigmentation and photosensitivity. *Br J Dermatol* 1984; **110**: 451–6.

5 Ferguson J, Addo HA, Jones S, *et al.* A study of cutaneous photosensitivity induced by amiodarone. *Br J Dermatol* 1985; **113**: 537–49.

6 Roupe G, Larkö O, Olsson SB, *et al.* Amiodarone photoreactions. *Acta Derm Venereol (Stockh)* 1987; **67**: 76–9.

7 Waitzer S, Butany J, From L, *et al.* Cutaneous ultrastructural changes and photosensitivity associated with amiodarone therapy. *J Am Acad Dermatol* 1987; **16**: 779–87.

8 Labouche F, Massé R, Jan A, *et al.* Pigmentations cutanées au cours de traitements par le chlorhydrate d'amiodarone. *Bull Soc Fr Dermatol Syphiligr* 1971; **78**: 27–30.

9 Korting HC, Kolz R, Schmoeckel C, Balda B-R. Amiodaronepigmentierung. Eine seltene, aber typische Medikamentnebenwirkung. *Hautarzt* 1981; **32**: 301–5.

10 Trimble JW, Mendelson DS, Fetter BE, *et al.* Cutaneous pigmentation secondary to amiodarone therapy. *Arch Dermatol* 1983; **119**: 914–18.

11 McGovern B, Garan H, Kelly E, Ruskin JN. Adverse reactions during treatment with amiodarone hydrochloride. *Br Med J* 1983; **287**: 175–9.

12 Miller RAW, McDonald ATJ. Dermal lipofuscinosis associated with amiodarone therapy. Report of a case. *Arch Dermatol* 1984; **120**: 646–9.

13 Holt DW, Adams PC, Campbell RWF, *et al.* Amiodarone and its desethyl-metabolite: tissue distribution and ultrastructural changes in amiodarone treated patients. *Br J Clin Pharmacol* 1984; **17**: 195–6.

14 Török L, Szekeres L, Lakatos A, Szücs M. Amiodaronebedingte Hyperpigmentierung. *Hautarzt* 1986; **37**: 507–10.

15 Heger JJ, Prystowsky EN, Zipes DP. Relationships between amiodarone dosage, drug concentrations, and adverse side effects. *Am Heart J* 1983; **106**: 931–5.

16 Rappersberger K, Konrad K, Wieser E, *et al.* Morphological changes in peripheral blood cells and skin in amiodarone-treated patients. *Br J Dermatol* 1986; **114**: 189–96.

17 Staubli M, Zimmerman A, Bircher J. Amiodarone-induced vasculitis and polyserositis. *Postgrad Med J* 1985; **61**: 245–7.

18 Bencini PL, Crosti C, Sala F, *et al.* Toxic epidermal necrolysis and amiodarone. *Arch Dermatol* 1985; **121**: 838.

19 Morgan DJR. Adverse reactions profile: 3. Amiodarone. *Drug Ther Bull* 1991; **31**: 104–11.

Digoxin

Allergic reactions are very rare, but exanthematic erythema, urticaria, bullous eruptions and thrombocytopenic purpura are documented.

In one patient a psoriasiform rash occurred, confirmed by later re-exposure [1].

1 David M, Livni E, Stern E, *et al.* Psoriasiform eruption induced by digoxin: confirmed by re-exposure. *J Am Acad Dermatol* 1981; **5**: 702–3.

Procainamide

This drug is well known to precipitate a lupus-like syndrome [1–6], perhaps as a result of binding of the hydroxylamine metabolite of procainamide to complement component C4, with resultant impaired complement-mediated clearance of immune complexes [5,6]. A lichenoid eruption followed the occurrence of drug-induced lupus erythematosus (LE) in one case [7]. Urticarial vasculitis has been reported [8].

1 Dubois EL. Procainamide induction of a systemic lupus erythematosus-like syndrome. Presentation of six cases, review of the literature, and analysis and follow up of reported cases. *Medicine* 1969; **48**: 217–18.
2 Blomgren SE, Condemi JJ, Vaughan JH. Procainamide-induced lupus erythematosus. Clinical and laboratory observations. *Am J Med* 1972; **52**: 338–48.
3 Whittle TS Jr, Ainsworth SK. Procainamide-induced systemic lupus erythematosus. Renal involvement with deposition of immune complexes. *Arch Pathol Lab Med* 1976; **100**: 469–74.
4 Tan EM, Rubin RL. Autoallergic reactions induced by procainamide. *J Allergy Clin Immunol* 1984; **74**: 631–4.
5 Sim E, Stanley L, Gill EW, Jones A. Metabolites of procainamide and practolol inhibit complement components C3 and C4. *Biochem J* 1988; **251**: 323–6.
6 Sim E. Drug-induced immune complex disease. *Complement Inflamm* 1989; **6**: 119–26.
7 Sherertz EF. Lichen planus following procainamide-induced lupus erythematosus. *Cutis* 1988; **42**: 51–3.
8 Knox JP, Welykyj SE, Gradini R, Massa MC. Procainamide-induced urticarial vasculitis. *Cutis* 1988; **42**: 469–72.

Quinidine

An eczematous photosensitivity is well described [1–5]; fever is common. Thrombocytopenic purpura may be induced, resulting from antibodies to drug–platelet conjugates [6,7]. Urticarial, scarlatiniform and morbilliform eruptions occur; the latter may proceed to generalized exfoliative dermatitis if the drug is continued. Fixed, and lichenoid eruptions [8–14], often light-induced, are recorded, as well as an acneiform rash [15]. Livedo reticularis has been documented; the mechanism is unknown, although recent sunlight exposure was a feature common to all cases [16–18]. Drug-induced LE [19–21] and Henoch–Schönlein vasculitis [22,23] have been seen. Psoriasis may be exacerbated [24]. Localized blue–grey pigmentation of the shins, hard palate, nails, nose, ears, and forearms has been recorded [25].

1 Berger TG, Sesody SJ. Quinidine-induced lichenoid photodermatitis. *Cutis* 1982; **29**: 595–8.

2 Marx JL, Eisenstat BA, Gladstein AH. Quinidine photosensitivity. *Arch Dermatol* 1983; **119**: 39−43.

3 Armstrong RB, Leach EE, Whitman G, *et al*. Quinidine photosensitivity. *Arch Dermatol* 1985; **121**: 525−8.

4 Jeanmougin M, Sigal M, Djian B, *et al*. Photo-allergie à la quinidine. *Ann Dermatol Vénéréol (Paris)* 1986; **113**: 985−7.

5 Schürer NY, Lehmann P, Plewig G. Chinidininduzierte Photoallergie. Eine klinische und experimentelle Studie. *Hautarzt* 1991; **42**: 158−61.

6 Christie DJ, Weber RW, Mullen PC, *et al*. Structural features of the quinidine and quinine molecules necessary for binding of drug-induced antibodies to human platelets. *J Lab Clin Med* 1984; **104**: 730−40.

7 Gary M, Ilfeld D, Kelton JG. Correlation of a quinidine-induced platelet-specific antibody with development of thrombocytopenia. *Am J Med* 1985; **79**: 253−5.

8 Anderson TE. Lichen planus following quinidine therapy. *Br J Dermatol* 1967; **79**: 500.

9 Pegum JS. Lichenoid quinidine eruption. *Br J Dermatol* 1968; **80**: 343.

10 Maltz BL, Becker LE. Quinidine-induced lichen planus. *Int J Dermatol* 1980; **19**: 96−7.

11 Bonnetblanc J-M, Bernard P, Catanzano G, Souyri N. Éruptions lichénoides photinduites aux quinidiniques. *Ann Dermatol Vénéréol (Paris)* 1987; **114**: 957−61.

12 Wolf R, Dorfman B, Krakowski A. Quinidine induced lichenoid and eczematous photodermatitis. *Dermatologica* 1987; **174**: 285−9.

13 De Larrard G, Jeanmougin M, Moulonguet I, *et al*. Toxidermie lichénoide alopéciante à la quinidine. *Ann Dermatol Vénéréol (Paris)* 1988; **115**: 1172−4.

14 Jeanmougin M, Elkara-Marrak H, Pons A, *et al*. Éruption lichénoïde photoinduite à l'hydroxyquinidine. *Ann Dermatol Vénéréol (Paris)* 1987; **114**: 1397−9.

15 Burckhart CG. Quinidine-induced acne. *Arch Dermatol* 1981; **117**: 603−4.

16 Marion DF, Terrien CM. Photosensitive livedo reticularis. *Arch Dermatol* 1973; **108**: 100−1.

17 De Groot WP, Wuite J. Livedo racemosa-like photosensitivity reaction during quinidine durettes medication. *Dermatologica* 1974; **148**: 371−6.

18 Bruce S, Wolf JE Jr. Quinidine-induced photosensitive livedo reticularis-like eruption. *J Am Acad Dermatol* 1985; **12**: 332−6.

19 Lavie CJ, Biundo J, Quinet RJ, Waxman J. Systemic lupus erythematosus (SLE) induced by quinidine. *Arch Intern Med* 1985; **145**: 446−8.

20 McCormack GD, Barth WF. Quinidine induced lupus syndrome. *Semin Arthritis Rheum* 1985; **15**: 73−9.

21 Cohen MG, Kevat S, Prowse MV, *et al*. Two distinct quinidine-induced rheumatic syndromes. *Ann Intern Med* 1988; **108**: 369−71.

22 Aviram A. Henoch−Schönlein syndrome associated with quinidine. *JAMA* 1980; **243**: 432−4.

23 Zax RH, Hodge SJ, Callen JP. Cutaneous leukocytoclastic vasculitis. Serial histopathologic evaluation demonstrates the dynamic nature of the infiltrate. *Arch Dermatol* 1990; **126**: 69−72.

24 Baker H. The influence of chloroquine and related drugs on psoriasis and keratoderma blenorrhagicum. *Br J Dermatol* 1966; **78**: 161−6.

25 Mahler R, Sissons W, Watters K. Pigmentation induced by quinidine therapy. *Arch Dermatol* 1986; **122**: 1062−4.

9.2 β-Adrenoceptor blocking agents

This group of drugs shares in common certain potential side-effects [1,2]. Peripheral ischaemia may be aggravated, and cold extremities and Raynaud's phenomenon [3] may present as new symptoms. Peripheral gangrene and peripheral skin necrosis [4,5] have been reported. An LE-like syndrome [6], and eczematous or lichenoid

[1,2] eruptions may be induced rarely. Psoriasis vulgaris is occasionally aggravated or precipitated by a number of β-blockers including atenolol, oxprenolol, practolol (discontinued) and propranolol [7−10]. Cross-sensitivity is not usual [11], but cross-reactivity between atenolol, oxprenolol, and propranolol, has been reported [12]. Peyronie's disease (induratio penis plastica) has been attributed to labetalol, metoprolol and propranolol [13,14]. β-Blockers may enhance anaphylactic reactions caused by other allergens, and may make resuscitation more difficult [15−17]. Alopecia has been attributed to topical ophthalmic β-blockers, especially timolol [18].

1 Felix RH, Ive FA, Dahl MGC. Skin reactions to beta-blockers. *Br Med J* 1975; i: 626.
2 Hödl S. Nebenwirkungen der Betarezeptorenblocker an der Haut. Übersicht und eigene Beobachtungen. *Hautarzt* 1985; **36**: 549−57.
3 Marshall AJ, Roberts CJC, Barritt DW. Raynaud's phenomenon as a side effect of beta-blockers in hypertension. *Br Med J* 1976; i: 1498−9.
4 Gokal R, Dornan TL, Ledingham JGG. Peripheral skin necrosis complicating beta-blockade. *Br Med J* 1979; i: 721−2.
5 Hoffbrand BI. Peripheral skin necrosis complicating beta-blockade. *Br Med J* 1979; i: 1082.
6 Hughes GRV. Hypotensive agents, beta-blockers, and drug-induced lupus. *Br Med J* 1982; **284**: 1358−9.
7 Arntzen N, Kavli G, Volden G. Psoriasis provoked by β-blocking agents. *Acta Derm Venereol (Stockh)* 1984; **64**: 346−8.
8 Abel EA, Dicicco LM, Orenberg EK, *et al*. Drugs in exacerbation of psoriasis. *J Am Acad Dermatol* 1986; **15**: 1007−22.
9 Heng MCY, Heng MK. Beta-adrenoceptor antagonist-induced psoriasiform eruption. Clinical and pathogenetic aspects. *Int J Dermatol* 1988; **27**: 619−27.
10 Gold MH, Holy AK, Roenigk HH Jr. Beta-blocking drugs and psoriasis. A review of cutaneous side effects and retrospective analysis of their effects on psoriasis. *J Am Acad Dermatol* 1988; **19**: 837−41.
11 Furhoff A-K, Norlander M, Peterson C. Cross-sensitivity between practolol and other beta-blockers? *Br Med J* 1976; i: 831.
12 Van Joost T, Smitt JHS. Skin reactions to propranolol and cross sensitivity to β-adrenoreceptor blocking agents. *Arch Dermatol* 1981; **117**: 600−1.
13 Yudkin JS. Peyronie's disease in association with metoprolol. *Lancet* 1977; ii: 1355.
14 Jones HA, Castleden WM. Peyronie's disease. *Med J Aust* 1981; ii: 514−15.
15 Hannaway PJ, Hopper GDK. Severe anaphylaxis and drug-induced beta-blockade. *N Engl J Med* 1983; **308**: 1536.
16 Toogood JH. Risk of anaphylaxis in patients receiving beta-blocker drugs. *J Allergy Clin Immunol*; 1988; **81**: 1−5.
17 Hepner MJ, Ownby DR, Anderson JA, *et al*. Risk of systemic reactions in patients taking beta-blocker drugs receiving allergen immunotherapy injections. *J Allergy Clin Immunol* 1990; **86**: 407−11.
18 Fraunfelder FT, Meyer SM, Menacker SJ. Alopecia possibly secondary to topical ophthalmic β-blockers. *JAMA* 1990; **263**: 1493−4.

Acebutolol

Rashes with mixed lichenoid and LE-like features have been reported [1]. The LE-syndrome may have pleuro-pulmonary features [2].

Atenolol

Conjunctivitis and a peri-ocular dermatitis [3], as well as a psoriasiform rash [4], pseudolymphomatous reaction [5] and vasculitis [6] are recorded.

Cetamolol

A psoriasiform eruption has been documented [7].

Labetalol

Mixed eruptions with psoriasiform and pityriasis rubra pilaris-like changes [8], a bullous lichenoid eruption [9], and an SLE-like syndrome [10] are documented.

Metoprolol

Various psoriasiform or eczematous rashes may follow long-term therapy [11,12]. Conjunctivitis and peri-ocular dermatitis have occurred [3]. Peyronie's disease appears to be a rare but confirmed side-effect and may be reversible. Telogen effluvium has been noted [13].

Oxprenolol

This drug, like practolol, has caused an oculocutaneous syndrome [14]. An eruption combining well-defined, eroded or scaly, red rings with a lichenoid histology [15,16] is recognized. Acute psoriasis with arthropathy has been described [17]. Peripheral skin necrosis associated with Raynaud's phenomenon, an LE syndrome, various patterns of dermatitis [3], and generalized pigmentation [18] are all documented.

Practolol

This drug has been withdrawn, but is discussed in view of its important side-effect profile. It caused an oculocutaneous syndrome comprising dry eyes and scarring, fibrosis and metaplasia of the conjunctiva; a psoriasiform, lichenoid or mixed eruption with a characteristic histology; pleural and pericardial reactions; fibrinous peritonitis and serous otitis media [19,20]. Subsequent treatment with another β-blocker did not elicit cross-sensitivity reactivation of the syndrome [21]. Ocular cicatricial pemphigoid was seen [22], and exacerbation of psoriasis was recorded [23].

Pindolol

Psoriasiform [24], and lichenoid rashes with pemphigus-like antibodies demonstrated by immunofluorescence, have been seen, as well as an SLE syndrome [25].

Propranolol

This is probably the most widely used β-blocker and many adverse cutaneous reactions have been reported [26–29].` Rashes may be lichenoid [30], psoriasiform [29] or generalized and exfoliative. Other miscellaneous reported reactions have been alopecia [31], erythema multiforme [32] and a cheilostomatitis with ulceration of the lips. Peyronie's disease has developed. Generalized pustular psoriasis [33] and pemphigus [34] have occurred.

1 Taylor AEM, Hindson C, Wacks H. A drug eruption due to acebutolol with combined lichenoid and lupus erythematosus features. *Clin Exp Dermatol* 1982; **7**: 219–21.

2 Record NB. Acebutolol-induced pleuropulmonary lupus syndrome. *Ann Intern Med* 1981; **95**: 326–7.

3 Van Joost T, Middelkamp Hup H, Ros FE. Dermatitis as a side-effect of long-term topical treatment with certain beta-blocking agents. *Br J Dermatol* 1979; **101**: 171–6.

4 Gawkrodger DJ, Beveridge GW. Psoriasiform reaction to atenolol. *Clin Exp Dermatol* 1984; **9**: 92–4.

5 Henderson CA, Shamy HK. Atenolol-induced pseudolymphoma. *Clin Exp Dermatol* 1990; **15**: 119–20.

6 Wolf R, Ophir J, Elman M, Krakowski A. Atenolol-induced cutaneous vasculitis. *Cutis* 1989; **43**: 231–3.

7 White WB, Schulman P, McCabe EJ. Psoriasiform cutaneous eruptions induced by cetamolol hydrochloride. *Arch Dermatol* 1986; **122**: 857–8.

8 Finlay AY, Waddington E, Savage RL, *et al.* Cutaneous reactions to labetalol. *Br Med J* 1978; **i**: 987.

9 Gange RW, Wilson Jones E. Bullous lichen planus caused by labetalol. *Br Med J* 1978; **i**: 816–17.

10 Brown RC, Cooke M, Losowsky MS. SLE syndrome, probably induced by labetalol. *Postgrad Med J* 1981; **57**: 189–90.

11 Neumann HAM, van Joost T, Westerhof W. Dermatitis as a side-effect of long-term metoprolol. *Lancet* 1979; **ii**: 745.

12 Neumann HAM, van Joost T. Adverse reactions of the skin to metoprolol and other beta-adrenergic-blocking agents. *Dermatologica* 1981; **162**: 330–5.

13 Graeber CW, Lapkin RA. Metoprolol and alopecia. *Cutis* 1981; **28**: 633–4.

14 Holt PJA, Waddington E. Oculocutaneous reaction to oxprenolol. *Br Med J* 1975; **ii**: 539–40.

15 Levene GM, Gange RW. Eruption during treatment with oxprenolol. *Br Med J* 1978; **i**: 784.

16 Gange RW, Levene GM. A distinctive eruption in patients receiving oxprenolol. *Clin Exp Dermatol* 1979; **4**: 87–97.

17 MacFarlane DG, Settas L. Acute psoriatic arthropathy precipitated by oxprenolol. *Ann Rheum Dis* 1984; **43**: 102–4.

18 Harrower ADB, Strong JA. Hyperpigmentation associated with oxprenolol administration. *Br Med J* 1977; **ii**: 296.

19 Felix RH, Ive FA, Dahl MGC. Cutaneous and ocular reactions to practolol. *Br Med J* 1974; **iv**: 321–4.

20 Wright P. Untoward effects associated with practolol administration: oculomucocutaneous syndrome. *Br Med J* 1975; **i**: 595–8.

21 Furhoff A-K, Norlander M, Peterson C. Cross-sensitivity between practolol and other beta-blockers? *Br Med J* 1976; **i**: 831.

22 Van Joost T, Crone RA, Overdijk AD. Ocular cicatricial pemphigoid associated with practolol therapy. *Br J Dermatol* 1976; **94**: 447–50.

23 Søndergaard J, Wadskov S, Ærenlund-Jensen H, Mikkelsen HI. Aggravation of psoriasis and occurrence of psoriasiform cutaneous eruptions induced by practolol (Eraldin®). *Acta Derm Venereol (Stockh)* 1976; **56**: 239–43.

24 Bonerandi J-J, Follana J, Privat Y. Apparition d'un psoriasis au cours d'un traitement par bêta-bloquants (Pindolol). *Ann Dermatol Syphiligr (Paris)* 1976; **103**: 604–6.

25 Bensaid J, Aldigier J-C, Gualde N. Systemic lupus erythematosus syndrome induced by pindolol. *Br Med J* 1979; **i**: 1603–4.

26 Ærenlund-Jensen H, Mikkelsen HI, Wadskov S, Søndergaard J. Cutaneous reactions to propranolol (Inderal). *Acta Med Scand* 1976; **199**: 363–7.

27 Cochran REI, Thomson J, McQueen A, Beevers DG. Skin reactions associated with propranolol. *Arch Dermatol* 1976; **112**: 1173–4.

28 Scribner MD. Propranolol therapy. *Arch Dermatol* 1977; **113**: 1303.

29 Faure M, Hermier C, Perrot H. Accidents cutanés provoqués par le propranolol. *Ann Dermatol Vénéréol (Paris)* 1979; **106**: 161–5.

30 Hawk JLM. Lichenoid drug eruption induced by propranolol. *Clin Exp Dermatol* 1980; **5**: 93–6.

31 Hilder RJ. Propranolol and alopecia. *Cutis* 1979; **24**: 63–4.

32 Pimstone B, Joffe B, Pimstone N, *et al.* Clinical response to long-term propranolol therapy in hyperthyroidism. *S Afr Med J* 1969; **43**: 1203–5.

33 Hu C-H, Miller AC, Peppercorn R, Farber EM. Generalized pustular psoriasis provoked by propranolol. *Arch Dermatol* 1985; **121**: 1326–7.

34 Godard W, Lambert D, Gavanou J, Chapuis J-L. Pemphigus induit après traitement par l'association propranolol-méprobamate. *Ann Dermatol Vénéréol (Paris)* 1980; **107**: 1213–16.

9.3 Antihypertensive drugs and vasodilators

The dermatological side-effects of antihypertensive agents have been reviewed [1].

1 Thestrup-Pedersen K. Adverse reactions in the skin from antihypertensive drugs. *Dan Med Bull* 1987; **34**: 3–5.

Angiotensin-converting enzyme (ACE) inhibitors

In addition to dermatological problems, these drugs may be nephrotoxic, cause cough and electrolyte disturbances, and are teratogenic [1]. Angioedema has been reported with captopril, enalapril maleate, and lisinopril [2]. Anaphylactoid reactions have been reported during haemodialysis with AN69 membranes in patients receiving ACE inhibitors; the role of bacterial contamination of dialysate is controversial [3–5].

Captopril

Dermatological complications occur in between 4% [6] and 12% [7] of patients treated with captopril, and less commonly with other ACE inhibitors; side-effects are more likely with renal impairment. Loss of sense of taste, or a metallic taste (augesia), ulceration of the tongue and aphthous stomatitis [8] are reported. Early changes within the first months [9–11] include pruritus, urticaria [12] and angioedema, which occurs in about 1 in 1000 patients and may occasionally be fatal [13], pityriasis rosea-like [14] and morbilliform rashes. These are dose dependent and have a good prognosis. Late changes [9–11] consist of pemphigus-like [15–18] and lichenoid eruptions [19−23]. A gyrate subacute type lupus-like eruption has been recorded [24]. Antinuclear antibodies may develop [25,26]. Oral changes may be due to a leucocytoclastic vasculitis [27], and a serum sickness-like syndrome has been induced [28]. Psoriasis has been reported to be exacerbated or triggered [29,30].

Severe reactions [31−34] have included exfoliative dermatitis, and marrow depression with neutropenia or agranulocytosis [35]. Lymphadenopathy may be induced [36]. Alopecia [37] and an acquired IgA deficiency [38] have been reported. The merits of skin testing in the prediction of captopril reactions have been discussed [39]. It has been postulated that toxic effects are related to the presence of a sulphydryl group, since enalapril (another ACE inhibitor lacking this group) has been safely substituted in captopril hypersensitivity [40].

Enalapril

A single report of pemphigus foliaceus has appeared; part of the structure of this drug is identical to that of captopril, although it does not contain a sulphydryl group [41].

Lisinopril

Vasculitis has been recorded [42].

1 Ferner RE. Adverse effects of angiotensin-converting-enzyme inhibitors. *Adverse Drug React Bull* 1990; **141**: 528−31.
2 Orfan N, Patterson R, Dykewicz MS. Severe angioedema related to ACE inhibitors in patients with a history of idiopathic angioedema. *JAMA* 1990; **264**: 1287−9.
3 Verresen L, Waer M, Vanrenterghem Y, Michielsen P. Angiotensin-converting-enzyme inhibitors and anaphylactoid reactions to high-flux membrane dialysis. *Lancet* 1990; **336**: 1360−2.
4 Tielemans C, Madhoun P, Lenears M, *et al*. Anaphylactoid reactions during hemodialysis on AN69 membranes in patients receiving ACE inhibitors. *Kidney Int* 1990; **38**: 982−4.
5 Verresen L, Waer M, Vanrenterghem Y, Michielsen P. Anaphylactoid reactions, haemodialysis, and ACE inhibitors. *Lancet* 1991; **337**: 1294.
6 Williams GH. Converting-enzyme inhibitors in the treatment of hypertension. *N Engl J Med* 1988; **319**: 1517−25.
7 Wilkin JK, Hammond JJ, Kirkendall WM. The captopril-induced eruption. A possible mechanism: cutaneous kinin potentiation. *Arch Dermatol* 1980; **116**: 902−5.
8 Seedat YK. Aphthous ulcers of mouth from captopril. *Lancet* 1979; **ii**: 1297−8.
9 Clement M. Captopril-induced eruptions. *Arch Dermatol* 1981; **117**: 525−6.
10 Luderer JR, Lookingbill DP, Schneck DW, *et al*. Captopril-induced skin eruptions. *J Clin Pharmacol* 1982; **22**: 151−9.
11 Daniel F, Foix C, Barbet M, *et al*. Captopril-induced eruptions: Occurrence over a three-year period. *Ann Dermatol Vénéréol (Paris)* 1983; **110**: 441−6.
12 Wood SM, Mann RD, Rawlins MD. Angio-oedema and urticaria associated with angiotensin converting enzyme inhibitors. *Br Med J* 1987; **294**: 91−2.
13 Slater EE, Merrill DD, Guess HA, *et al*. Clinical profile of angioedema associated with angiotensin converting-enzyme inhibition. *JAMA* 1988; **260**: 967−70.
14 Wilkin JK, Kirkendall WM. Pityriasis rosea-like rash from captopril. *Arch Dermatol* 1982; **118**: 186−7.

15 Parfrey PS, Clement M, Vandenburg MJ, Wright P. Captopril-induced pemphigus. *Br Med J* 1980; **281**: 194.

16 Clement M. Captopril-induced eruptions. *Arch Dermatol* 1981; **117**: 525−6.

17 Katz RA, Hood AF, Anhalt GJ. Pemphigus-like eruption from captopril. *Arch Dermatol* 1987; **123**: 20−1.

18 Korman NJ, Eyre RW, Stanley JR. Drug-induced pemphigus: autoantibodies directed against the pemphigus antigen complexes are present in penicillamine and captopril-induced pemphigus. *J Invest Dermatol* 1991; **96**: 273−6.

19 Reinhardt LA, Wilkin JK, Kirkendall WM. Lichenoid eruption produced by captopril. *Cutis* 1983; **31**: 98−9.

20 Bravard P, Barbet M, Eich D, *et al.* Éruption lichénoïde au captopril. *Ann Dermatol Vénéréol (Paris)* 1983; **110**: 433−8.

21 Flageul B, Foldes C, Wallach D, *et al.* Captopril-induced lichen planus pemphigoides with pemphigus-like features. A case report. *Dermatologica* 1986; **173**: 248−55.

22 Bretin N, Dreno B, Bureau B, Litoux P. Immunohistological study of captopril-induced late cutaneous reactions. *Dermatologica* 1988; **177**: 11−15.

23 Rotstein E, Rotstein H. Drug eruptions with lichenoid histology produced by captopril. *Australas J Dermatol* 1989; **30**: 9−14.

24 Patri P, Nigro A, Rebora A. Lupus erythematosus-like eruption from captopril. *Acta Derm Venereol (Stockh)* 1985; **65**: 447−8.

25 Reidenberg MM, Case DB, Drayer DE, *et al.* Development of antinuclear antibodies in patients treated with high doses of captopril. *Arthritis Rheum* 1984; **27**: 579−81.

26 Kallenberg CGM. Autoantibodies during captopril treatment. *Arthritis Rheum* 1985; **28**: 597−8.

27 Viraben R, Adoue D, Dupre A, Touron P. Erosions and ulcers of the mouth. *Arch Dermatol* 1982; **118**: 959.

28 Hoorntje SJ, Weening JJ, Kallenberg GGM, *et al.* Serum-sickness-like syndrome with membranous glomerulopathy in patient on captopril. *Lancet* 1979; **ii**: 1297.

29 Hauschild TT, Bauer R, Kreysel HW. Erstmanifestation einer eruptiv-exanthematischen Psoriasis vulgaris unter Captoprilmedikation. *Hautarzt* 1986; **37**: 274−7.

30 Wolf R, Dorfman B, Krakowski A. Psoriasiform eruption induced by captopril and chlorthalidone. *Cutis* 1987; **40**: 162−4.

31 Solinger AM. Exfoliative dermatitis from captopril. *Cutis* 1982; **29**: 473−4.

32 Goodfield MJ, Millard LG. Severe cutaneous reactions to captopril. *Br Med J* 1985; **290**: 1111.

33 Furness PN, Goodfield MJ, MacLennan KA, *et al.* Severe cutaneous reactions to captopril and enalopril; histological study and comparison with early mycosis fungoides. *J Clin Pathol* 1986; **39**: 902−7.

34 O'Neill PG, Rajan N, Charlat ML, Bolli R. Captopril-related exfoliative dermatitis. *Texas Med* 1989; **85**: 40−1.

35 Edwards CRW, Drury P, Penketh A, Damluji SA. Successful reintroduction of captopril following neutropenia. *Lancet* 1981; **i**: 723.

36 Åberg H, Mörlin C, Frithz G. Captopril-associated lymphadenopathy. *Br Med J* 1981; **283**: 1297−8.

37 Motel PJ. Captopril and alopecia: A case report and review of known cutaneous reactions in captopril use. *J Am Acad Dermatol* 1990; **23**: 124−5.

38 Hammarström L, Smith CIE, Berg U. Captopril-induced IgA deficiency. *Lancet* 1991; **337**: 436.

39 Smit AJ, van der Laan S, De Monchy J, *et al.* Cutaneous reactions to captopril. Predictive values of skin tests. *Clin Allergy* 1984; **14**: 413−19.

40 Gavras I, Gavras H. Captopril and enalapril. *Ann Intern Med* 1983; **98**: 556−7.

41 Shelto RM. Pemphigus foliaceus associated with enalapril. *J Am Acad Dermatol* 1991; **24**: 503−4.

42 Barlow RJ, Schulz EJ. Lisinopril-induced vasculitis. *Clin Exp Dermatol* 1988; **13**: 117−20.

Calcium channel blockers

Cutaneous reactions are rare and have been reported in 5.8 per million prescriptions of nifedipine, 16.6 per million prescriptions of verapamil, and 6.5 per million prescriptions of diltiazem [1,2]. Pruritus, maculopapular rashes, and urticaria/angioedema have been described with all three drugs, as have Stevens−Johnson syndrome and erythema multiforme; toxic epidermal necrolysis has occurred with diltiazem. There is a suggestion that the more severe reactions are commoner with diltiazem. Peripheral oedema as a side-effect is common to the dihydropyridine calcium antagonists, including nifedipine, nicardipine, isradipine, and amlodipine; it occurs in 7−30% of patients depending on the specific drug, but is usually mild [3].

Diltiazem

Hyperplastic gingivitis has been documented [4]. Toxic erythema [5,6], erythema multiforme [7], a photosensitive eruption [8], vasculitis [9] and vasculitic leg ulcers [10], a generalized pustular dermatitis [11], and exfoliative dermatitis in a patient with psoriasis [12] are recorded. Generalized lymphadenopathy has occurred [13].

Nicardipine

Erythromelalgia is recorded [14].

Nifedipine

Headache, tachycardia and flushing are common side-effects. Gingival hyperplasia is well recognized [15]. Burning sensations, erythema, painful oedema and erythromelalgia have been described [16−19]. There have been isolated reports of a fixed drug reaction [20], a generalized bullous eruption, vasculitis [21], photosensitivity [22,23] in one case confirmed by rechallenge [23], gynaecomastia [24], erysipelas-like lesions on the shins with erythematous plaques on the trunk [25] and exfoliative dermatitis [26].

Verapamil

Erythema multiforme has been reported [27].

1 Stern R, Khalsa JH. Cutaneous adverse reactions associated with calcium channel blockers. *Arch Intern Med* 1989; **149**: 829−32.
2 Sadick NS, Katz AS, Schreiber TL. Angioedema from calcium channel blockers. *J Am Acad Dermatol* 1989; **21**: 132−3.
3 Maclean D, MacConnachie AM. Selected side-effects: 1. Peripheral oedema with dihydropyridine calcium antagonists. *Prescribers' J* 1991; **31**: 4−6.
4 Giustiniani S, Robustelli della Cuna F, Marieni M. Hyperplastic gingivitis during diltiazem therapy. *Int J Cardiol* 1987; **15**: 247−9.

5 Wakeel RA, Gavin MP, Keefe M. Severe toxic erythema caused by diltiazem. *Br Med J* 1988; **296**: 1071.

6 Hammentgen R, Lutz G, Köhler U, Nitsch J. Makulopapulöses Exanthem bei Diltiazem-Therapie. *Dtsch Med Wochenschr* 1988; **113**: 1283–5.

7 Berbis P, Alfonso MJ, Levy JL, Privat Y. Diltiazem associated erythema multiforme. *Dermatologica* 1990; **179**: 90.

8 Hashimoto M, Tanaka S, Horio T. Photosensibility due to diltiazem hydrochloride. *Acta Dermatol (Kyoto)* 1979; **74**: 181–4.

9 Sheehan-Dare RA, Goodfield MJ. Severe cutaneous vasculitis induced by diltiazem. *Br J Dermatol* 1988; **119**: 134.

10 Carmichael AJ, Paul CJ. Vasculitic leg ulcers associated with diltiazem. *Br Med J* 1988; **297**: 562.

11 Lambert DG, Dalac S, Beer F, *et al.* Acute generalized exanthematous pustular dermatitis induced by diltiazem. *Br J Dermatol* 1988; **118**: 308–9.

12 Larvijsen APM, Van Dijke C, Vermeer B-J. Diltiazem-associated exfoliative dermatitis in a patient with psoriasis. *Acta Derm Venereol (Stockh)* 1986; **66**: 536–8.

13 Scolnick B, Brinberg D. Diltiazem and generalized lymphadenopathy. *Ann Intern Med* 1985; **102**: 558.

14 Levesque H, Moore N, Wolfe LM, Courtoid H. Erythromelalgia induced by nicardipine (inverse Raynaud's phenomenon ?). *Br Med J* 1989; **298**: 1252–3.

15 Benini PL, Crosti C, Sala F, *et al.* Gingival hypoplasia by nifedipine. Report of a case. *Acta Derm Venereol (Stockh)* 1985; **65**: 362–5.

16 Bridgman JF. Erythematous edema of the legs due to nifedipine. *Br Med J* 1978; **i**: 578.

17 Fisher JR, Padnick MB, Olstein S. Nifedipine and erythromelalgia. *Ann Intern Med* 1983; **98**: 671–2.

18 Brodmerkel GJ Jr. Nifedipine and erythromelalgia. *Ann Intern Med* 1983; **99**: 415.

19 Alcalay J, David M, Sandbank M. Cutaneous reactions to nifedipine. *Dermatologica* 1987; **175**: 191–3.

20 Alcalay J, David M. Generalized fixed drug eruptions associated with nifedipine. *Br Med J* 1986; **292**: 450.

21 Brenner S, Brau S. Vasculitis following nifedipine. *Harefuah* 1985; **108**: 139–40.

22 Thomas SE, Wood ML. Photosensitivity reactions associated with nifedipine. *Br Med J* 1986; **292**: 992.

23 Zenarola P, Gatti S, Lomuto M. Photodermatitis due to nifedipine: report of 2 cases. *Dermatologica* 1991; **182**: 196–8.

24 Clyne CAC. Unilateral gynaecomastia and nifedipine. *Br Med J* 1986; **292**: 380.

25 Leibovici V, Zlotogorski A, Heyman A, *et al.* Polymorphous drug eruption due to nifedipine. *Cutis* 1988; **41**: 367.

26 Reynolds BJ, Jones SK, Crossley J, Harman RRM. Exfoliative dermatitis due to nifedipine. *Br J Dermatol* 1989; **121**: 401–4.

27 Kürkçüoglu N, Alaybeyi F. Erythema multiforme after verapamil treatment. *J Am Acad Dermatol* 1991; **24**: 511–12.

Centrally acting antihypertensive drugs

Clonidine

Hypersensitivity rashes occur in up to 5% of patients. A pityriasis rosea-like and LE-like syndrome, exacerbation of psoriasis [1] and an isolated instance of anogenital cicatricial pemphigoid [2] have been documented. Transdermally administered clonidine has caused allergic contact dermatitis.

1 Wilkin JK. Exacerbation of psoriasis during clonidine therapy. *Arch Dermatol* 1981; **117**: 4.
2 Van Joost T, Faber WR, Manuel HR. Drug-induced anogenital cicatricial pemphigoid. *Br J Dermatol* 1980; **102**: 715–18.

Methyldopa

An eczematous eruption of discoid or seborrhoeic pattern is characteristic, is more likely to occur in previously eczematous subjects, and persists until the drug is stopped [1]. Eczema of the palms and soles has also been described and may become widespread. The reaction is probably allergic as it may be dose related. Purpuric, erythematous and lichenoid rashes occur, sometimes in association with fever and other allergic symptoms [2,3]. Lichenoid eruptions may be ulcerated [4,5] and persistent ulceration of the tongue has been described. Fixed eruptions are very rare. A lupus-like syndrome is documented [6,7] and an autoimmune haemolytic anaemia is well known [5]. Psoriasis may be precipitated.

1 Church R. Eczema provoked by methyldopa. *Br J Dermatol* 1974; **91**: 373–8.
2 Stevenson CJ. Lichenoid eruptions due to methyldopa. *Br J Dermatol* 1971; **85**: 600.
3 Burry JN, Kirk J. Lichenoid drug reaction from methyldopa. *Br J Dermatol* 1974; **91**: 475–6.
4 Burry JN. Ulcerative lichenoid eruption from methyldopa. *Arch Dermatol* 1976; **112**: 880.
5 Furhoff A-K. Adverse reactions with methyldopa — a decade's reports. *Acta Med Scand* 1978; **203**: 425–8.
6 Harrington TM, Davis DE. Systemic lupus-like syndrome induced by methyldopa therapy. *Chest* 1981; **79**: 696–7.
7 Dupont A, Six R. Lupus-like syndrome induced by methyldopa. *Br Med J* 1982; **285**: 693–4.

Adrenergic neurone blocking agents

Guanethidine

Hypersensitivity eruptions are very rare but polyarteritis nodosa has been attributed to this drug [1].

1 Dewar HA, Peaston MJT. Three cases resembling polyarteritis nodosa arising during treatment with guanethidine. *Br Med J* 1964; **ii**: 609–11.

Vasodilator antihypertensive drugs

Diazoxide

Transient flushing is common. During long-term treatment up to half the patients develop hirsutism without other signs of virilization [1]. A clinical picture resembling hypertrichosis lanuginosa may develop [2,3]. Oedema occurs in at least 10% of patients; photosensitivity is very uncommon but well recognized. Lichenoid [3,4] and other rashes occur rarely.

1 Burton JL, Schutt WH, Caldwell JW. Hypertrichosis due to diazoxide. *Br J Dermatol* 1975; **93**: 707–11.
2 Koblenzer PJ, Baker J. Hypertrichosis lanuginosa associated with diazoxide therapy in prepubertal children: a clinicopathologic study. *Ann N Y Acad Sci* 1968; **150**: 373–82.
3 Menter MA. Hypertrichosis lanuginosa and a lichenoid eruption due to diazoxide therapy. *Proc R Soc Med* 1973; **66**: 326–7.
4 Okun R, Russell RP, Wilson WR. Use of diazoxide with trichlormethiazide for hypertension. *Arch Intern Med* 1963; **112**: 882–6.

Hydralazine

The LE-like syndrome due to this drug is well known [1–7]. Hydralazine binds to complement component C4 and inhibits its function; this may impair clearance of immune complexes, and predispose to development of an LE syndrome [6,7]. Orogenital ulceration may be part of the picture [8] and the syndrome has presented as a leg ulcer [9]. Cutaneous vasculitis may be severe and necrotizing [10,11]. An association between a hydralazine-induced lupus syndrome and the development of Sweet's syndrome has been noted rarely [12]. Fixed drug eruption has been reported [13]. Characteristic lung changes are attributed to the drug [14].

1 Alarcon-Segovia D, Wakin KG, Worthington JW, *et al.* Clinical and experimental studies on the hydralazine syndrome and its relationship to systemic lupus erythematosus. *Medicine* 1967; **46**: 1–33.
2 Batchelor JR, Welsh KI, Mansilla Tinoco R, *et al.* Hydralazine-induced systemic lupus erythematosus: influence of HLA-DR and sex upon susceptibility. *Lancet* 1980; **i**: 1107–9.
3 Dubroff LM, Reid R Jr, Papalian M. Molecular models for hydralazine-related systemic lupus erythematosus. *Arthritis Rheum* 1981; **24**: 1082–5.
4 Perry HM Jr. Possible mechanisms of the hydralazine-related lupus-like syndrome. *Arthritis Rheum* 1981; **24**: 1093–105.
5 Mansilla Tinoco R, Harland SJ, Ryan P, *et al.* Hydralazine, antinuclear antibodies, and the lupus syndrome. *Br Med J* 1982; **284**: 936–9.
6 Sim E, Law S-KA. Hydralazine binds covalently to complement component C4. Different reactivity of C4A and C4B gene products. *FEBS Lett* 1985; **184**: 323–7.
7 Sim E. Drug-induced immune complex disease. *Complement Inflamm* 1989; **6**: 119–26.
8 Neville E, Graham PY, Brewis RA. Orogenital ulcers, SLE and hydralazine. *Postgrad Med J* 1981; **57**: 378–9.
9 Kissin MW, Williamson RCN. Hydralazine-induced SLE-like syndrome presenting as a leg ulcer. *Br Med J* 1979; **ii**: 1330.
10 Bernstein RM, Egerton-Vernon J, Webster J. Hydralazine-induced cutaneous vasculitis. *Br Med J* 1980; **280**: 156–7.
11 Peacock A, Weatherall D. Hydralazine-induced necrotising vasculitis. *Br Med J* 1981; **282**: 1121–2.
12 Servitje O, Ribera M, Juanola X, Rodriguez-Moreno J. Acute neutrophilic dermatosis associated with hydralazine-induced lupus. *Arch Dermatol* 1988; **123**: 1435–6.
13 Sehgal VN, Gangwani OP. Hydralazine-induced fixed drug eruption. *Int J Dermatol* 1986; **25**: 394.
14 Bass BH. Hydralazine lung. *Thorax* 1981; **36**: 695–6.

Minoxidil

This arterial vasodilator causes hypertrichosis, especially of the arms and face, which may be unacceptable to women [1,2]; the hair disappears slowly after the drug is withdrawn. Fluid retention may require diuretic therapy to control it. Thrombocytopenia [3], bullous eruptions [4] and erythema multiforme or Stevens—Johnson syndrome [5] have been described.

1 Burton JL, Marshall A. Hypertrichosis due to minoxidil. *Br J Dermatol* 1979; **101**: 593—5.
2 Ryckmanns F. Hypertrichose durch Minoxidil. *Hautarzt* 1980; **31**: 205—6.
3 Peitzmann SJ, Martin C. Thrombocytopenia and minoxidil. *Ann Intern Med* 1980; **92**: 874.
4 Rosenthal T, Teicher A, Swartz J, Boichis H. Minoxidil-induced bullous eruption. *Arch Intern Med* 1978; **138**: 1856—7.
5 DiSantis DJ, Flanagan J. Minoxidil-induced Stevens—Johnson syndrome. *Arch Intern Med* 1981; **141**: 1515.

Nitrate vasodilators

Glyceryl and penta-erythritol tetranitrate

Reactions to nitrate vasodilators are rare, but erythroderma with cross-reactivity to glyceryl trinitrate has been caused by this drug [1].

1 Ryan FP. Erythroderma due to peritrate and glyceryl trinitrate. *Br J Dermatol* 1972; **87**: 498—500.

9.4 Diuretics

Carbonic anhydrase inhibitor

Acetazolamide

This has caused hirsutism in a child [1]. Hypersensitivity reactions are rare.

1 Weiss IS. Hirsutism after chronic administration of acetazolamide. *Am J Ophthalmol* 1974; **78**: 327—8.

Loop diuretics

Bumetanide

Occasional hypersensitivity rashes occur. Pseudoporphyria has been reported with this sulphonamide-derived drug [1].

Ethacrynic acid

A Henoch—Schönlein type of vasculitis has been documented.

Frusemide

Reactions are rare; only two patients of 3830 receiving this medication in a recent study developed cutaneous complications [2]. Phototoxic blistering has followed very high dosage (2.0 g daily) in chronic renal failure [3] but erythema multiforme [4,5], bullous pemphigoid [6,7], other bullous haemorrhagic eruptions [8] and an acquired blistering disorder with skin fragility [9] have apparently been precipitated by conventional dosage. The skin changes may mimic those of porphyria. Several cases of generalized exfoliative dermatitis have been documented. Anaphylaxis [10], a necrotizing vasculitis [11] and an eruption resembling Sweet's syndrome [12] have been reported. Cross-reactivity between frusemide, hydrochlorothiazide and sulphonamides is recorded, but the use of one of these drugs in a patient known to have allergy to another involves only low risk [13].

1 Leitao EA, Person JR. Bumetanide-induced pseudoporphyria. *J Am Acad Dermatol* 1990; **23**: 129–30.
2 Bigby M, Jick S, Jick H, Arndt K. Drug-induced cutaneous reactions. A report from the Boston Collaborative Drug Surveillance Program on 15 438 consecutive inpatients, 1975 to 1982. *JAMA* 1986; **256**: 3358–63.
3 Burry JN, Lawrence JR. Phototoxic blisters from high frusemide dosage. *Br J Dermatol* 1976; **94**: 493–9.
4 Gibson TP, Blue P. Erythema multiforme and furosemide therapy. *JAMA* 1970; **212**: 1709.
5 Zugerman C, La Voo EJ. Erythema multiforme caused by oral furosemide. *Arch Dermatol* 1980; **116**: 518–19.
6 Fellner MI, Katz JM. Occurrence of bullous pemphigoid after furosemide therapy. *Arch Dermatol* 1976; **112**: 75–7.
7 Castel T, Gratacos R, Castro J, *et al.* Bullous pemphigoid induced by frusemide. *Clin Exp Dermatol* 1981; **6**: 635–8.
8 Ebringer A, Adam WR, Parkin JD. Bullous haemorrhagic eruption associated with frusemide. *Med J Aust* 1969; **1**: 768–71.
9 Kennedy AC, Lyell A. Acquired epidermolysis bullosa due to high dose frusemide. *Br Med J* 1976; **i**: 1509–10.
10 Hansbrough JR, Wedner HJ, Chaplin DD. Anaphylaxis to intravenous furosemide. *J Allergy Clin Immunol* 1987; **80**: 538–41.
11 Hendricks WM, Ader RS. Furosemide-induced cutaneous necrotizing vasculitis. *Arch Dermatol* 1977; **113**: 375.
12 Cobb MW. Furosemide-induced eruption simulating Sweet's syndrome. *J Am Acad Dermatol* 1989; **21**: 339–43.
13 Sullivan TJ. Cross-reactions among furosemide, hydrochlorothiazide, and sulfonamides. *JAMA* 1991; **265**: 120–1.

Potassium sparing diuretics

Spironolactone

This drug, used for the treatment of acne vulgaris and hirsutism [1], may cause gynaecomastia (Fig. 9.2) [2–4], gastrointestinal upset, hyperkalaemia, and rarely agranulocytosis [1]. Spironolactone has an antiandrogen effect [4] and may result in loss of libido and impotence, or menstrual irregularities. A lupus-like syndrome [5], annular lupus erythematosus [6], erythema annulare centrifugum [7], and a lichenoid eruption [8] have been seen.

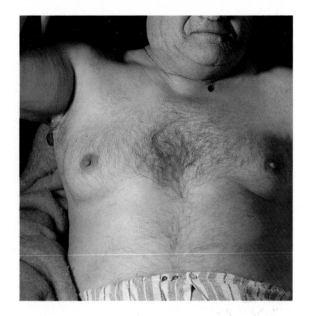

Figure 9.2 Gynaecomastia related to spironolactone.

1 Shaw JC. Spironolactone in dermatologic therapy. *J Am Acad Dermatol* 1991; **24**: 236–43.
2 Clarke E. Spironolactone therapy and gynecomastia. *JAMA* 1965; **193**: 157–8.
3 Loriaux DL, Meuard R, Taylor A, *et al*. Spironolactone and endocrine dysfunction. *Ann Intern Med* 1976; **85**: 630–6.
4 Rose LI, Underwood RH, Newmark SR, *et al*. Pathophysiology of spironolactone-induced gynecomastia. *Ann Intern Med* 1977; **87**: 398–403.
5 Uddin MS, Lynfield YL, Grosberg SJ, Stiefler R. Cutaneous reaction to spironolactone resembling lupus erythematosus. *Cutis* 1979; **24**: 198–200.
6 Leroy D, Dompmartin A, Le Jean S, *et al*. Toxidermie à l'aldactone® a type d'érytheme annulaire centrifuge lupique. *Ann Dermatol Vénéréol (Paris)* 1987; **114**: 1237–40.
7 Carsuzaa F, Pierre C, Dubegny M. Érytheme annulaire centrifuge à l'aldactone. *Ann Dermatol Vénéréol (Paris)* 1987; **114**: 375–6.
8 Downham TF III. Spironolactone-induced lichen planus. *JAMA* 1978; **240**: 1138.

Thiazides and related diuretics

Photosensitivity (Figs 9.3 & 9.4) is uncommon, probably occurring in between 1 in 1000 and 1 in 100 000 prescriptions [1], but well known [1–7]. Hydrochlorothiazide causes considerably more reactions than bendroflumethiazide. The mechanism is unknown, and both phototoxic [1,4,7] and photo-allergic [2,3] mechanisms have been proposed. The commonest reaction is lichenoid, but petechial and erythematous eruptions may occur in exposed skin. Xerostomia has been reported, as has a vasculitis [8]. An eruption resembling subacute cutaneous LE has been described in patients taking a combination of hydrochlorothiazide and triamterene [9,10] and with hydrochlorothiazide alone [11]. Other side-effects include hypokalaemia, short-term elevation of low density lipoprotein cholesterol, impotence, a diabetogenic effect, and exacerbation of gout [12].

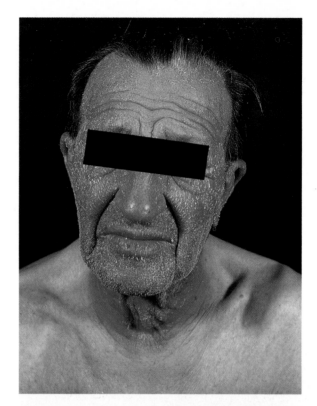

Figure 9.3 Photosensitive eruption
due to a thiazide.

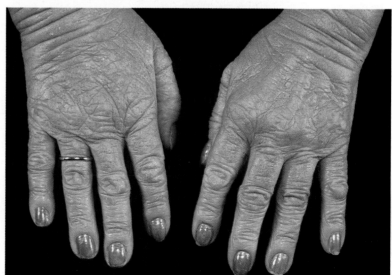

Figure 9.4 Photosensitive lichenoid
eruption due to a thiazide. (Courtesy
of Dr D.H. McGibbon, St John's
Institute of Dermatology, London.)

Chlorthalidone

Pseudoporphyria has been documented with this thiazide-related
diuretic [13]. Psoriasis has been triggered in a patient also receiving
captopril [14].

1 Diffey BL, Langtry J. Phototoxic potential of thiazide diuretics in normal
subjects. *Arch Dermatol* 1989; **125**: 1355–8.

2 Harber LC, Lashinsky AM, Baer RL. Photosensitivity to chlorothiazide and hydrochlorothiazide. *N Engl J Med* 1959; **261**: 1378−81.

3 Torinuki W. Photosensitivity due to hydrochlorothiazide. *J Dermatol (Tokyo)* 1980; **7**: 293−6.

4 Rosén K, Swanbeck G. Phototoxic reactions from some common drugs provoked by a high-intensity UVA lamp. *Acta Derm Venereol (Stockh)* 1982; **62**: 246−8.

5 Hawk JLM. Photosensitizing agents used in the United Kingdom. *Clin Exp Dermatol* 1984; **9**: 300−2.

6 Robinson HN, Morison WL, Hood AF. Thiazide diuretic therapy and chronic photosensitivity. *Arch Dermatol* 1985; **121**: 522−4.

7 Addo HA, Ferguson J, Frain-Bell W. Thiazide-induced photosensitivity: a study of 33 subjects. *Br J Dermatol* 1987; **116**: 749−60.

8 Björnberg A, Gisslén H. Thiazides: a cause of necrotising vasculitis? *Lancet* 1965; **ii**: 982−3.

9 Berbis P, Vernay-Vaisse C, Privat Y. Lupus cutané subaigu observé au cours d'un traitement par diurétiques thiazidiques. *Ann Dermatol Vénéréol (Paris)* 1986; **113**: 1245−8.

10 Darken M, McBurney EI. Subacute cutaneous lupus erythematosus-like drug eruption due to combination diuretic hydrochlorothiazide and triamterene. *J Am Acad Dermatol* 1988; **18**: 38−42.

11 Reed BR, Huff JC, Jones SK, *et al*. Subacute cutaneous lupus erythematosus associated with hydrochlorothiazide therapy. *Ann Intern Med* 1985; **103**: 49−51.

12 Orme M. Thiazides in the 1990s. The risk:benefit ratio still favours the drug. *Br Med J* 1990; **300**: 1168−9.

13 Baker EJ, Reed KD, Dixon SL. Chlorthalidone-induced pseudopophyria: clinical and microscopic findings of a case. *J Am Acad Dermatol* 1989; **21**: 1026−9.

14 Wolf R, Dorfman B, Krakowski A. Psoriasiform eruption induced by captopril and chlorthalidone. *Cutis* 1987; **40**: 162−4.

9.5 Miscellaneous cardiovascular drugs

Dopamine

This positive inotropic agent has caused local skin necrosis, due to extravasation at the site of an intravenous cannula [1], and acral gangrene secondary to distal vasoconstriction [2]. Localized pilo-erection and vasoconstriction proximal to the site of infusion have been documented [3].

1 Green SI, Smith JW. Dopamine gangrene. *N Engl J Med* 1976; **294**: 114.

2 Boltax RS, Dineen JP, Scarpa FJ. Gangrene resulting from infiltrated dopamine solution. *N Engl J Med* 1977; **296**: 823.

3 Ross M. Dopamine-induced localized cutaneous vasoconstriction and pilo-erection. *Arch Dermatol* 1991; **127**: 586−7.

Vasopressin

This drug, when used intravenously for control of bleeding oesophageal varices or as a local vasoconstrictor agent, has caused cutaneous necrosis at sites of extravasation (Fig. 9.5), and occasionally at distant sites, with a bullous eruption [1].

1 Korenberg RJ, Landau-Price D, Penneys NS. Vasopressin-induced bullous disease and cutaneous necrosis. *J Am Acad Dermatol* 1986; **15**: 393−8.

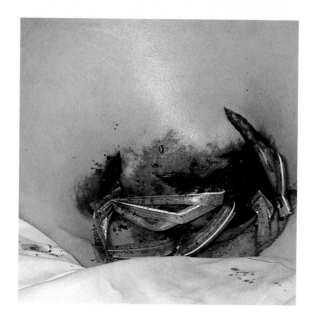

Figure 9.5 Severe cutaneous necrosis at site of injection of vasopressin.

9.6 β-Agonist drugs

Albuterol

Patchy erythema of the hands developed in a pregnant patient following infusion [1].

Salbutamol

Lupus-like acral erythema developed after infusion in three pregnant patients with premature labour [2].

Salmeterol

An urticarial reaction which recurred on challenge was attributed to this drug administered from a metered dose inhaler [3].

1 Morin Leport LRM, Loisel JC, Feuilly C. Hand erythema due to infusion of sympathomimetics. *Br J Dermatol* 1990; **122**: 116–17.
2 Reygagne P, Lacour JP, Ortonne J-P. Palmar and plantar erythema due to infusion of sympathomimetics in pregnant women. *Br J Dermatol* 1991; **124**: 210.
3 Hatton MQF, Allen MB, Mellor EJ, Cooke NJ. Salmeterol rash. *Lancet* 1991; **337**: 1169–70.

9.7 Antimuscarinic bronchodilators

Aminophylline

This drug is a mixture of theophylline and ethylenediamine. Urticaria, generalized erythema and exfoliative dermatitis have followed systemic administration, probably as a result of reactions to the ethylenediamine component, rather than of theophylline itself [1]. Cross-reactions may occur with ethylenediamine in antihistamines and topical preparations [1,2]. Patch tests may or may not be positive [3].

1 Gibb W, Thompson PJ. Allergy to aminophylline. *Br Med J* 1983; **287**: 501.
2 Elias JA, Levinson AI. Hypersensitivity reactions to ethylenediamine in aminophylline. *Am Rev Respir Dis* 1981; **123**: 550–2.
3 Kradjan WA, Lakshminarayan S. Allergy to aminophylline: lack of predictability by skin testing. *Am J Hosp Pharm* 1981; **38**: 1031–3.

9.8 Miscellaneous respiratory system drugs

Sodium cromoglycate

Hypersensitivity reactions are rare, but urticaria, angioedema and anaphylactic shock are recorded [1].

1 Scheffer AL, Rocklin RE, Goetzl EJ. Immunologic components of hypersensitivity reactions to cromolyn sodium. *N Engl J Med* 1975; **293**: 1220–4.

Pseudoephedrine

This drug present in nasal decongestants has caused a fixed drug eruption [1] and recurrent pseudo-scarlatina [2].

1 Shelly WB, Shelly ED. Non-pigmenting fixed drug reaction pattern: Examples caused by sensitivity to pseudoephedrine hydrochloride and tetrahydrozoline. *J Am Acad Dermatol* 1987; **17**: 403–7.
2 Taylor BJ, Duffill MB. Recurrent pseudoscarlatina and allergy to pseudoephedrine hydrochloride. *Br J Dermatol* 1988; **118**: 827–9.

Chapter 10
Metals and Metal Antagonists

10.1 Metals

Arsenic

Bullous eruptions, photosensitivity, exfoliative dermatitis and alopecia may be acute manifestations of arsenic toxicity. Occupational exposure may occur, especially in agriculture. Fowler's solution (containing 1% potassium arsenite) and sodium arsenate were used in the past for psoriasis; as little as 0.19 g has been carcinogenic and the interval between exposure and tumour induction may be as long as 47 years [1]. Subjects with an abnormally high retention of ingested arsenic may be at particular risk [2]. The cutaneous manifestations of arsenic exposure, including pigmentation, palmoplantar punctate keratoses (Fig. 10.1) and intra-epidermal (Bowen's disease), basal cell (Fig. 10.2) or squamous carcinomata of the skin, are well known [1—8]. Keratoses and tumours may be present without pigmentation. In one series of patients, there was a dose-related development of palmar and plantar keratoses in 40%, and carcinomas of the skin in 8%, of patients who received arsenic in the form of Fowler's solution for 6—26 years; the minimum latent period before development of keratoses was 2.5 years, and the

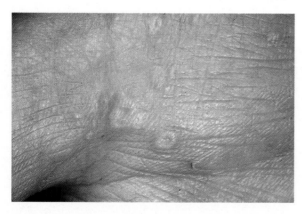

Figure 10.1 Arsenical keratoses of the palm. (Courtesy of St John's Institute of Dermatology, London.)

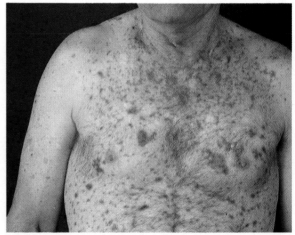

Figure 10.2 Multiple keratoses, areas of Bowen's disease, and basal cell cancers related to arsenic exposure.

average was 6 years [3]. Bowen's disease occurred within 10 years, and invasive carcinomas within 20 years, in another series [7]. Arsenic contamination of well water in Taiwan resulted in numerous affected individuals with arsenical keratoses and cutaneous carcinomas [5]. Carcinomas may arise in the arsenical keratoses [5]. Cutaneous electron microscopic changes are said to be characteristic [8]. The diagnostic significance of the skin arsenic content is disputed. A 42-year-old man who took arsenic for 35 years for psoriasis developed melanoderma, keratoses, muscular dystrophies, hyperlipidaemia, testicular atrophy, gynaecomastia, skin tumours and an obliterating angiitis of leg vessels which led to amputation [4]. The role of arsenic in causing internal malignancy is the subject of controversy [7,9,10].

1 Evans S. Arsenic and cancer. *Br J Dermatol* 1977; **97** (Suppl 15): 13–14.
2 Bettley FR, O'Shea JA. The absorption of arsenic and its relation to carcinoma. *Br J Dermatol* 1975; **92**: 563–8.
3 Fierz U. Katamnestische Untersuchungen über die Nebenwirkungen der Therapie mit anorganischem Arsen bei Hautkrankheiten. *Dermatologica* 1965; **131**: 41–58.
4 Meyhofer W, Knoth W. Über die Auswirkung einer langjährigen antipsoriatischen Arsentherapie auf mehrere Organe unter besonderer Berücksichtigung andrologischer Befunde. *Hautarzt* 1966; **117**: 309–13.
5 Yeh S. Skin cancer in chronic arsenicism. *Hum Pathol* 1973; **4**: 469–85.
6 Weiss J, Jänner M. Multiple Basaliome und Menigiom nach mehrjähriger Arsentherapie. *Hautarzt* 1980; **31**: 654–6.
7 Miki Y, Kawatsu T, Matsuda K, *et al.* Cutaneous and pulmonary cancers associated with Bowen's disease. *J Am Acad Dermatol* 1982; **6**: 26–31.
8 Ohyama K, Sonoda K, Kuwahara H. Electron microscopic observations of arsenical keratoses and Bowen's disease associated with chronic arsenicism. *Dermatologica* 1982; **64**: 161–6.
9 Reymann F, Møller R, Nielsen A. Relationship between arsenic intake and internal malignant neoplasms. *Arch Dermatol* 1978; **114**: 378–81.
10 Callen JP, Headington J. Bowen's and non-Bowen's squamous intraepidermal neoplasia of the skin. Relationship to internal malignancy. *Arch Dermatol* 1980; **116**: 422–6.

Gold

The use of gold in rheumatoid arthritis is associated with a 30% incidence of reactions [1,2]; most of these are minor, but about 15% may be severe or even fatal [3]. Possession of the HLA-DR3 and B8 phenotypes predisposes to thrombocytopenia, leucopenia and nephrotoxicity, DR4 is linked to leucopenia, and HLA-B7 is associated with cutaneous adverse reactions [2]. In addition, an impaired ability to sulphoxidize carbocisteine is associated with increased gold toxicity.

Dermatological complications

Rashes and mouth ulcers are common [1,2,4–6], representing about 50% of all complications with parenteral gold and 35% with oral gold. Localized or generalized pruritus is an important warning sign of potential toxicity. Gold reactions may simulate exanthematic eruptions, erythema multiforme, pityriasis rosea, seborrhoeic dermatitis (Fig. 10.3), or lichen planus (Fig. 10.4); a mixture of these patterns, sometimes with discoid eczematoid lesions, is characteristic [5]. Lichen planus is often of the hypertrophic variety especially on the scalp, and severe and irreversible alopecia may follow. There may be striking and persistent postinflammatory hyperpigmentation. Permanent nail dystrophy has followed onycholysis [7]. In one study, eczematous or lichenoid rashes persisted up to 11 months after cessation of therapy [8]. Histology was characterized by a sparse dermal perivascular infiltrate, predominantly of CD4$^+$ HLA-DR$^+$ T-helper lymphocytes, an increase in the number of dermal Langerhans cells and of epidermal macrophage-like cells, and Langerhans cell apposition to mononuclear cells. A patient with a lichenoid and seborrhoeic dermatitis-like rash on gold sodium thiomalate therapy had a positive intradermal test to gold thiomalate; patch tests were positive to thiomalate (the thiol carrier of gold thiomalate), but negative to gold itself [9]. Interestingly, the same patient subsequently developed a seborrhoeic dermatitis-like eruption, but not a lichenoid eruption, whilst on auranofin; this time, patch tests were positive to both auranofin and to gold. A previous contact dermatitis from gold jewellery may be reactivated [10]. Other reactions documented include erythema nodosum [11], severe hypersensitivity reactions [12], vasculitis [13], polyarteritis, a sys-

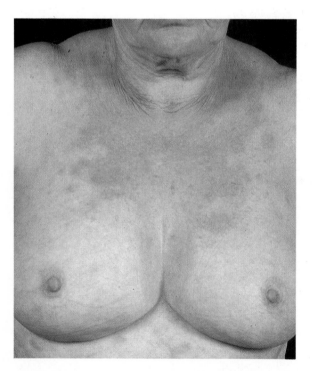

Figure 10.3 Seborrhoeic dermatitis-like rash related to gold therapy.

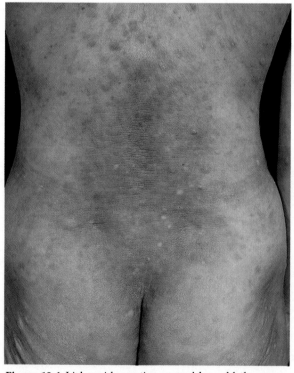

Figure 10.4 Lichenoid eruption caused by gold therapy.

temic lupus-like syndrome, generalized exfoliative dermatitis, and toxic epidermal necrolysis. Psoriasis was reported to be exacerbated in a patient with arthritis treated with gold [14].

Prolonged administration may cause a distinct grey, blue or purple pigmentation of exposed skin (chrysiasis) which is a dose-dependent reaction; gold granules are seen within dermal endothelial cells and macrophages [15,16]. Even in the absence of pigmentation, gold can be detected histochemically in the skin up to 20 years after therapy. An unusual late cutaneous reaction involved appearance of widespread keloid-like angiofibromatoid lesions [17].

Systemic side-effects

A benign vasodilatory 'nitritoid' reaction, consisting of flushing, light-headedness and transient hypotension, may occur immediately after the first injection of gold [2]. Non-vasomotor effects including arthralgia, myalgia and constitutional symptoms within the first 24 hours, are recognized. Mucous membrane symptoms include loss of taste, metallic taste, stomatitis and glossitis, and diarrhoea. Punctate stomatitis may occur with or without skin lesions. Gold is also deposited in the cornea and may cause a keratitis with ulceration. A polyneuropathy is recorded. In general, auranofin is less toxic than intramuscular gold [2]. Eosinophilia is common and may sometimes herald another complication; serum IgE may be raised [18]. Other immunological reactions are rare although pulmonary fibrosis is recorded [19]. Blood dyscrasias, especially thrombocytopenic purpura, and occasionally fatal neutropenia or aplastic anaemia, occur in a small proportion of cases and usually present within the first 6 months of therapy. Jaundice occurs in about 3% of cases, and may result from idiosyncratic intrahepatic cholestasis [20]. Proteinuria and renal damage are well known.

1 Thomas I. Gold therapy and its indications in dermatology. A review. *J Am Acad Dermatol* 1987; **16**: 845–54.
2 Pullar T. Adverse reactions profile: 1. Gold. *Prescribers' J* 1991; **31**: 22–6.
3 Girdwood RH. Death after taking medicaments. *Br Med J* 1974; i: 501–4.
4 Almeyda J, Baker H. Drug reactions XII. Cutaneous reactions to anti-rheumatic drugs. *Br J Dermatol* 1970; **83**: 707–11.
5 Penneys NS, Ackerman AB, Gottlieb NL. Gold dermatitis: A clinical and histopathological study. *Arch Dermatol* 1974; **109**: 372–6.
6 Penneys NS. Gold therapy: Dermatologic uses and toxicities. *J Am Acad Dermatol* 1979; **1**: 315–20.
7 Voigt K, Holzegel K. Bleibende nagelveränderungen nach Goldtherapie. *Hautarzt* 1977; **28**: 421–3.
8 Ranki A, Niemi K-M, Kanerva L. Clinical, immunohistochemical, and electron-microscopic findings in gold dermatitis. *Am J Dermatopathol* 1989; **11**: 22–8.
9 Ikezawa Z, Kitamura K, Nakajima H. Gold sodium thiomalate (GTM) induces hypersensitivity to thiomalate, the thiol carrier of GTM. *J Dermatol (Tokyo)* 1990; **17**: 550–4.
10 Rennie T. Local gold toxicity. *Br Med J* 1976; ii: 1294.
11 Stone RL, Claflin A, Penneys NS. Erythema nodosum following gold sodium thiomalate therapy. *Arch Dermatol* 1973; **107**: 603–4.
12 Walzer RA, Feinstein R, Shapiro L, Einbinder J. Severe hypersensitivity

reaction to gold. Positive lymphocyte transformation test. *Arch Dermatol* 1972; **106**: 231−4.

13 Roenigk HR, Handel D. Gold vasculitis. *Arch Dermatol* 1974; **109**: 253−5.

14 Smith DL, Wernick R. Exacerbation of psoriasis by chrysotherapy. *Arch Dermatol* 1991; **127**: 268−70.

15 Beckett VL, Doyle JA, Hadley GA, *et al*. Chrysiasis resulting from gold therapy in rheumatoid arthritis: Identification of gold by X-ray microanalysis. *Mayo Clin Proc* 1982; **57**: 773−5.

16 Pelachyk IM, Bergfeld WF, McMahon JT. Chrysiasis following gold therapy for rheumatoid arthritis. *J Cutan Pathol* 1984; **11**: 491−4.

17 Herbst WM, Hornstein OP, Grießmeyer G. Ungewöhnliche kutane Angiofibromatose nach Goldtherapie einer primär chronischen Polyarthritis. *Hautarzt* 1989; **40**: 568−72.

18 Davis P, Ezeoke A, Munro J, *et al*. Immunological studies on the mechanism of gold hypersensitivity reactions. *Br Med J* 1973; **iii**: 676−8.

19 Morley TF, Komansky HJ, Adelizzi RA, *et al*. Pulmonary gold toxicity. *Eur J Respir Dis* 1984; **65**: 627−32.

20 Favreau M, Tannebaum H, Lough J. Hepatic toxicity associated with gold therapy. *Ann Intern Med* 1977; **87**: 717−19.

Iron

Iron-induced brownish discoloration has been noted at the site of local injection (local siderosis) [1].

1 Bork K. Lokalisierte kutane Siderose nach intramuskulären Eiseninjekition. *Hautarzt* 1984; **35**: 598−9.

Mercury

Mercury-containing teething powders have long been banned, but occasional occupational or environmental exposure can occur. Mercury amalgam in dental fillings has caused buccal pigmentation (see section 3.33, drug-induced oral conditions, Fig. 3.76, p. 132). Stomatitis may occur as a toxic reaction. Allergic reactions may be scarlatiniform or morbilliform, and can progress to generalized exfoliative dermatitis. Pink disease or acrodynia, a distinctive pattern of reaction to chronic exposure to mercury in young infants and children, is now very rare [1]. Painful extremities, pinkish acral discoloration, peeling of the palms and soles, gingivitis and various systemic complications may occur. Acrodynia developed in a child following inhalation of mercury-containing vapours from phenylmercuric acetate contained in latex paint [2]. (See also Chapter 19, Fig. 19.1, p. 355 for information on exogenous ochronosis from topical mercury-containing preparations.)

1 Dinehart SM, Dillard R, Raimer SS, *et al*. Cutaneous manifestations of acrodynia (pink disease). *Arch Dermatol* 1988; **124**: 107−9.

2 From the MMWR. Mercury exposure from interior latex paint − Michigan. *Arch Dermatol* 1990; **126**: 577.

Ingestion, or topical application, of silver preparations to the oral mucosa or upper respiratory tract, can produce slate-blue discoloration, especially of exposed skin, including oral and conjunctival mucosae [1–8]. Topical application may also cause systemic argyria, in which visceral organs are also discoloured [9]. Localized argyria can result from earring backs becoming embedded [10]. In some patients, the nail beds of the fingers but not the toes may show bluish discoloration [11]. Silver granules are found free within the dermis; the melanin may be increased in the epidermis or within melanophages [12,13].

1 Pariser RJ. Generalized argyria. Clinicopathologic features and histochemical studies. *Arch Dermatol* 1978; **114**: 373–7.
2 Reymond J-L, Stoebner P, Amblard P. Argyrie cutanée. Étude en microscopie electronique et en microanalyse X de 4 cas. *Ann Dermatol Vénéréol (Paris)* 1980; **107**: 251–5.
3 Johansson EA, Kanerva L, Niemi K-M, *et al.* Generalized argyria with low ceruloplasmin and copper levels in the serum. A case report with clinical and microscopical findings and a trial of penicillamine treatment. *Clin Exp Dermatol* 1982; **7**: 169–76.
4 Pezzarossa E, Alinovi A, Ferrari C. Generalized argyria. *J Cutan Pathol* 1983; **10**: 361–3.
5 Gherardi R, Brochard P, Chamak B, *et al.* Human generalized argyria. *Arch Pathol Lab Med* 1984; **108**: 181–2.
6 Jurecka W. Generalisierte Argyrose. *Hautarzt* 1986; **37**: 628–31.
7 Mittag H, Knecht J, Arnold R, *et al.* Zur Frage der Argyrie. Ein klinische, analytisch-chemische und mikromorphologische Untersuchung. *Hautarzt* 1987; **38**: 670–7.
8 Tanner LS, Gross DJ. Generalized argyria. *Cutis* 1990; **45**: 237–9.
9 Marshall IP, Schneider RP. Systemic argyria secondary to topical silver nitrate. *Arch Dermatol* 1977; **113**: 1077–9.
10 van den Nieuwenhijsen IJ, Calame JJ, Bruynzeel DP. Localized argyria caused by silver earrings. *Dermatologica* 1988; **177**: 189–91.
11 Plewig G, Lincke H, Wolff HH. Silver-blue nails. *Acta Derm Venereol (Stockh)* 1977; **57**: 413–19.
12 Hönigsmann H, Konrad K, Wolff K. Argyrose (Histologie und Ultrastruktur). *Hautarzt* 1973; **24**: 24–30.
13 Shelley WB, Shelley ED, Burmeister V. Argyria: The intradermal 'photograph', a manifestation of passive photosensitivity. *J Am Acad Dermatol* 1987; **16**: 211–17.

10.2 Metal antagonists

Desferrioxamine

Itching, erythema and urticaria are occasionally seen [1]. An indurated erythema with oedema lasting 2 weeks has been reported following infusion [2].

1 Bousquet J, Navarro M, Robert G, *et al.* Rapid desensitisation for desferrioxamine anaphylactoid reactions. *Lancet* 1983; **ii**: 859–60.
2 Venencie P-Y, Rain B, Blanc A, Tertian G. Toxidermie a la déféroxamine (Desféral). *Ann Dermatol Vénéréol (Paris)* 1988; **115**: 1174.

Penicillamine

There is a fourfold increase in toxicity with this drug in patients with rheumatoid arthritis with a genetically determined poor capacity to sulphoxidate the structurally related mucolytic agent, carbocisteine [1,2]. In addition, penicillamine toxicity is independently associated with HLA phenotype [1–3]. HLA-DR3 and B8 are associated with renal toxicity, DR3, B7 and DR2 with haematological toxicity, and A1 and DR4 with thrombocytopenia. Cutaneous adverse reactions are linked to HLA-DRw6.

1 Emery P, Panayi GS, Huston G, *et al*. D-Penicillamine induced toxicity in rheumatoid arthritis: the role of sulphoxidation status and HLA-DR3. *J Rheumatol* 1984; **11**: 626–32.
2 Dasgupta B. Adverse reactions profile: 2. Penicillamine. *Prescribers' J* 1991; **31**: 72–7.
3 Wooley PH, Griffin J, Panayi GS, *et al*. HLA-DR antigens and toxic reaction to sodium aurothiomalate and D-penicillamine in patients with rheumatoid arthritis. *N Engl J Med* 1980; **303**: 300–2.

Dermatological complications

The cutaneous side-effects of this chelating agent are of three distinct types, namely acute hypersensitivity reactions occurring early during treatment, late reactions including disturbances of autoimmune mechanisms, and lathyrogenic effects on connective tissue [1–5]. Hypersensitivity reactions are common and consist of urticarial or morbilliform rashes appearing within the first few weeks; the eruption clears on drug withdrawal and does not always recur on re-exposure.

1 Dasgupta B. Adverse reactions profile: 2. Penicillamine. *Prescribers' J* 1991; **31**: 72–7.
2 Katz R. Penicillamine-induced skin lesions. Occurrence in a patient with hepatolenticular degeneration (Wilson's disease). *Arch Dermatol* 1967; **95**: 196–8.
3 Greer KE, Askew FC, Richardson DR. Skin lesions induced by penicillamine. *Arch Dermatol* 1976; **112**: 1267–9.
4 Sternlieb I, Fisher M, Scheinberg IH. Penicillamine-induced skin lesions. *J Rheumatol* 1981; **8** (Suppl. 7): 149–54.
5 Levy RS, Fisher M, Alter JN. Penicillamine: Review and cutaneous manifestations. *J Am Acad Dermatol* 1983; **8**: 548–58.

Autoimmune syndromes caused by penicillamine are well documented. The development of pemphigus during the treatment of both Wilson's disease and rheumatoid arthritis with penicillamine was first noted in the French literature [1,2]. Since then, there have been numerous case reports [3–15]; about 7% of patients receiving penicillamine for more than 6 months develop drug-induced pemphigus [3]. (The reader is referred to section 3.21, p. 104, for further discussion of penicillamine-induced pemphigus.) Direct immunofluorescence findings mimic the idiopathic disorder, with epidermal intracellular deposition of immunoreactants [6]. Most patients develop pemphigus foliaceus (Fig. 3.59, p. 106), although there have been isolated reports of pemphigus vulgaris [4], and of pemphigus erythematosus with both epidermal intracellular, and subepidermal deposition of IgG [5,7]. In some patients clinical appearances may resemble dermatitis herpetiformis [11,12]. Oral lesions may be indistinguishable from those seen in the idiopathic disease, causing cheilosis, glossitis and stomatitis [13]. Painful erosive vulvovaginitis may lead to scarring. Penicillamine-induced pemphigus usually subsides rapidly after cessation of the drug; occasionally it may be more persistent [3] and fatalities have occurred [14,15]. A curious bullous dermatosis without the features of pemphigus has been described recently [16]. Other autoimmune manifestations include a bullous pemphigoid-like reaction [17], cicatricial pemphigoid [18,19], both discoid [20] and systemic [21,22], lupus erythematosus [23], dermatomyositis [24−27], and both morphea and systemic sclerosis [28,29]. Pre-existing lichen planus [30] may be exacerbated, and lichenoid eruptions develop *de novo* [31,32]. Alopecia, facial dryness and scaling, nail changes and hypertrichosis are recorded. The yellow nail syndrome has been reported frequently in association with penicillamine [33].

1 Degos R, Touraine R, Belaïch S, *et al*. Pemphigus chez un malade traité par pénicillamine pour maladie de Wilson. *Bull Soc Fr Dermatol Syphiligr* 1969; **76**: 751−3.
2 Benveniste M, Crouzet J, Homberg JC, *et al*. Pemphigus induits par la D-pénicillamine dans la polyarthrite rhumatoïde. *Nouv Presse Med* 1975; **4**: 3125−8.
3 Marsden RA, Ryan TJ, Vanhegan RI, *et al*. Pemphigus foliaceus induced by penicillamine. *Br Med J* 1976; **ii**: 1423−4.
4 From E, Frederiksen P. Pemphigus vulgaris following D-penicillamine. *Dermatologica* 1976; **152**: 358−62.
5 Thorvaldsen J. Two cases of penicillamine-induced pemphigus erythematosus. *Dermatologica* 1979; **159**: 167−70.
6 Santa Cruz DJ, Prioleau PG, Marcus MD, Uitto J. Pemphigus-like lesions induced by D-penicillamine. Analysis of clinical, histopathological, and immunofluorescence features in 34 cases. *Am J Dermatopathol* 1981; **3**: 85−92.
7 Yung CW, Hambrick GW Jr. D-Penicillamine-induced pemphigus syndrome. *J Am Acad Dermatol* 1982; **6**: 317−24.
8 Bahmer FA, Bambauer R, Stenger D. Penicillamine-induced pemphigus foliaceus-like dermatosis. A case with unusual features, successfully treated by plasmapheresis. *Arch Dermatol* 1985; **121**: 665−8.
9 Kind P, Goerz G, Gleichmann E, Plewig G. Penicillamininduzierter Pemphigus. *Hautarzt* 1987; **38**: 548−52.
10 Civatte J. Durch Medikamente induzierte Pemphigus-Erkrankungen. *Dermatol Monatsschr* 1989; **175**: 1−7.
11 Marsden RA, Dawber RPR, Millard PR, Mowat AG. Herpetiform pemphigus induced by penicillamine. *Br J Dermatol* 1977; **97**: 451−2.
12 Weltfriend S, Ingber A, David M, Sandbank M. Pemphigus herpetiformis nach D-Penicillamin bei einem Patienten mit HLA B8. *Hautarzt* 1988; **39**: 587−8.
13 Eisenberg E, Ballow M, Wolfe SH, *et al*. Pemphigus-like mucosal lesions: a side effect of penicillamine therapy. *Oral Surg* 1981; **51**: 409−14.
14 Sparrow GP. Penicillamine pemphigus and the nephrotic syndrome occurring simultaneously. *Br J Dermatol* 1978; **98**: 103−5.
15 Matkaluk RM, Bailin PL. Penicillamine-induced pemphigus foliaceus. A fatal outcome. *Arch Dermatol* 1981; **117**: 156−7.

16 Fulton RA, Thomson J. Penicillamine-induced bullous dermatosis. *Br J Dermatol* 1982; **107** (Suppl 22): 95–6.

17 Brown MD, Dubin HV. Penicillamine-induced bullous pemphigoid-like eruption. *Arch Dermatol* 1987; **123**: 1119–20.

18 Pegum JS, Pembroke AC. Benign mucous membrane pemphigoid associated with penicillamine treatment. *Br Med J* 1977; **i**: 1473.

19 Shuttleworth D, Graham-Brown RAC, Hutchinson PE, Jolliffe DS. Cicatricial pemphigoid in D-penicillamine treated patients with rheumatoid arthritis — a report of three cases. *Clin Exp Dermatol* 1985; **10**: 392–7.

20 Burns DA, Sarkany I. Penicillamine induced discoid lupus erythematosus. *Clin Exp Dermatol* 1979; **4**: 389–92.

21 Walshe JM. Penicillamine and the SLE syndrome. *J Rheumatol* 1981; **8** (Suppl 7): 155–60.

22 Chalmers A, Thompson D, Stein HE, *et al*. Systemic lupus erythematosus during penicillamine therapy for rheumatoid arthritis. *Ann Intern Med* 1982; **97**: 659–63.

23 Tsankov NK, Lazarov AZ, Vasileva S, Obreshkova EV. Lupus erythematosus-like eruption due to D-penicillamine in progressive systemic sclerosis. *Int J Dermatol* 1990; **29**: 571–4.

24 Simpson NB, Golding JR. Dermatomyositis induced by penicillamine. *Acta Derm Venereol (Stockh)* 1979; **59**: 543–4.

25 Wojnorowska F. Dermatomyositis induced by penicillamine. *J R Soc Med* 1980; **73**: 884–6.

26 Carroll GC, Will RK, Peter JB, *et al*. Penicillamine induced polymyositis and dermatomyositis. *J Rheumatol* 1987; **14**: 995–1001.

27 Wilson CL, Bradlow A, Wojnarowska F. Cutaneous problems with drug therapy in rheumatoid arthritis. *Int J Dermatol* 1991; **30**: 148–9.

28 Bernstein RM, Hall MA, Gostelow BE. Morphea-like reaction to D-penicillamine therapy. *Ann Rheum Dis* 1981; **40**: 42–4.

29 Miyagawa S, Yoshioka A, Hatoko M, *et al*. Systemic sclerosis-like lesions during long-term penicillamine therapy for Wilson's disease. *Br J Dermatol* 1987; **116**: 95–100.

30 Powell FC, Rogers RS III, Dickson ER. Lichen planus, primary biliary cirrhosis and penicillamine. *Br J Dermatol* 1982; **107**: 616.

31 Seehafer JR, Rogers RS III, Fleming R, Dickson ER. Lichen planus-like lesions caused by penicillamine in primary biliary cirrhosis. *Arch Dermatol* 1981; **117**: 140–2.

32 Van Hecke E, Kint A, Temmerman L. A lichenoid eruption induced by penicillamine. *Arch Dermatol* 1981; **117**: 676–7.

33 Ilchyshyn A, Vickers CFH. Yellow nail syndrome associated with penicillamine therapy. *Acta Derm Venereol (Stockh)* 1983; **63**: 554–5.

Prolonged high dose therapy for more than a year, as for Wilson's disease, has effects on collagen and elastin, resulting from inhibition of the condensation of soluble tropocollagen to insoluble collagen. There is anisodiametricity of connective tissue fibres, resulting in the 'lumpy-bumpy elastic fibre' [1–3]. The skin becomes wrinkled and thin, aged looking and abnormally fragile; asymptomatic violaceous, friable, haemorrhagic macules, papules and plaques develop on pressure sites, and minor trauma causes ecchymoses [4]. There may be light-blue anetoderma-like lesions [5], and small white papules at venepuncture sites. Lymphangiectasis may develop [4]. Blisters may occur, with a picture resembling epidermolysis bullosa with scarring and milia formation [6]. Cutis laxa, and elastosis perforans serpiginosa (Fig. 10.5) [7–12], which may be verruciform [7,10], are described. Lesions resembling pseudoxanthoma elasticum have been documented rarely [13–16].

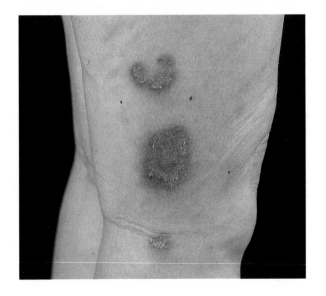

Figure 10.5 Elastosis perforans serpiginosa due to D-penicillamine in a patient treated for 26 years for Wilson's disease. (Courtesy of Professor K. Wolff, Vienna.)

1 Bardach H, Gebhart W, Niebauer G. 'Lumpy-bumpy' elastic fibers in the skin and lungs of a patient with a penicillamine-induced elastosis perforans serpiginosa. *J Cutan Pathol* 1979; **6**: 243–52.

2 Gebhart W, Bardach H. The 'lumpy-bumpy' elastic fiber: A marker for long-term administration of penicillamine. *Am J Dermatopathol* 1981; **3**: 33–9.

3 Hashimoto K, McEvoy B, Belcher R. Ultrastructure of penicillamine-induced skin lesions. *J Am Acad Dermatol* 1981; **4**: 300–15.

4 Goldstein JB, McNutt S, Hambrick GW. Penicillamine dermatopathy with lymphangiectases. A clinical, immunohistologic, and ultrastructural study. *Arch Dermatol* 1989; **125**: 92–7.

5 Davis W. Wilson's disease and penicillamine-induced anetoderma. *Arch Dermatol* 1977; **113**: 976.

6 Beer WE, Cooke KB. Epidermolysis bullosa induced by penicillamine. *Br J Dermatol* 1967; **79**: 123–5.

7 Guilane J, Benhamou JP, Molas G. Élastome perforant verruciforme chez un malade traité par pénicillamine pour maladie de Wilson. *Bull Soc Fr Derm Syph* 1972; **79**: 450–3.

8 Gloor M, Bersch A. Elastoma intrapapillare perforans verruciforme (Lutz-Miescher) als Folge einer Langzeittherapie mit D-Penizillamin. *Hautarzt* 1982; **33**: 291–3.

9 Reymond JL, Stoebner P, Zambelli P, *et al*. Penicillamine induced elastosis perforans serpiginosa: an ultrastructural study of two cases. *J Cutan Pathol* 1982; **9**: 352–7.

10 Sfar Z, Lakhua M, Kamoun MR, *et al*. Deux cas d'élastomes verruciforme après administration prolongée de D-pénicillamine. *Ann Dermatol Vénéréol (Paris)* 1982; **109**: 813–14.

11 Price RG, Prentice RSA. Penicillamine-induced elastosis perforans serpiginosa. Tip of the iceberg? *Am J Dermatopathol* 1986; **8**: 314–20.

12 Sahn EE, Maize JC, Garen PD, *et al*. D-Penicillamine-induced elastosis perforans serpiginosa in a child with juvenile rheumatoid arthritis. Report of a case and review of the literature. *J Am Acad Dermatol* 1989; **20**: 979–88.

13 Meyrick Thomas RH, Light N, Stephens AD, *et al*. Pseudoxanthoma elasticum-like skin changes induced by penicillamine. *J R Soc Med* 1984; **77**: 794–8.

14 Meyrick Thomas RH, Kirby JDT. Elastosis perforans serpiginosa and pseudoxanthoma elasticum-like skin change due to D-penicillamine. *Clin Exp Dermatol* 1985; **10**: 386–91.

15 Light N, Meyrick Thomas RH, Stephens A, *et al*. Collagen and elastin changes in D-penicillamine-induced pseudoxanthoma elasticum. *Br J Dermatol* 1986; **114**: 381–8.

16 Burge S, Ryan T. Penicillamine-induced pseudo-pseudoxanthoma elasticum in a patient with rheumatoid arthritis. *Clin Exp Dermatol* 1988; **13**: 255−8.

Systemic complications

Penicillamine may induce impaired taste sensation in up to 25% of patients, but other gastrointestinal effects are usually minor. Important non-dermatological complications [1,2] include marrow suppression, and various renal problems such as reversible proteinuria in up to 30% of patients on therapy for more than 6 months, established nephrotic syndrome and Goodpasture's syndrome. Thrombocytopenia occurs in up to 3% of patients, and may be either of gradual or precipitous onset. Immunological abnormalities include acquired IgA deficiency [3] and development of myasthenia gravis [4]. The bones may be involved in the connective tissue disorder. A chronic broncho-alveolitis is recognized [5]. Breast enlargement and breast gigantism [6] are documented.

1 Dasgupta B. Adverse reactions profile: 2. Penicillamine. *Prescribers' J* 1991; **31**: 72−7.
2 Levy RS, Fisher M, Alter JN. Penicillamine: Review and cutaneous manifestations. *J Am Acad Dermatol* 1983; **8**: 548−58.
3 Hjalmarson O, Hanson L-Å, Nilsson L-Å. IgA deficiency during D-penicillamine treatment. *Br Med J* 1977; **i**: 549.
4 Garlepp MJ, Dawkins RL, Christiansen FT. HLA antigens and acetylcholine receptor antibodies in penicillamine induced myasthenia gravis. *Br Med J* 1983; **286**: 338−40.
5 Murphy KC, Atkins CJ, Offer RC, *et al*. Obliterative bronchiolitis in two rheumatoid arthritis patients treated with penicillamine. *Arthritis Rheum* 1981; **24**: 557−60.
6 Passas C, Weinstein A. Breast gigantism with penicillamine therapy. *Arthritis Rheum* 1978; **21**: 167−8.

Tiopronin (*N*-(2-mercaptopropionyl)glycine)

This drug, used in Japan for the treatment of liver disease, mercury intoxication, cataracts and allergic dermatoses, dissociates disulphide bonds like, penicillamine. Morbilliform, urticarial and lichenoid eruptions, bullous in one case, have occurred [1].

1 Hsiao L, Yoshinaga A, Ono T. Drug-induced bullous lichen planus in a patient with diabetes mellitus and liver disease. *J Am Acad Dermatol* 1986; **15**: 103−5.

Chapter 11
Anticoagulants, Fibrinolytic Agents, and Antiplatelet Drugs

11.1 Oral anticoagulants

Adverse reactions to oral anticoagulant drugs have been reviewed [1,2].

1 Baker H, Levene GM. Drug reactions V. Cutaneous reactions to anticoagulants. *Br J Dermatol* 1969; **81**: 236–8.
2 Hirsh J. Oral anticoagulant drugs. *N Engl J Med* 1991; **324**: 1865–75.

Coumarins

There may be cross-sensitivity across the group of acenocoumarol, phenprocoumon, and warfarin [1].

Phenprocoumon

A patient on long-term anticoagulation therapy developed repeated episodes of skin and subcutaneous fat necrosis related to episodes of over-anticoagulation with acquired functional deficiency of protein C, thought to be due to hepatic dysfunction resulting from congestive cardiac failure [2].

Warfarin

Haemorrhage is the commonest adverse reaction. Maculopapular rashes occur [1]. Rarely, an oral loading dose may lead to one or more areas of painful erythema and ecchymosis, which rapidly progress to central blistering and massive cutaneous and sub-cutaneous necrosis [3–9]; if extensive, the condition may be fatal [3]. The lesions usually start between the second and fourteenth day of treatment (usually third to fifth day), tend to be symmetrical, and occur over fatty areas, e.g. the breasts, buttocks, thighs, calves and abdomen. Most patients have been women, but lesions of the penis may occur [5]. Warfarin necrosis has been associated with the heterozygous state for deficiency of protein C, a vitamin K-dependent serine protease [7–9]. Activated protein C is a potent anticoagulant that selectively inactivates cofactors Va and VIIIa and inhibits platelet coagulant activity by inactivation of platelet factor Va. Continued coumarin therapy does not aggravate the condition, but resumption

[247]

of therapy with loading doses may lead to new lesions [6]. The condition is preventable by vitamin K_1 injections. Other side-effects are rare, and include urticaria [10], dermatitis, gastrointestinal upset, purple erythema of the dependent parts (the purple toe syndrome) [11–13], acral purpura [14], and alopecia [15].

Oral anticoagulants and quinidine act synergistically to depress vitamin K-sensitive hepatic clotting synthesis [16]. Their combined use can precipitate serious hypoprothrombinaemic haemorrhage. Azapropazone displaces warfarin from protein binding sites and also alters renal clearance of *R* and *S* isomers of warfarin; this may lead to effective warfarin overdosage [17]. Itraconazole may potentiate the action of warfarin [18].

1 Kruis-de Vries MH, Stricker BHC, Coenraads PJ, Nater JP. Maculopapular rash due to coumarin derivatives. *Dermatologica* 1989; **178**: 109–11.
2 Teepe RGC, Broekmans AW, Vermeer BJ, *et al.* Recurrent coumarin-induced skin necrosis in a patient with an acquired functional protein C deficiency. *Arch Dermatol* 1986; **122**: 1408–12.
3 Lacy JP, Goodin RR. Warfarin induced necrosis of skin. *Ann Intern Med* 1975; **82**: 381–2.
4 Schleicher SM, Fricker MP. Coumarin necrosis. *Arch Dermatol* 1980; **116**: 444–5.
5 Weinberg AC, Lieskovsky G, McGehee WG, Skinner DG. Warfarin necrosis of the skin and subcutaneous tissue of the male external genitalia. *J Urol* 1983; **130**: 352–4.
6 Slutzki S, Bogokowsky H, Gilboa Y, Halpern Z. Coumadin-induced skin necrosis. *Int J Dermatol* 1984; **23**: 117–19.
7 Kazmier FJ. Thromboembolism, coumarin necrosis, and protein C. *Mayo Clin Proc* 1985; **60**: 673–4.
8 Gladson CL, Groncy P, Griffin JH. Coumarin necrosis, neonatal purpura fulminans, and protein C deficiency. *Arch Dermatol* 1988; **123**: 1701a–1706a.
9 Auletta MJ, Headington JT. Purpura fulminans. A cutaneous manifestation of severe protein C deficiency. *Arch Dermatol* 1988; **124**: 1387–91.
10 Sheps ES, Gifford RW. Urticaria after administration of warfarin sodium. *Am J Cardiol* 1959; **3**: 118–20.
11 Feder W, Auerbach R. 'Purple toes': An uncommon sequela of oral coumarin drug therapy. *Ann Intern Med* 1961; **55**: 911–17.
12 Akle CA, Joiner CL. Purple toe syndrome. *J R Soc Med* 1981; **74**: 219.
13 Lebsack CS, Weibert RT. Purple toes syndrome. *Postgrad Med* 1982; **71**: 81–4.
14 Stone MS, Rosen T. Acral purpura: an unusual sign of coumarin necrosis. *J Am Acad Dermatol* 1986; **14**: 797–802.
15 Umlas J, Harken DE. Warfarin-induced alopecia. *Cutis* 1988; **42**: 63–4.
16 Koch-Weser J. Quinidine-induced hypoprothrombinemic hemorrhage in patients on chronic warfarin therapy. *Ann Intern Med* 1968; **68**: 511–17.
17 Win N, Mitchell DC. Azapropazone and warfarin. *Br Med J* 1991; **302**: 969–70.
18 Yeh J, Soo SC, Summerton C, Richardson C. Potentiation of action of warfarin by itraconazole. *Br Med J* 1990; **301**: 669.

Indandiones

Hypersensitivity reactions occur in up to 0.3% of patients within 3 months of onset of treatment of phenindione. Scarlatiniform, eczematous, erythema multiforme-like or generalized exfoliative eruptions are seen [1,2]. Alopecia and a stomatitis may accompany the rash. Brownish-yellow or orange discoloration of the palmar or finger skin on handling the tablets develops after contact with soap alkali [3]. Cutaneous necrosis occurs rarely.

1 Hollman A, Wong HO. Phenindione sensitivity. *Br Med J* 1964; **ii**: 730−2.
2 Copeman PWM. Phenindione toxicity. *Br Med J* 1965; **ii**: 305.
3 Silverton NH. Skin pigmentation by phenindione. *Br Med J* 1966; **i**: 675.

11.2 Heparin: parenteral anticoagulant

The most frequent side-effect is haemorrhage [1,2]. Other common side-effects include osteoporosis and (temporary) telogen effluvium 6−16 weeks after administration. Hypoaldosteronism may occur. Hypersensitivity reactions including urticaria and anaphylactic shock are well documented but very uncommon [3]. Vasospastic reactions, including pain, cyanosis and severe itching or burning plantar sensations, are described.

Erythematous infiltrated plaques developing 3−21 days after commencement of heparin therapy [4−9] may closely mimic contact dermatitis both clinically (Fig. 11.1) and histologically (Fig. 11.2), and patch tests may be positive [7,8]. A subcutaneous provocation test may be a useful diagnostic measure. Low molecular weight heparin analogues may be satisfactorily substituted in some patients with this reaction [4], but are not always tolerated [6]; a panel of different low molecular weight heparin preparations should be checked by subcutaneous provocation tests before re-institution of heparin therapy. Chlorocresol may be responsible for some reactions attributed to heparin [6,9], including anaphylactoid reactions.

Skin necrosis occurring 6−8 days after onset of subcutaneous heparin (Fig. 11.3) is rare, but may occur at injection sites and

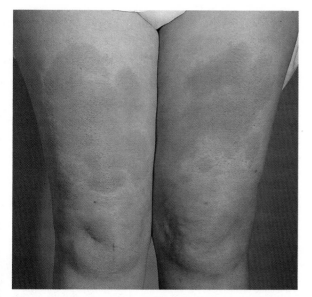

Figure 11.1 Erythematous infiltrated plaques resulting from allergy to heparin.

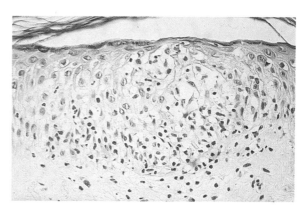

Figure 11.2 Eczematous histology with epidermal spongiosis and lymphocyte exocytosis in heparin reaction.

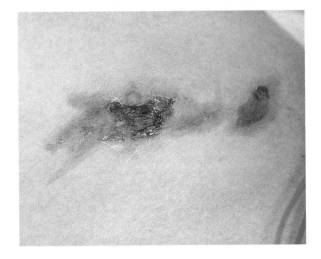

Figure 11.3 Heparin necrosis.

occasionally at distal sites elsewhere [10−16]. Diabetic women on high-dose antibiotics are predisposed to this complication. A scleroderma-like evolution has been recorded [13]. Clinically the skin necrosis resembles that of coumarin necrosis [16]. It may occur with use of low molecular weight heparin [14].

Heparin may cause an allergic thrombocytopenia [17−21]. Thrombocytopenia is usually asymptomatic, but may be associated with arterial or venous thrombosis in about 0.4% of cases [18]; thrombo-embolism may occasionally be lethal [19]. Thrombocytopenia usually begins between 3 and 15 days after initiation of therapy, may occur within hours in previously exposed patients, and is thought to be caused by an IgG−heparin immune complex involving both the Fab and Fc portions of the IgG molecule [18]. Heparin-induced anti-endothelial cell antibodies, which recognize heparin-like glycans on the cell surface of platelets and endothelial cells, may lead to platelet aggregation and endothelial cell expression of procoagulant tissue factor, with resultant thrombocytopenia and thrombosis [21]. Thrombocytopenia may occur with both unfractionated and with low molecular weight heparin [20]. The heparinoid Org 10172, which has minimal cross-reactivity with heparin, has been used successfully in patients with heparin-induced thrombocytopenia [22].

1 Tuneu A, Moreno A, de Moragas JM. Cutaneous reactions secondary to heparin injections. *J Am Acad Dermatol* 1985; **12**: 1072−7.
2 Hirsh J. Heparin. *N Engl J Med* 1991; **324**: 1565−74.
3 Curry N, Bandana EJ, Pirofsky B. Heparin sensitivity: report of a case. *Arch Intern Med* 1973; **132**: 744−5.
4 Zimmermann R, Harenberg J, Weber E, *et al.* Behandlung bei heparininduzierter kutaner Reaktion mit einem niedermolekularen Heparin-Analog. *Dtsch Med Wochenschr* 1984; **109**: 1326−8.
5 Ulrick PJ, Manoharan A. Heparin-induced skin reaction. *Med J Aust* 1987; **140**: 287−9.
6 Klein GF, Kofler H, Wol H, Fritsch PO. Eczema-like, erythematous, infiltrated plaques: A common side effect of subcutaneous heparin therapy. *J Am Acad Dermatol* 1989; **21**: 703−7.

7 Guillet G, Delaire P, Plantin P, Guillet MH. Eczema as a complication of heparin therapy. *J Am Acad Dermatol* 1989; **21**: 1130.

8 Bircher AJ, Flückiger R, Buchner SA. Eczematous infiltrated plaques to subcutaneous heparin: a type IV allergic reaction. *Br J Dermatol* 1990; **123**: 507–14.

9 Ainley EJ, Mackie IG, MacArthur D. Adverse reaction to chlorocresol-preserved heparin. *Lancet* 1977; **i**: 705.

10 Shelley WB, Säyen JJ. Heparin necrosis: an anticoagulant-induced cutaneous infarct. *J Am Acad Dermatol* 1982; **7**: 674–7.

11 Levine LE, Bernstein JE, Soltani K, *et al*. Heparin-induced skin necrosis unrelated to injection sites; a sign of potentially lethal complications. *Arch Dermatol* 1983; **119**: 400–3.

12 Mathieu A, Avril MF, Schlumberger M, *et al*. Un cas de nécrose cutanée induite par l'héparine. *Ann Dermatol Vénéréol (Paris)* 1984; **111**: 733–4.

13 Barthelemy H, Hermier C, Perrot H. Nécrose cutanée avec évolution scléridermiforme après l'injection souscutanée d'heparinate de calcium. *Ann Dermatol Vénéréol (Paris)* 1985; **112**: 245–7.

14 Cordoliani F, Saiag P, Guillaume J-C, *et al*. Nécrose cutanés étendues induites par la fraxiparine. *Ann Dermatol Vénéréol (Paris)* 1987; **114**: 1366–8.

15 Rongioletti F, Pisani S, Ciaccio M, Rebora A. Skin necrosis due to intravenous heparin. *Dermatologica* 1989; **178**: 47–50.

16 Gold JA, Watters AK, O'Brien E. Coumadin versus heparin necrosis. *J Am Acad Dermatol* 1987; **16**: 148–50.

17 Cines DB, Kaywin P, Mahin Bina AT, *et al*. Heparin-associated thrombocytopenia. *N Engl J Med* 1980; **303**: 788–95.

18 Warkentin TE, Kelton JG. Heparin-induced thrombocytopenia. *Annu Rev Med* 1989; **40**: 31–44.

19 Jaffray B, Welch GH, Cooke TG. Fatal venous thrombosis after heparin therapy. *Lancet* 1991; **337**: 561.

20 Eichinger S, Kyrle PA, Brenner B, *et al*. Thrombocytopenia associated with low-molecular-weight heparin. *Lancet* 1991; **337**: 1425–6.

21 Cine DB, Tomaski A, Tannenbaum S. Immune endothelial cell injury in heparin-associated thrombocytopenia. *N Engl J Med* 1987; **316**: 581–9.

22 Chong BJ, Ismail F, Cade J, *et al*. Heparin-induced thrombocytopenia: studies with a new low molecular weight heparinoid, Org 10172. *Blood* 1989; **73**: 1592–6.

11.3 Protamine: heparin antagonist

This low molecular weight protein, derived from salmon sperm and/or testes, is used for neutralization of heparin anticoagulation after cardiac surgery. Idiosyncratic responses or those related to complement generation of anaphylatoxins are recorded [1]. IgE-dependent anaphylaxis may occur in diabetics treated with protamine-containing insulin [2].

1 Sussman GL, Dolovich J. Prevention of anaphylaxis. *Semin Dermatol* 1989; **8**: 158–65.

2 Sarche MB, Paolillo M, Chacon RS, *et al*. Protamine as a cause of generalized allergic reactions to NPH insulin. *Lancet* 1982; **i**: 1243.

11.4 Fibrinolytic drugs

Haemorrhage is the most common untoward effect from use of thrombolysins [1].

Alteplase (tissue plasminogen activator)

Painful purpura occurring within hours of administration has been recorded [2].

Anistreplase

Anistreplase anisoylated plasminogen streptokinase activator complex given for an acute myocardial infarction was associated with leucocytoclastic vasculitis [3].

Streptokinase

Allergic reactions have been reported in up to 6% of patients, ranging from minor skin rashes to anaphylaxis [4−6]. This drug has been reported in association with a hypersensitivity vasculitis [7,8], serum sickness with leucocytoclastic vasculitis [9,10] and a lymphocytic angiitis [11].

1 Chesebro JH, Knatterud G, Roberts R, *et al*. Thrombolysis in myocardial infarction (TIMI) trial, phase I: a comparison between intravenous tissue plasminogen activator and intravenous streptokinase. *Circulation* 1987; **76**: 142−54.
2 DeTrana C, Hurwitz RM. Painful purpura: an adverse effect to a thrombolysin. *Arch Dermatol* 1990; **126**: 690−1.
3 Burrows N, Russell Jones R. Rash after treatment with anistreplase. *Br Heart J* 1990; **64**: 289−90.
4 Sharma GVRK, Sella G, Parisi AF, *et al*. Thrombolytic therapy. *N Engl J Med* 1982; **306**: 1268−76.
5 Dykewicz MS, McGratt KG, Davison R, *et al*. Identification of patients at risk for anaphylaxis due to streptokinase. *Arch Intern Med* 1986; **146**: 305−7.
6 ISIS-2 (Second International Study of Infarct Survival). Collaborative Group. Randomized trial of intravenous streptokinase, oral aspirin, both, or neither among 17 187 cases of suspected acute myocardial infarction: ISIS-2. *Lancet* 1988; **ii**: 349−60.
7 Ong ACM, Handler CE, Walker JM. Hypersensitivity vasculitis complicating intravenous streptokinase therapy in acute myocardial infarction. *Int J Cardiol* 1988; **21**: 71−3.
8 Thompson RF, Stratton MA, Heffron WA. Hypersensitivity vasculitis associated with streptokinase. *Clin Pharmacol* 1985; **4**: 383−8.
9 Patel A, Prussick R, Buchanan WW, Sauder DN. Serum sickness-like illness and leukocytoclastic vasculitis after intravenous streptokinase. *J Am Acad Dermatol* 1991; **24**: 652−3.
10 Totto WG, Romano T, Benian GM, *et al*. Serum sickness following streptokinase therapy. *Am J Rheum* 1982; **138**: 143−4.
11 Sorber WA, Herbst V. Lymphocytic angiitis following streptokinase therapy. *Cutis* 1988; **42**: 57−8.

11.5 Antiplatelet drugs

Ticlopidine

This antiplatelet drug, indicated for coronary artery disease, cerebrovascular disease, peripheral vascular disease and diabetic retinopathy, is a thienopyridine derivative [1,2]. Gastrointestinal symptoms, thrombocytopenia with minor bleeding including bruising, neutropenia, rashes in 10–15% of patients, and hepatic dysfunction in 4% of cases, have been reported. Thrombotic thrombocytopenic purpura has also been documented [3].

1 McTavish D, Faulds D, Goa KL. Ticlopidine. An updated review of its pharmacology and therapeutic use in platelet-dependent disorders. *Drugs* 1990; **40**: 238–59.
2 Editorial. Ticlopidine. *Lancet* 1991; **337**: 459–60.
3 Page Y, Tardy B, Zeni F, *et al*. Thrombotic thrombocytopenic purpura related to ticlopidine. *Lancet* 1991; **337**: 774–6.

Chapter 12
Vitamins

12.1 Vitamin A

Generalized peeling may be a delayed manifestation of acute intoxication [1]. Chronic intoxication produces the following epithelial problems: pruritus, erythema, hyperkeratosis, dryness of mouth, nose and eyes, epistaxis, fissuring, dryness and scaling of the lips, peeling of the palms and soles, and alopecia. A yellow–orange skin discoloration, photosensitivity, and nail changes have also been observed [2–5]. Headache, pseudotumour cerebri, anaemia, hepatomegaly and skeletal pain may be present. Cortical hyperostoses and periosteal reaction of tubular bone [6], and more rarely premature epiphyseal closure and change in the contour of long bones [7], are seen.

1 Nater P, Doeglas HMG. Halibut liver poisoning in 11 fishermen. *Acta Derm Venereol (Stockh)* 1970; **50**: 109–13.
2 Oliver TK. Chronic vitamin A intoxication. Report of a case in an older child and a review of the literature. *Am J Dis Child* 1959; **95**: 57–67.
3 Muenter MD, Perry HO, Ludwig J. Chronic vitamin A intoxication in adults. Hepatic, neurologic and dermatologic complications. *Am J Med* 1971; **50**: 129–36.
4 Teo ST, Newth J, Pascoe BJ. Chronic vitamin A intoxication. *Med J Aust* 1973; **2**: 324–6.
5 Bobb R, Kieraldo JH. Cirrhosis due to hypervitaminosis A. *West J Med* 1978; **128**: 244–6.
6 Frame B, Jackson CE, Reynolds WA, Umphrey JE. Hypercalcemia and skeletal effects in chronic hypervitaminosis A. *Ann Intern Med* 1974; **80**: 44–8.
7 Ruby LK, Mital MA. Skeletal deformities following chronic hypervitaminosis A. *J Bone Joint Surg* 1974; **56**: 1283–7.

12.2 Retinoids

The cutaneous and systemic side-effects of these synthetic vitamin A-related compounds resemble those of hypervitaminosis A, and have been extensively reviewed [1–7].

1 Orfanos CE, Braun-Falco O, Farber EM, *et al.* (eds) *Retinoids. Advances in Basic Research and Therapy.* Springer-Verlag, Berlin, 1981.
2 Foged E, Jacobsen F. Side-effects due to Ro 10-3959 (Tigason). *Dermatologica* 1982; **164**: 395–403.
3 Windhorst DB, Nigra T. General clinical toxicology of oral retinoids. *J Am Acad Dermatol* 1982; **4**: 675–82.

4 Cunliffe WJ, Miller AJ, (eds) *Retinoid Therapy. A Review of Clinical and Laboratory Research*. MTP Press Ltd, Lancaster, 1984.
5 Saurat JH, (ed) *Retinoids: New Trends in Research and Therapy*. Karger, Basel, 1985.
6 Yob EH, Pochi PE. Side effects and long-term toxicity of synthetic retinoids. *Arch Dermatol* 1987; **123**: 1375−8.
7 Bigby M, Stern RS. Adverse reactions to isotretinoin. A report from the Adverse Drug Reaction Reporting System. *J Am Acad Dermatol* 1988; **18**: 543−52.

Acitretin

The side-effects of this principal metabolite of etretinate are similar to those of the parent compound [1−5], comprising cheilitis, conjunctivitis, peeling of the palms and soles, xerosis, myalgia and alopecia; elevated serum triglyceride, cholesterol and liver transaminase levels are seen. Alopecia is particularly frequent [4], and scaling of the palms and soles appears more prominent than with etretinate [5]. Persistent levels of etretinate have been detected in plasma following changing therapy to acitretin [6].

1 Geiger J-M, Czarnetzki BM. Acitretin (Ro 10-1670, Etretin): overall evaluation of clinical studies. *Dermatologica* 1988; **176**: 182−90.
2 Gupta AK, Goldfarb MT, Ellis CN, Voorhees JJ. Side-effect profile of acitretin therapy in psoriasis. *J Am Acad Dermatol* 1989; **21**: 1088−93.
3 Ruzicka T, Sommerburg C, Braun-Falco O, *et al.* Efficiency of acitretin in combination with UV-B in the treatment of severe psoriasis. *Arch Dermatol* 1990; **126**: 482−6.
4 Murray HE, Anhalt AW, Lessard R, *et al.* A 12-month treatment of severe psoriasis with acitretin: Results of a Canadian open multicenter study. *J Am Acad Dermatol* 1991; **24**: 598−602.
5 Blanchet-Bardon C, Nazzaro V, Rognin C, *et al.* Acitretin in the treatment of severe disorders of keratinization. Results of an open study. *J Am Acad Dermatol* 1991; **24**: 982−6.
6 Lambert WE, De Leenheer AP, De Bersaques JP, Kint A. Persistent etretinate levels in plasma after changing the therapy to acitretin. *Arch Dermatol Res* 1990; **282**: 343−4.

Etretinate

Dermatological complications

The side-effects are dose dependent, and resemble those associated with isotretinoin therapy [1−3]. With dosage over 0.5 mg/kg, cheilitis with dryness, scaling and fissuring of the lips is almost universal. There may be pruritus, a dry mouth, dry nose, epistaxis, meatitis, desquamation (Fig. 12.1) including on the face, hands (Fig. 12.2) and feet, and reduced tolerance of sunlight [4] and therapeutic products such as tar or dithranol. Pseudoporphyria has been reported in a renal transplant recipient treated with etretinate to suppress cutaneous neoplasia [5]. A 'retinoid dermatitis' resembling asteatotic eczema may develop in up to 50% of patients [6]. Increased stickiness of the palms and soles, possibly due to

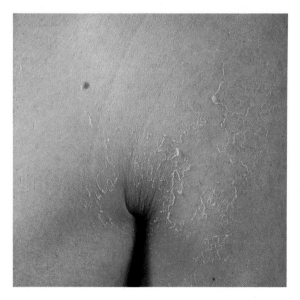 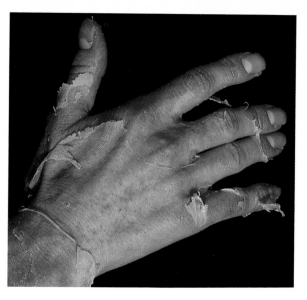

Figure 12.1 Fine desquamation in a patient treated with etretinate. (Courtesy of Professor H. Hönigsmann, Vienna.)

Figure 12.2 Sheet-like desquamation due to etretinate.

increased quantities of carcino-embryonic antigen and other glyco-proteins in eccrine sweat [7], has been reported. Mucosal erosions, conjunctivitis, paronychia, and alopecia [8] or curling or kinking of hair are all well documented. Intertriginous erosions have also been described [9]. Oedema [10], excess granulation tissue [11] and multiple pyogenic granulomata [12] develop rarely. Erythroderma has been reported [13].

Prolonged therapy may lead to skin fragility [14,15]; blistering, erosions and scarring have been reported in one patient [16]. Softening of the nails is seen [17], and chronic paronychia, onycho-lysis, onychomadesis, nail shedding, onychoschizia and fragility may occur [18,19]. Parakeratotic digitate keratoses appearing after treatment of disseminated superficial actinic porokeratosis may arise as a result of etretinate-resistant regions in the ring of the cornoid lamella [20]. There has been a single case of generalization of palmoplantar pustulosis following cessation of etretinate therapy [21].

1 Foged E, Jacobsen F. Side-effects due to Ro 10-3959 (Tigason). *Dermatologica* 1982; **164**: 395–403.
2 Ellis CN, Voorhees JJ. Etretinate therapy. *J Am Acad Dermatol* 1987; **16**: 267–91.
3 Halioua B, Saurat J-H. Risk:benefit ratio in the treatment of psoriasis with systemic retinoids. *Br J Dermatol* 1990; **122** (Suppl 36): 135–50.
4 Collins MRL, James WD, Rodman OG. Etretinate photosensitivity. *J Am Acad Dermatol* 1986; **14**: 274.
5 McDonagh AJG, Harrington CI. Pseudoporphyria complicating etretinate therapy. *Clin Exp Dermatol* 1989; **14**: 437–8.
6 Taieb A, Maleville J. Retinoid dermatitis mimicking 'eczéma craquelé'. *Acta Derm Venereol (Stockh)* 1985; **65**: 570.

7 Penneys NS, Hernandez D. A sticky problem with etretinate. *N Engl J Med* 1991; **325**: 521.

8 Berth-Jones J, Shuttleworth D, Hutchinson PE. A study of etretinate alopecia. *Br J Dermatol* 1990; **122**: 751−5.

9 Shelley ED, Shelley WB. Inframammary, intertriginous, and decubital erosion due to etretinate. *Cutis* 1991; **47**: 111−13.

10 Allan S, Christmas T. Severe edema associated with etretinate. *J Am Acad Dermatol* 1988; **19**: 140.

11 Hodak E, David M, Feuerman EJ. Excess granulation tissue during etretinate therapy. *J Am Acad Dermatol* 1984; **11**: 1166−7.

12 Williamson DM, Creenwood R. Multiple pyogenic granulomata occurring during etretinate therapy. *Br J Dermatol* 1983; **109**: 615−17.

13 Levin J, Almeyda J. Erythroderma due to etretinate. *Br J Dermatol* 1985; **112**: 373.

14 Williams ML, Elias PM. Nature of skin fragility in patients receiving retinoids for systemic effect. *Arch Dermatol* 1981; **117**: 611−19.

15 Neild VS, Moss RF, Marsden RA, *et al*. Retinoid-induced skin fragility in a patient with hepatic disease. *Clin Exp Dermatol* 1985; **10**: 459−65.

16 Ramsay B, Bloxham C, Eldred A, *et al*. Blistering, erosions and scarring in a patient on etretinate. *Br J Dermatol* 1989; **121**: 397−400.

17 Lindskov R. Soft nails after treatment with aromatic retinoids. *Arch Dermatol* 1982; **118**: 535−6.

18 Baran R. Action thérapeutique et complications du rétinoïde aromatique sur l'appareil unguéal. *Ann Dermatol Vénéréol* (Paris) 1982; **109**: 367−71.

19 Baran R. Etretinate and the nails (study of 130 cases): possible mechanisms of some side-effects. *Clin Exp Dermatol* 1986; **11**: 148−52.

20 Carmichael AJ, Tan CY. Digitate keratoses − a complication of etretinate used in the treatment of disseminated superficial actinic porokeratosis. *Clin Exp Dermatol* 1990; **15**: 370−1.

21 Miyagawa S, Muramatsu T, Shirai T. Generalization of palmoplantar pustulosis after withdrawal of etretinate. *J Am Acad Dermatol* 1991; **24**: 305−6.

Systemic side-effects

Benign intracranial hypertension is recorded [1]. Minor disturbances of tests of liver function are not uncommon, and may not always be reversible [2,3]. Fatal liver necrosis occurred in a patient with ichthyosiform erythroderma [4], but other factors may have been relevant. Several studies involving liver biopsies have indicated good tolerance of etretinate without significant hepatotoxic side-effects [5−7]; in one study patients were followed for 3 years [7]. Etretinate, like isotretinoin, can cause triglyceride and cholesterol increases [8−11] but to a lesser extent [10]. There have been isolated reports of possible etretinate-related thrombocytopenia [12]. Retinal toxicity has been postulated [13], although a recent report has not confirmed this [14]. Erectile dysfunction has been documented occasionally [15].

Skeletal abnormalities such as periosteal thickening, vertebral hyperostosis, disc degeneration, osteoporosis, and calcification of spinal ligaments occur in a significant number of adults receiving long-term therapy for disorders of keratinization, but the severity of the changes is minor [16,17]. Radiological evidence of thinning of long bones may be seen in children [18], and premature epiphyseal closure has been recorded [19].

1 Viraben R, Mathieu C. Benign intracranial hypertension during etretinate therapy for mycosis fungoides. *J Am Acad Dermatol* 1985; **13**: 515−17.

2 Schmidt H, Foged E. Some hepatotoxic side effects observed in patients treated with aromatic retinoid (Ro 10-9359). In Orfanos CE, Braun-Falco O, Farber EM, *et al.* (eds) *Retinoids. Advances in Basic Research and Therapy.* Springer-Verlag, Berlin, 1981, pp 359−62.

3 Van Voorst Vader P, Houthoff H, Eggink H, Gips C. Etretinate (Tigason) hepatitis in two patients. *Dermatologica* 1984; **168**: 41−6.

4 Thune P, Mørk NJ. A case of centrolobular necrosis of the liver due to aromatic retinoid − Tigason (Ro-10-9359). *Dermatologica* 1980; **160**: 405−8.

5 Foged E, Bjerring P, Kragballe K, *et al.* Histologic changes in the liver during etretinate treatment. *J Am Acad Dermatol* 1984; **11**: 580−3.

6 Zachariae H, Foged E, Bjerring P, *et al.* Liver biopsy during etretinate (Tigason®) treatment. In Saurat JH (ed.) *Retinoids: New Trends in Research and Therapy.* Karger, Basel, 1985, pp 494−7.

7 Roenigk HH Jr. Retinoids: effect on the liver. In Saurat JH (ed.) *Retinoids: New Trends in Research and Therapy.* Karger, Basel, 1985, pp 476−88.

8 Ellis CN, Swanson NA, Grekin RC, *et al.* Etretinate therapy causes increases in lipid levels in patients with psoriasis. *Arch Dermatol* 1982; **118**: 559−62.

9 Michaëlsson G, Bergquist A, Vahlquist A, Vessby B. The influence of Tigason (R 10-9359) on the serum lipoproteins in man. *Br J Dermatol* 1981; **105**: 201−5.

10 Vahlquist C, Michaëlsson G, Vahlquist A, Vessby B. A sequential comparison of etretinate (Tigason) and isotretinoin (Roaccutane) with special regard to their effects on serum lipoproteins. *Br J Dermatol* 1985; **112**: 69−76.

11 Marsden J. Hyperlipidaemia due to isotretinoin and etretinate: possible mechanisms and consequences. *Br J Dermatol* 1986; **114**: 401−7.

12 Naldi L, Rozzoni M, Finazzi G, *et al.* Etretinate therapy and thrombocytopenia. *Br J Dermatol* 1991; **124**: 395.

13 Weber U, Melink B, Goerz G, Michaelis L. Abnormal retinal function associated with long-term etretinate? *Lancet* 1988; i: 235−6.

14 Pitts JF, MacKie RM, Dutton GN, *et al.* Etretinate and visual function: a 1-year follow-up study. *Br J Dermatol* 1991; **125**: 53−5.

15 Reynolds OD. Erectile dysfunction in etretinate treatment. *Arch Dermatol* 1991; **127**: 425−6.

16 DiGiovanna JJ, Gerber LH, Helfgott RK, *et al.* Extraspinal tendon and ligament calcification associated with long-term therapy with etretinate. *N Engl J Med* 1986; **315**: 1177−82.

17 Halkier-Sørensen L, Andresen J. A retrospective study of bone changes in adults treated with etretinate. *J Am Acad Dermatol* 1989; **20**: 83−7.

18 Halkier-Sørensen L, Laurberg G, Andresen J. Bone changes in children on long-term treatment and etretinate. *J Am Acad Dermatol* 1987; **16**: 999−1006.

19 Prendiville J, Bingham EA, Burrows D. Premature epiphyseal closure − a complication of etretinate therapy in children. *J Am Acad Dermatol* 1986; **15**: 1259−62.

Teratogenicity

Etretinate is, like isotretinoin, grossly teratogenic, and because of its deposition in body fat stores it is excreted only very slowly, especially in the obese [1]. Detectable serum levels have been found in some patients more than 2 years following discontinuation of therapy. It is therefore recommended that female patients of child-bearing years should be advised to prevent pregnancy not only during the course of treatment, but also for at least 2 years after stopping therapy; if pregnancy is contemplated after this period of time, estimation of circulating levels of retinoid metabolites should be obtained.

1 DiGiovanna JJ, Zech LA, Ruddel ME, *et al.* Etretinate: persistent serum levels after long-term therapy. *Arch Dermatol* 1989; **125**: 246−51.

Isotretinoin (13-*cis*-retinoic acid)

Dermatological complications [1,2]

Erythema and scaling of the face (Fig. 12.3), generalized xerosis, skin fragility, pruritus, epistaxis, dry nose and dry mouth may be seen in up to 80% of cystic acne patients. A dose-related cheilitis (Fig. 12.4) occurs in over 90%, while conjunctivitis occurs in about 40% of patients. Transient exacerbation of acne may occur, especially in the early stages of therapy. Exuberant granulation tissue, or pyogenic granuloma at the site of healing acne lesions (Fig. 12.5), has been reported frequently [3−7].

Rashes including erythema, and thinning of the hair (in rare cases persistent) occur in less than 10% of patients. Both isotretinoin and etretinate may cause curliness or kinking of hair [8]. The following have occurred in approximately 5% of cases: peeling of the palms and soles, skin infections, and possible increased susceptibility to sunburn. Phototesting confirmed photosensitivity in

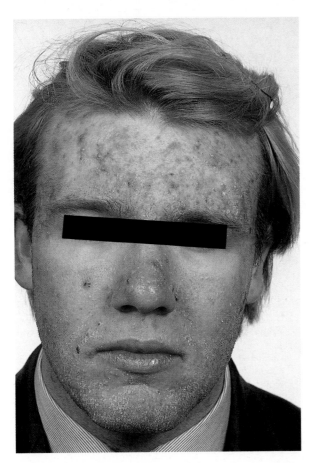

Figure 12.3 Erythema and scaling of the face in a patient with acne treated with isotretinoin.

[259]

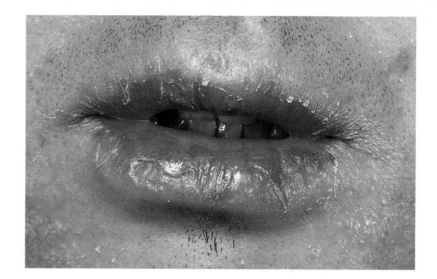

Figure 12.4 Cheilitis resulting from isotretinoin.

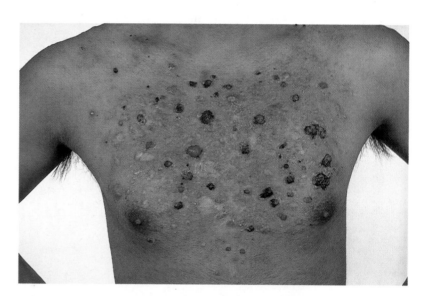

Figure 12.5 Multiple pyogenic granulomata in a patient with acne treated with isotretinoin.

some patients in one [9] but not another [10] study. A photo-aggravated allergic reaction has been documented in which the patient had positive patch tests to isotretinoin [11].

1 Yob EH, Pochi PE. Side effects and long-term toxicity of synthetic retinoids. *Arch Dermatol* 1987; **123**: 1375–8.
2 Bigby M, Stern RS. Adverse reactions to isotretinoin. A report from the Adverse Drug Reaction Reporting System. *J Am Acad Dermatol* 1988; **18**: 543–52.
3 Campbell JP, Grekin RC, Ellis CN, *et al*. Retinoid therapy is associated with excess granulation tissue responses. *J Am Acad Dermatol* 1983; **9**: 708–13.
4 Exner JH, Dahod S, Pochi PE. Pyogenic granuloma-like acne lesions during isotretinoin therapy. *Arch Dermatol* 1983; **119**: 808–11.
5 Valentic JP, Barr RJ, Weinstein GD. Inflammatory neovascular nodules associated with oral isotretinoin treatment of severe acne. *Arch Dermatol* 1983; **119**: 871–2.

6 Stary A. Acne conglobata: Ungewöhnlicher Verlauf unter 13-*cis*-Retinsäuretherapie. *Hautarzt* 1986; **37**: 28–30.

7 Blanc D, Zultak M, Wendling P, Lonchampt F. Eruptive pyogenic granulomas and acne fulminans in two siblings treated with isotretinoin. A possible common pathogenesis. *Dermatologica* 1988; **177**: 16–18.

8 Bunker CB, Maurice PDL, Dowd PM. Isotretinoin and curly hair. *Clin Exp Dermatol* 1990; **15**: 143–5.

9 Ferguson J, Johnson BE. Photosensitivity due to retinoids: clinical and laboratory studies. *Br J Dermatol* 1986; **115**: 275–83.

10 Wong RC, Gilber M, Woo TY, *et al*. Photosensitivity and isotretinoin therapy. *J Am Acad Dermatol* 1986; **15**: 1095–6.

11 Auffret N, Bruley C, Brunetiere RA, *et al*. Photoaggravated allergic reaction to isotretinoin. *J Am Acad Dermatol* 1990; **23**: 321–2.

Systemic side-effects

Headache is not uncommon, and anorexia, nausea and vomiting are much more common than with etretinate, as are lethargy and fatigue [1]. Isotretinoin therapy has been associated with benign intracranial hypertension [2]; in some cases there was concomitant use of tetracyclines, so this combination should be avoided. A variety of central nervous system reactions have been reported, but may bear no relationship to therapy. Depression with recurrence following rechallenge has been recorded [3]. Patients treated for disorders of keratinization have developed corneal opacities which improved when the drug was withdrawn [4]. Dry eyes with decreased tolerance of contact lenses, and decreased night vision have been documented rarely, as have cataracts and other visual disturbances [5–7]. Transient chest pain is uncommon. Non-specific urogenital findings, and non-specific gastrointestinal symptoms, have occurred in approximately 5% of cases. Isotretinoin therapy has been associated with onset of inflammatory bowel disease [8] and with impairment of pulmonary function in patients with systemic sclerosis [9,10].

Approximately 16% of patients develop musculoskeletal symptoms, including arthralgia, of mild to moderate degree; cases of acute knee aseptic arthritis have been documented [11]. High-dose prolonged therapy in a child for epidermolytic hyperkeratosis was associated with premature closure of epiphyses [12]. A high prevalence of skeletal hyperostosis has been noted in patients on prolonged (1 year or more), relatively high dose (2 mg/kg/day), isotretinoin therapy for disorders of keratinization [13–17]. The syndrome of diffuse idiopathic interstitial hyperostosis (DISH) includes ossification of ligaments and accretion of bone on to vertebral bodies, especially of the cervical spine. Mild osteoporosis has also been seen. X-ray changes have been minimal in prospective studies of patients with cystic acne treated with a single course of isotretinoin at recommended doses [18–20]. Nasal bone osteophytosis has been described with short-term therapy for acne [21].

Mild to moderate elevation of liver enzymes occurs in about 15% of cases; in some patients these return to normal despite continued administration of the drug. A single report of fatty liver developing in a patient, with low-normal levels of α_1-antitrypsin, on low dose isotretinoin has been reported [22]. Elevated sedimentation rates occur in about 40% of patients. Between 10 and 20% of patients show decreased red blood cell parameters and white blood cell counts, elevated platelet counts, and pyuria. There has been a single report of thrombocytopenia [23].

Roaccutane induces reversible changes in serum lipids in a significant number of treated subjects [24–29]. A dose-related increase in triglycerides occurs in about 25% of individuals according to the Roche data sheet; 5 of 135 cystic acne patients, and 32 of 298 patients treated for all diagnoses showed triglyceride levels above 500 mg%. In another study, 17% of patients taking isotretinoin for 20 weeks exhibited hypertriglyceridaemia, but in 15% this was only of mild to moderate degree [27]. About 15% showed a mild to moderate decrease in serum high density lipoprotein (HDL) levels, and 7% experienced minimal elevations of serum cholesterol during therapy; some patients had increases in low-density lipoprotein cholesterol [27]. Lipid abnormalities peaked within 4 weeks in men, but not until 12 weeks in women. If sustained over a long period, these alterations in lipoproteins might be risk factors for coronary artery disease. Patients with an increased tendency to develop hypertriglyceridaemia include those with diabetes mellitus, obesity, increased alcohol intake, or a familial history. Some patients have been able to reverse triglyceride elevation by reduction in weight, restriction of dietary fat and alcohol, and reduction in dose while continuing the drug. An obese male patient with Darier's disease developed elevated triglycerides and subsequent eruptive xanthomas [30].

1 Windhorst DB, Nigra T. General clinical toxicology of oral retinoids. *J Am Acad Dermatol* 1982; **4**: 675–82.
2 Anon. Adverse effects with isotretinoin. *J Am Acad Dermatol* 1984; **10**: 519–20.
3 Scheinman PL, Peck GL, Rubinow DR, *et al.* Acute depression from isotretinoin. *J Am Acad Dermatol* 1990; **23**: 1112–14.
4 Cunningham WJ. Use of isotretinoin in the ichthyoses. In Cunliffe WJ, Miller AJ (eds) *Retinoid Therapy. A Review of Clinical and Laboratory Research.* MTP Press Ltd, Lancaster, 1984, pp 321–5.
5 Fraunfelder FT, La Braico JM, Meyer SM. Adverse ocular reactions possibly associated with isotretinoin. *Am J Ophthalmol* 1985; **100**: 534–7.
6 Brown RD, Gratten CEH. Visual toxicity of synthetic retinoids. *Br J Ophthalmol* 1989; **73**: 286–8.
7 Gold JA, Shupack JL, Nemec MA. Ocular side effects of the retinoids. *Int J Dermatol* 1989; **28**: 218–25.
8 Gold MH, Roenigk HH. The retinoids and inflammatory bowel disease. *Arch Dermatol* 1988; **124**: 325–6.
9 Bunker CB, Sheron N, Maurice PDL, *et al.* Isotretinoin and eosinophilic pleural effusion. *Lancet* 1989; **i**: 435–6.
10 Bunker CB, Maurice PDL, Little S, *et al.* Isotretinoin and lung function in systemic sclerosis. *Clin Exp Dermatol* 1991; **16**: 11–13.
11 Matsuoka LY, Wortsman J, Pepper JJ. Acute arthritis during isotretinoin treatment for acne. *Arch Intern Med* 1984; **144**: 1870–1.

12 Milstone LM, McGuire J, Ablow RC. Premature epiphyseal closure in a child receiving oral 13-*cis*-retinoic acid. *J Am Acad Dermatol* 1982; **7**: 663–6.

13 Pittsley R, Yoder K. Retinoid hyperostosis. Skeletal toxicity associated with long-term administration of 13-*cis*-retinoic acid for refractory ichthyosis. *N Engl J Med* 1983; **308**: 1012–14.

14 Ellis CN, Madison KC, Pennes DR, *et al*. Isotretinoin is associated with early skeletal radiographic changes. *J Am Acad Dermatol* 1984; **10**: 1024–9.

15 Gerber L, Helfgott R, Gross E, *et al*. Vertebral abnormalities associated with synthetic retinoid use. *J Am Acad Dermatol* 1984; **10**: 817–23.

16 Pennes D, Ellis C, Madison K, *et al*. Early skeletal hyperostosis secondary to 13-*cis*-retinoic acid. *Am J Roentg* 1984; **142**: 979–83.

17 McGuire J, Milstone L, Lawson J. Isotretinoin administration alters juvenile and adult bone. In Saurat JH (ed.) *Retinoids: New Trends in Research and Therapy*. Karger, Basel, 1985, pp 419–39.

18 Ellis CN, Pennes DR, Madison KC, *et al*. Skeletal radiographic changes during retinoid therapy. In Saurat JH (ed.) *Retinoids: New Trends in Research and Therapy*. Karger, Basel, 1985, pp 440–4.

19 Kilcoyne RF, Cope R, Cunningham W, *et al*. Minimal spinal hyperostosis with low-dose isotretinoin therapy. *Invest Radiol* 1986; **21**: 41–4.

20 Carey BM, Parkin GJS, Cunliffe WJ, Pritlove J. Skeletal toxicity with iso-tretinoin therapy: a clinico-radiological evaluation. *Br J Dermatol* 1988; **119**: 609–14.

21 Novick NL, Lawson W, Schwartz IS. Bilateral nasal bone osteophytosis associated with short-term oral isotretinoin therapy for cystic acne vulgaris. *Am J Med* 1984; **77**: 736–9.

22 Taylor AEM, Mitchison H. Fatty liver following isotretinoin. *Br J Dermatol* 1991; **124**: 505–6.

23 Johnson TM, Rainin R. Isotretinoin-induced thrombocytopenia. *J Am Acad Dermatol* 1987; **17**: 838–9.

24 Nigra TP, Katz RA, Jorgensen H. Elevation of serum triglyceride levels from oral 13-*cis*-retinoic acid. In Orfanos CE, Braun-Falco O, Farber EM, *et al*. (eds) *Retinoids. Advances in Basic Research and Therapy*. Springer-Verlag, Berlin, 1981, pp 363–9.

25 Lyons F, Laker MF, Marsden JR, *et al*. Effect of oral 13-*cis*-retinoic acid on serum lipids. *Br J Dermatol* 1982; **107**: 591–5.

26 Zech LA, Gross EG, Peck GL, Brewer HB. Changes in plasma cholesterol and triglyceride levels after treatment with oral isotretinoin. A prospective study. *Arch Dermatol* 1983; **119**: 987–93.

27 Bershad S, Rubinstein A, Paterniti JR Jr, *et al*. Changes in plasma lipids and lipoproteins during isotretinoin therapy for acne. *N Engl J Med* 1985; **313**: 981–5.

28 Gollnick H, Schwartzkopff W, Pröschle W, *et al*. Retinoids and blood lipids: an update and review. In Saurat JH (ed.) *Retinoids: New Trends in Research and Therapy*. Karger, Basel, 1985, pp 445–60.

29 Marsden J. Hyperlipidaemia due to isotretinoin and etretinate: possible mechanisms and consequences. *Br J Dermatol* 1986; **114**: 401–7.

30 Dicken CH, Connolly SM. Eruptive xanthomas associated with isotretinoin (13-*cis*-retinoic acid). *Arch Dermatol* 1980; **16**: 951–2.

Teratogenicity

Major human fetal abnormalities related to Roaccutane therapy during pregnancy have been documented [1–4]. The most frequently reported abnormalities involve the central nervous system (micro-cephaly or hydrocephalus and cerebellar malformation), cardio-vascular system (anomalies of the great vessels); microtia or absence of external ears, microphthalmia, and facial dysmorphia; thymus gland abnormalities have also been reported. There is an increased risk of spontaneous abortion. Women of child-bearing potential should sign a consent form and be instructed that they should not be pregnant when Roaccutane therapy is started (preferably on the second or third day of the next normal menstrual period), and should use effective contraception during, and for one month after stopping, therapy. Roaccutane has a much shorter half life than etretinate, so that pregnancy is permissible 1 month after stopping therapy. Analysis of data voluntarily reported to Hoffmann-La Roche Inc. in the US enabled prospective study of 88 patients who had completed or discontinued isotretinoin therapy prior to becoming pregnant; 90% of all pregnancies occurred within 2 months after cessation of therapy, and 64% within 1 month [5]. There were no significant increases in the rates of spontaneous abortion or of congenital malformations among the live births. There appears to be no adverse effect of isotretinoin on male reproductive function [6,7].

1 Hill RM. Isotretinoin teratogenicity. *Lancet* 1984; i: 1465.
2 Stern RS, Rosa F, Baum C. Isotretinoin and pregnancy. *J Am Acad Dermatol* 1984; **10**: 851−4.
3 Chen DT, Human pregnancy experience with the retinoids. In Saurat JH (ed.) *Retinoids: New Trends in Research and Therapy.* Karger, Basel, 1985, pp 398−406.
4 Rosa FW, Wilk AL, Kelsey FO. Teratogen update: vitamin A cogeners. The outcome of pregnancies in patients who had taken isotretinoin *Teratology* 1986; **33**: 355−64.
5 Dai WS, Hsu M-A, Itri L. Safety of pregnancy after discontinuation of isotretinoin. *Arch Dermatol* 1989; **125**: 362−5.
6 Schill W-B, Wagner A, Nikolowski J, Plewig G. Aromatic retinoid and 13-*cis*-retinoic acid: spermatological investigations. In Orfanos CE, Braun-Falco O, Farber EM, *et al.* (eds) *Retinoids, Advances in Basic Research and Therapy.* Springer-Verlag, Berlin, 1981, pp 389−95.
7 Töröck L, Kása M. Spermatological and endocrinological examinations connected with isotretinoin treatment. In Saurat JH (ed.) *Retinoids: New Trends in Research and Therapy.* Karger, Basel, 1985, pp 407−10.

Tretinoin

Oral tretinoin administered as differentiation therapy of acute promyelocytic leukaemia was associated with mild skin rashes, the nature of which was unspecified [1].

1 Warrell RP, Frankel SR, Miller WH, *et al.* Differentiation therapy of acute promyelocytic leukemia with tretinoin (all-*trans*-retinoic acid). *N Engl J Med* 1991; **324**: 1385−93.

12.3 Vitamin B

Vitamin B$_1$

Anaphylaxis following intravenous administration has occurred [1].

Vitamin B₆ (pyridoxine)

Vasculitis is recorded [2], as is a pseudoporphyria syndrome with megadosage [3].

Nicotinic acid

Flushing is common; other transient rashes, urticaria, pruritus, scaling, hyperpigmentation and an acanthosis nigricans-like eruption [4,5] are all documented. Persistent rashes and hair loss have rarely occurred.

1 Kolz R, Lonsdorf G, Burg G. Unverträgslichkeitsreaktionen nach parenteraler Gabe von Vitamin B₁. *Hautarzt* 1980; **31**: 657−9.
2 Ruzicka T, Ring J, Braun-Falco O. Vasculitis allergica durch Vitamin B₆. *Hautarzt* 1984; **35**: 197−9.
3 Baer R, Stilman MA. Cutaneous skin changes probably due to pyridoxine abuse. *J Am Acad Dermatol* 1984; **10**: 527−8.
4 Tromovitch TA, Jacobs PH, Kern S. Acanthosis nigricans-like lesions from nicotinic acid. *Arch Dermatol* 1964; **89**: 222−3.
5 Elgart ML. Acanthosis nigricans and nicotinic acid. *J Am Acad Dermatol* 1981; **5**: 709−10.

12.4 Vitamin C (ascorbic acid)

Patients with cutaneous and respiratory allergy have been described.

12.5 Vitamin E (α-tocopherol)

White hair developed at injection sites in infants given intramuscular vitamin E for epidermolysis bullosa, probably due to quinones formed during vitamin E degradation [1].

1 Sehgal VN. Vitamin E − A melanotoxic agent. A preliminary report. *Dermatologica* 1972; **145**: 56−9.

12.6 Vitamin K

Skin reactions with vitamin K have been reviewed [1−4]. Eruption may occur after a single intramuscular injection of 10 mg of vitamin K₁. The pruritic erythematous macular lesions or plaques, localized to the site of injection, appear 4−16 days later, and may last for up to 6 months [1−6]. Patch and intradermal skin tests may be positive, suggesting an immunological basis. Most, but not all [3,6], cases have occurred in patients with liver disease. In addition, a proportion of these reactions progress to produce scleroderma-like changes [7−10]. An annular erythema has been documented [11].

1 Barnes HM, Sarkany I. Adverse skin reactions from vitamin K₁. *Br J Dermatol* 1976; **95**: 653−6.
2 Bullen AW, Miller JP, Cunliffe WJ, Losowsky MS. Skin reactions caused by vitamin K in patients with liver disease. *Br J Dermatol* 1978; **98**: 561−5.

3 Sanders MN, Winkelmann RK. Cutaneous reactions to vitamin K. *J Am Acad Dermatol* 1988; **19**: 699−704.

4 Mosser C, Janin-Mercier A, Souteyrand P. Les réactions cutanées apres administration parentérale de vitamine K. *Ann Dermatol Vénéréol (Paris)* 1987; **114**: 243−51.

5 Finkelstein H, Champion MC, Adam JE. Cutaneous hypersensitivity to vitamin K_1 injection. *J Am Acad Dermatol* 1987; **16**: 540−5.

6 Joyce JP, Hood AF, Weiss MM. Persistent cutaneous reaction to intramuscular vitamin K injection. *Arch Dermatol* 1988; **124**; 27−8.

7 Texier L, Gendre PH, Gauthier O, *et al.* Hypodermites sclérodermiformes lombo-fessières induites par des injections médicamenteuses intramusculaires associées a la vitamine K_1. *Ann Dermatol Syphiligr (Paris)* 1972; **99**: 363−71.

8 Janin-Mercier A, Mosser C, Souteyrand P, Bourges M. Subcutaneous sclerosis with fasciitis and eosinophilia after phytonadione injections. *Arch Dermatol* 1985; **121**: 1421−3.

9 Brunskill NJ, Berth-Jones J, Graham-Brown RAC. Pseudosclerodermatous reaction to phytomenadione injection (Texier's syndrome). *Clin Exp Dermatol* 1988; **13**: 276−8.

10 Pujol RM, Puig L, Moreno A, *et al.* Pseudoscleroderma secondary to phytonadione (vitamin K_1) injections. *Cutis* 1989; **43**: 365−8.

11 Kay MH, Duvic M. Reactive annular erythema after intramuscular vitamin K. *Cutis* 1986; **37**: 445−8.

Chapter 13
Hormones and Related Compounds

13.1 Adrenocorticotrophic hormone (ACTH) and corticosteroids

ACTH and systemic corticosteroids

The side-effects of these agents have been reviewed [1−10].

Cutaneous side-effects

These include acne, cutaneous thinning and atrophy, telangiectasia, striae distensae (Fig. 13.1), purpura and ecchymoses (Fig. 13.2), hypertrichosis, impaired wound healing, pigmentary changes, cushingoid (moon) facies, truncal adiposity [11], buffalo hump of the upper back, and potentiation of infections. Purpura and dermal thinning have been associated with high dose inhaled corticosteroids [12] as well as with oral therapy. Peri-oral dermatitis has been recorded in renal transplant recipients on corticosteroids and immunosuppressive therapy [13].

Panniculitis following short-term high dose steroid therapy in children manifests as subcutaneous nodules on the cheeks, arms and trunk [14]. Reversible panniculitis occurred in a child treated with steroids for hepatic encephalopathy [15]. Juxta-articular adiposis dolorosa developed in a patient treated with high doses of prednisone for the L-tryptophan-induced eosinophilia−myalgia syndrome [16]. Acanthosis nigricans may occur with corticosteroid therapy [17]. Immunosuppression with corticosteroids has been associated with the development of Kaposi's sarcoma during the treatment of temporal arteritis [18].

Systemic side-effects

These include fluid and electrolyte abnormalities, weight gain, oedema, hypertension, cardiac failure, peptic ulcer disease, pancreatitis, diabetes, muscular weakness, myopathy, tendon rupture, glaucoma, posterior subcapsular cataracts, mental changes including psychosis, osteoporosis, vertebral collapse, necrosis of the femoral head, growth suppression in children, opportunistic infection, masking of infection or reactivation of a dormant infection

[267]

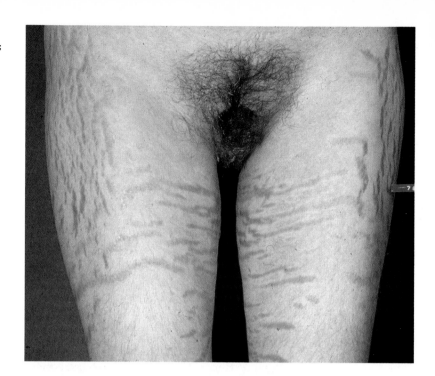

Figure 13.1 Striae distensae due to long-term systemic corticosteroid therapy for nephrotic syndrome.

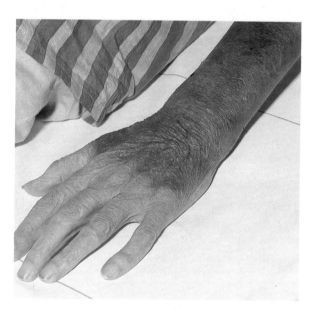

Figure 13.2 Purpura and atrophy due to prolonged systemic corticosteroid therapy for asthma.

(e.g. tuberculosis), polycythaemia, and suppression of the hypothalamic–pituitary axis.

ACTH

Allergic reactions to ACTH are recorded but are uncommon. Urticaria and dizziness, nausea and weakness are the most frequent, but severe anaphylactic shock has occurred. Synthetic ACTH is usually tolerated by patients sensitive to animal ACTH [19]. Depot preparations (tetracosactrin adsorbed on a zinc phosphate complex) have produced reactions [19,20] and may induce melanoderma [21].

Glucocorticosteroids

Allergic and immediate reactions to systemic glucocorticoids have been reviewed [22]. Urticarial reactions have followed the intra-arterial injection of prednisone, prednisolone or hydrocortisone [23], but are rare. Anaphylactoid reactions have been reported to topical and parenteral hydrocortisone, but may represent pseudo-allergic reactions rather than IgE-mediated immediate hypersensitivity [24,25]. Generalized skin reactions, including urticaria and maculopapular eruptions, developed in patients after therapy respectively with oral triamcinolone acetonide [26], or prednisone [27], or dexamethasone and betamethasone [28]; the patients were subsequently shown to be patch test positive to these corticosteroids. Systemic administration of hydrocortisone, and provocation of endogenous cortisol secretion by means of injection of the ACTH analogue tetracosactide, provoked dose-dependent allergic skin reactions at sites of previous allergic reactions to topical steroids in two patients with proven topical corticosteroids sensitivity (i.e. systemic allergic contact type dermatitis); in one case this was at a positive patch test site to hydrocortisone-17-butyrate [29]. Thus it has been postulated that high stress levels, which cause increased secretion of endogenous adrenal cortical hormones, could be implicated in exacerbations of eczema in corticosteroid-sensitive patients, and a persistent autoimmune skin reaction to cortisol might occur following topical sensitization to topical hydrocortisone [29]. The fact that systemic provocation testing with hydrocortisone results in a reaction confined to the skin in steroid-sensitive patients may be partly explained by the observation that, *in vitro*, only enriched Langerhans cells, and not peripheral blood mononuclear antigen-presenting cells, are capable of presenting corticosteroid to T cells of corticosteroid-sensitive subjects [30].

1 Lucky AW. Principles of the use of glucocorticosteroids in the growing child. *Pediatr Dermatol* 1984; **1**: 226−35.
2 Fritz KA, Weston WL. Systemic glucocorticosteroid therapy of skin disease in children. *Pediatr Dermatol* 1984; **1**: 236−45.
3 Davis GF. Adverse effects of corticosteroids: II. Systemic. *Clin Dermatol* 1986; **4**: 161−9.
4 Gallant C, Kenny P. Oral glucocorticoids and their complications. A review. *J Am Acad Dermatol* 1986; **14**: 161−77.
5 Seale PS, Compton MR. Side-effects of corticosteroid agents. *Med J Aust* 1986; **144**: 139−42.
6 Chosidow O, Étienne SD, Herson S, Puech AJ. Pharmacologie des corticoides. Notions classiques et nouvelles. *Ann Dermatol Vénéréol (Paris)* 1989; **116**: 147−66.
7 Fine R. Glucocorticoids (1989). *Int J Dermatol* 1990; **29**: 377−9.
8 Kyle V, Hazleman BL. Treatment of polymyalgia rheumatica and giant cell

arteritis: II. Relation between steroid dose and steroid associated side effects. *Ann Rheum Dis* 1989; **48**: 662−6.

9 Truhan AP, Ahmed AR. Corticosteroids: a review with emphasis on complications of prolonged systemic therapy. *Ann Allergy* 1989; **62**: 375−90.

10 Weiss MM. Corticosteroids in rheumatoid arthritis. *Semin Arthritis Rheum* 1989; **19**: 9−21.

11 Horber HH, Xurcher RM, Herren H, *et al*. Altered body fat distribution in patients with glucocorticoid treatment and in patients on long-term dialysis. *Am J Clin Nutr* 1986; **43**: 758−69.

12 Capewell S, Reynolds S, Shuttleworth D, *et al*. Purpura and dermal thinning associated with high dose inhaled corticosteroids. *Br Med J* 1990; **300**: 1548−51.

13 Adams SJ, Davison AM, Cunliffe WJ, Giles GR. Perioral dermatitis in renal transplant recipients maintained on corticosteroids and immunosuppressive therapy. *Br J Dermatol* 1982; **106**: 589−92.

14 Roenigk HH, Haserick JR, Arundell FD. Posteroid panniculitis. *Arch Dermatol* 1964; **90**: 387−91.

15 Saxena AK, Nigam PK. Panniculitis following steroid therapy. *Cutis* 1988; **42**: 341−2.

16 Greenbaum SS, Varga J. Corticosteroid-induced juxta-articular adiposis dolorosa. *Arch Dermatol* 1991; **127**: 231−3.

17 Brown J, Winkelmann RK. Acanthosis nigricans: A study of 90 cases. *Medicine* 1968; **47**: 33−51.

18 Leung F, Fam AG, Osoba D. Kaposi's sarcoma complicating corticosteroid therapy for temporal arteritis. *Am J Med* 1981; **71**: 320−2.

19 Patriarca G. Allergy to tetracosactrin-depot. *Lancet* 1971; **i**: 138.

20 Clee MD, Ferguson J, Browning MCK, *et al*. Glucocorticoid hypersensitivity in an asthmatic patient: presentation and treatment. *Thorax* 1985; **40**: 477−8.

21 Khan SA. Melanoderma caused by depot tetracosactrin. *Trans St John's Hosp Dermatol Soc* 1970; **56**: 168−71.

22 Preuss L. Allergic reactions to systemic glucocorticoids: a review. *Ann Allergy* 1985; **55**: 772−5.

23 Ashord RFU, Bailey A. Angioneurotic oedema and urticaria following hydrocortisone − a further case. *Postgrad Med J* 1980; **56**: 437.

24 King RA. A severe anaphylactoid reaction to hydrocortisone. *Lancet* 1960; **ii**: 1093−4.

25 Peller JS, Bardana EL Jr. Anaphylactoid reaction to corticosteroid: Case report and review of the literature. *Ann Allergy* 1985; **54**: 302−5.

26 Brambilla L, Boneschi V, Chiappino G, *et al*. Allergic reactions to topical desoxymethasone and oral triamcinolone. *Contact Dermatitis* 1989; **21**: 272−3.

27 De Corres LF, Bernaola G, Urrutia I, *et al*. Allergic dermatitis from systemic treatment with corticosteroids. *Contact Dermatitis* 1990; **22**: 104−5.

28 Maucher O, Faber M, Knipper H, *et al*. Kortikoidallergie. *Hautarzt* 1987; **38**: 577−82.

29 Lauerma AI, Reitamo S, Maibach HI. Systemic hydrocortisone/cortisol induces allergic skin reactions in presensitized subjects. *J Am Acad Dermatol* 1991; **24**: 182−5.

30 Lauerma AI, Räsänen L, Reunala T, Reitamo S. Langerhans cells but not monocytes are capable of antigen presentation *in vitro* in corticosteroid contact hypersensitivity. *Br J Dermatol* 1991; **123**: 699−705.

Topical corticosteroids

Local complications

The dermatological complications of topical corticosteroids have been reviewed [1−4]. Many of the adverse reactions are related to the potency of the preparation; thus in general, fluorinated steroids are associated with more significant side-effects. Topical steroids cause decreased epidermal kinetic activity [5], decreased dermal collagen and ground substance synthesis, and thinning of the dermis and epidermis [6–8]. Initial vasoconstriction of the superficial small vessels is followed by rebound vasodilatation, which becomes permanent in later stages. There are resultant striae, easy bruising, purpura, and hypertrichosis and telangiectasia (Fig. 13.3); stellate pseudoscars or ulcerated areas may be seen. Reversible hypopigmentation may develop. Local injection of a potent steroid may result in atrophy with telangiectasia (Fig. 13.4), and localized lipoatrophy may occur. Perilymphatic atrophy is recorded following intradermal steroid injection. Long-term daily use of a potent steroid, especially under plastic occlusion as for fingertip eczema, may result in acro-atrophy of terminal phalanges of the fingers [9,10].

Topical steroids may exacerbate acne, or lead to acne rosacea, with papules, pustules, and telangiectasia (Fig. 13.5), or perioral dermatitis (Fig. 13.6), characterized by erythema, papules and pustules at the perioral area [11–13]. They decrease the number and antigen-presenting capacity of epidermal Langerhans cells [14], and mask or potentiate skin infections, including fungal (tinea incognito) and bacterial infections and verruca vulgaris. Their withdrawal may provoke conversion of plaque to pustular type psoriasis [15]. Topical steroid therapy around the eye has been associated with development of glaucoma.

Topical corticosteroids may induce allergic contact dermatitis [16–22]. The allergen may be the steroid itself, or a preservative or a stabilizer such as ethylenediamine [3]. There may be cross-reactivity between different steroids [19,20]. Of an unselected series of 144 patients seen at the Contact Dermatitis Clinic at St John's

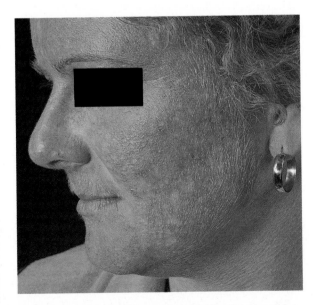

Figure 13.3 Telangiectasia and hypertrichosis induced by long-term topical corticosteroid therapy.

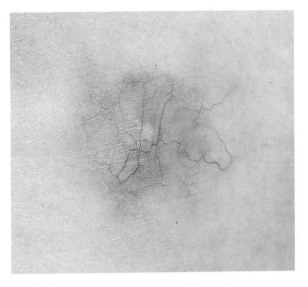

Figure 13.4 Cutaneous atrophy and telangiectasia due to local corticosteroid injection. (Courtesy of St John's Institute of Dermatology, London.)

[271]

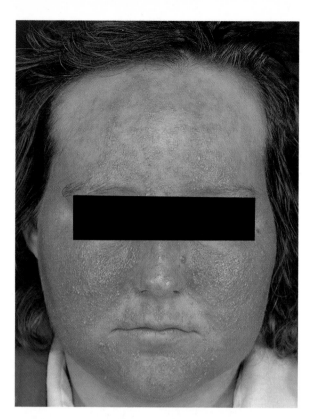

Figure 13.5 Acne rosacea-like rash due to topical corticosteroid therapy. (Courtesy of St John's Institute of Dermatology, London.)

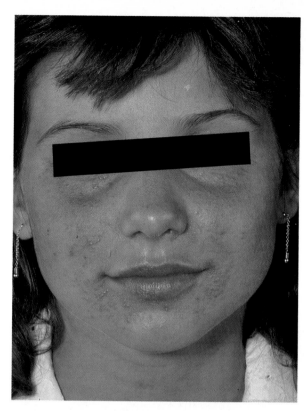

Figure 13.6 Perioral dermatitis due to topical corticosteroid therapy.

Dermatology Centre, 14% were patch test positive to one or more topical steroid preparations [19]. In another series, the incidence of allergy to hydrocortisone was 4.8% in unselected patients with a suspected allergic contact dermatitis [22].

Systemic side-effects

These occur particularly from the use of large amounts of high potency topical corticosteroids, especially under plastic occlusion [23,24]. Oedema from sodium retention occurs more frequently with halogenated corticosteroids [24]. Hypothalamic–pituitary axis suppression may occur [25,26]; a single application of 25 g of 0.05% clobetasol propionate ointment suppressed plasma cortisol for 96 hours [27]. Frank Cushing's syndrome [28–29] may result (Fig. 13.7), and growth retardation in children is a hazard [30]. Glycosuria and hyperglycaemia may rarely occur [31].

1 Miller JA, Munro DD. Topical corticosteroids: clinical pharmacology and therapeutic use. *Drugs* 1980; **19**: 119–34.
2 Behrendt H, Korting HC. Klinische Prüfung von erwünschten und unerwünschten Wirkungen topisch applizierbarer Glukokortikosteroide am Menschen. *Hautarzt* 1990: **41**: 2–8.

[272]

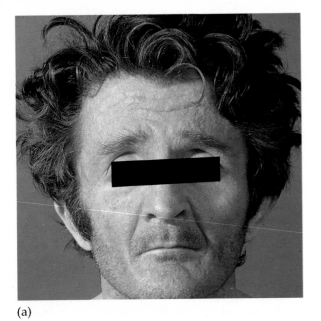 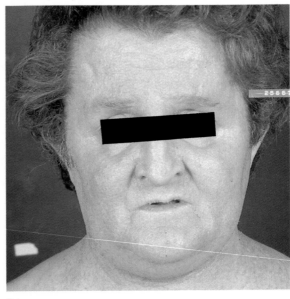

(a)   (b)

Figure 13.7 Patient with Darier's disease before (a) and after (b) extensive use of potent topical corticosteroids for 1 year; note Cushingoid facies in (b).

3 Coskey RJ. Adverse effects of corticosteroids: I. Topical and intralesional. *Clin Dermatol* 1986; **4**: 155–60.

4 Kligman AM. Adverse effects of topical corticosteroids. In Christophers E, Schöpf E, Kligman AM, Stoughton RB (eds) *Topical Corticosteroid Therapy: A Novel Approach to Safer Drugs*. Raven Press, New York, 1988, pp 181–7.

5 Marshall RC, Du Vivier RA. The effects on epidermal DNA synthesis of the butyrate esters of clobetasone and clobetasol, and the propionate ester of clobetasol. *Br J Dermatol* 1978; **98**: 355–9.

6 Smith JG, Wehr RF, Chalker DK. Corticosteroid-induced cutaneous atrophy and telangiectasia. *Arch Dermatol* 1976; **112**: 1115–17.

7 Winter GD, Burton HL. Experimentally induced steroid atrophy in the domestic pig and man. *Br J Dermatol* 1976; **94**: 107–9.

8 Lehmann P, Zheng P, Lacker RM, Kligman AM. Corticosteroid atrophy in human skin: a study by light, scanning and transmission electron microscopy. *J Invest Dermatol* 1983; **81**: 169–76.

9 Requena L, Zamora E, Martin L. Acroatrophy secondary to long-standing applications of topical steroids. *Arch Dermatol* 1990; **126**: 1013–14.

10 Wolf R, Tur E, Brenner S. Corticosteroid-induced 'disappearing digit'. *J Am Acad Dermatol* 1990; **23**: 755–6.

11 Sneddon I. Perioral dermatitis. *Br J Dermatol* 1972; **87**: 430–2.

12 Cotterill JA. Perioral dermatitis. *Br J Dermatol* 1979; **101**: 259–62.

13 Edwards EK Jr, Edwards ED Sr. Perioral dermatitis secondary to the use of a corticosteroid ointment as moustache wax. *Int J Dermatol* 1987; **26**: 649.

14 Ashworth J, Booker J, Breathnach SM. Effect of topical corticosteroid therapy on Langerhans cell function in human skin. *Br J Dermatol* 1988; **118**: 457–69.

15 Boxley JD, Dawber RPR, Summerly R. Generalised pustular psoriasis on withdrawal of clobetasol propionate ointment. *Br Med J* 1975; **2**: 225–6.

16 Reitamo S, Lauerma AI, Stubb S, *et al*. Delayed hypersensitivity to topical corticosteroids. *J Am Acad Dermatol* 1986; **14**: 582–9.

17 Dooms-Goossens AE, Degreef HJ, Marien KJC, Coopman SA. Contact allergy to corticosteroids: A frequently missed diagnosis? *J Am Acad Dermatol* 1989; **21**: 538–43.

18 Reitamo S, Lauerma AI, Förström L. Detection of contact hypersensitivity to topical corticosteroids with hydrocortisone-17-butyrate. *Contact Dermatitis* 1989; **21**: 159–65.

19 Ashworth J, White IR, Rycroft RJG, Cronin E. Contact sensitivity to topical corticosteroids. *Br J Dermatol* 1990; **123** (Suppl 37): 24.

20 Sasaki E. Corticosteroid sensitivity and cross-sensitivity. A review of cases 1967–1988. *Contact Dermatitis* 1990; **23**: 306–15.

21 Uter W. Allergische Reaktionen auf Glukokortikoide. *Dermatosen* 1990; **38**: 75–90.

22 Wilkinson SM, Cartwright PH, English JSC. Hydrocortisone: an important cutaneous allergen. *Lancet* 1991; **337**: 761–2.

23 Vickers CFH, Fritsch WC. A hazard of plastic film therapy. *Arch Dermatol* 1963; **87**: 633–5.

24 Fitzpatrick TB, Griswold MC, Hicks JH. Sodium retention and edema from percutaneous absorption of fluorocortisone acetate. *JAMA* 1955; **158**: 1149–52.

25 Carruthers JA, August PJ, Staughton RCD. Observations on the systemic effect of topical clobetasol propionate (Dermovate). *Br Med J* 1975; **4**: 203–4.

26 Weston WL, Fennessey PV, Morelli J, *et al.* Comparison of hypothalamus–pituitary–adrenal axis suppression from superpotent topical steroids by standard endocrine function testing and gas chromatographic mass spectrometry. *J Invest Dermatol* 1988; **90**: 532–5.

27 Hehir M, du Vivier A, Eilon L, *et al.* Investigation of the pharmacokinetics of clobetasol propionate and clobetasone butyrate after a single application of ointment. *Clin Exp Dermatol* 1983; **8**: 143–51.

28 May P, Stein ES, Ryler RJ, *et al.* Cushing syndrome from percutaneous absorption of triamcinolone cream. *Arch Intern Med* 1976; **136**: 612–13.

29 Himathongkam T, Dasanabhairochana P, Pitchayayothin N, Sriphrapradang A. Florid Cushing's syndrome and hirsutism induced by desoximetasone. *JAMA* 1978; **239**: 430–1.

30 Bode HH. Dwarfism following long-term topical corticosteroid therapy. *JAMA* 1980; **244**: 813–14.

31 Gomez EC, Frost P. Induction of glycosuria and hyperglycemia by topical corticosteroid therapy. *Arch Dermatol* 1976; **112**: 1559–62.

13.2 Oestrogens and related compounds

Oestrogens

Spider naevi and melanocytic naevi may develop under oestrogen therapy, as may chloasma. Stilboestrol therapy of pregnant women has been associated with female and male genital tract abnormalities in the offspring. Stilboestrol is a transplacental carcinogen and has caused adenocarcinoma of the vagina 20 years later in young women whose mothers took the drug in the first 18 weeks of pregnancy [1–5]. Acanthosis nigricans has resulted from diethylstilboestrol [6]. Hyperkeratosis of the nipples developed in a man treated for adenocarcinoma of the prostate with stilboestrol [7]. Porphyria cutanea tarda may also be precipitated [8,9].

1 Ulfelder H. The stilbestrol-adenosis-carcinoma syndrome. *Cancer* 1976; **38**: 426–31.

2 Poskanzer DC, Herbst AL. Epidemiology of vaginal adenosis and adenocarcinoma associated with exposure to stilbestrol *in utero*. *Cancer* 1977; **37**: 1892–5.

3 Monaghan JM, Sirisena LAW. Stilboestrol and vaginal clear-cell adenocarcinoma syndrome. *Br Med J* 1978; **i**: 1588–90.

4 Wingfield M. The daughters of stilboestrol. Grown up now but still at risk. *Br Med J* 1991; **302**: 1414–15.
5 Anonymous. Diethylstilboestrol — effects of exposure *in utero*. *Drug Ther Bull* 1991; **29**: 49–50.
6 Banuchi SR, Cohen L, Lorincz AL, Morgan J. Acanthosis nigricans following diethylstilbestrol therapy. *Arch Dermatol* 1974; **109**: 544–6.
7 Mold DE, Jegasothy BV. Estrogen-induced hyperkeratosis of the nipple. *Cutis* 1980; **26**: 95–6.
8 Becker FT. Porphyria cutanea tarda induced by estrogens. *Arch Dermatol* 1965; **92**: 252–6.
9 Roenigk HH, Gottlob ME. Estrogen-induced porphyria cutanea tarda. *Arch Dermatol* 1970; **102**: 260–6.

Oral contraceptives

Cutaneous complications of oral contraceptives have been reviewed [1–4]. These drugs combine an oestrogen with a progestogen. Candidiasis is common; the sexual partner may suffer penile irritation after coitus without physical signs or frank candidal balanoposthitis. Genital warts may increase. Facial hyperpigmentation known as chloasma (Fig. 13.8) is well recognized [5,6], as are hirsutism and acne. Gingival epithelial melanosis has been recorded [7]. Alopecia related to contraceptive therapy may be androgenic, or of postpartum telogen pattern following withdrawal of the drug. Erythema nodosum (Figs 3.70 & 3.71, p. 125) is a well recognized but rare complication [8,9].

The relapse of herpes gestationis is well documented [10]. Rare lichenoid, eczematous and fixed eruptions have been described, as has a lymphocytic cutaneous vasculitis, and an eruption resembling Sweet's syndrome [11]. Oral contraceptives have been implicated in both the provocation [12] and induction of remission of pityriasis lichenoides. A systemic lupus erythematosus-like reaction has also been reported [13]. An oral contraceptive-induced lupus erythematosus-like eruption, with erythematous lesions on the palms and feet in association with a weakly positive antinuclear factor and C1q deposition at the dermo-epidermal junction on direct immunofluorescence, developed in a patient and resolved on cessation of medication [14].

The jaundice rarely induced by these drugs resembles cholestatic jaundice of pregnancy. The hepatotoxic effects may result in provocation of variegate porphyria, porphyria cutanea tarda [15,16] and hereditary coproporphyria [17]; onycholysis may occur [16]. Photosensitivity unrelated to porphyrin disturbances has also been reported [18]. Benign hepatomas may also be a hazard [19].

1 Baker H. Drug reactions VIII. Adverse cutaneous reaction to oral contraceptives. *Br J Dermatol* 1969; **81**: 946–9.
2 Jelinek JE. Cutaneous complications of oral contraceptives. *Arch Dermatol* 1970; **101**: 181–6.
3 Coskey RJ. Eruptions due to oral contraceptives. *Arch Dermatol* 1977; **113**: 333–4.
4 Girard M. Évaluation des risques cutanés de la pilule. *Ann Dermatol Vénéréol (Paris)* 1990; **117**: 436–40.

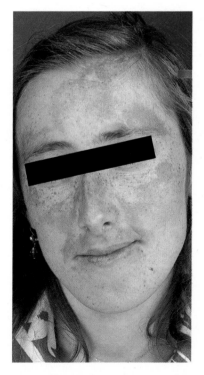

Figure 13.8 Chloasma due to an oral contraceptive (levonorgestrel–ethinyloestradiol).

5 Resnik S. Melasma induced by oral contraceptive drugs. *JAMA* 1967; **199**: 601.

6 Smith AG, Shuster S, Thody AJ, *et al*. Chloasma, oral contraceptives, and plasma immunoreactive beta-melanocyte-stimulating hormone. *J Invest Dermatol* 1977; **68**: 169−70.

7 Hertz RS, Beckstead PC, Brown WJ. Epithelial melanosis of the gingiva possibly resulting from the use of oral contraceptives. *J Am Dent Assoc* 1980; **100**: 713−14.

8 Posternal F, Orusco MMM, Laugier P. Eythème noueux et contraceptifs oraux. *Bull Derm* 1974; **81**: 642−5.

9 Bombardieri S, Di Munno O, Di Punzio C, Pasero G. Erythema nodosum associated with pregnancy and oral contraceptives. *Br Med J* 1977; **i**: 1509−10.

10 Morgan JK. Herpes gestationis influenced by an oral contraceptive. *Br J Dermatol* 1968; **80**: 456−8.

11 Tefany FJ, Georgouras K. A neutrophilic reaction of Sweet's syndrome type associated with the oral contraceptive. *Australas J Dermatol* 1991; **32**: 55−9.

12 Hollander A, Grotts IA. Mucha−Habermann disease following estrogen−progesterone therapy. *Arch Dermatol* 1973; **107**: 465.

13 Garrovich M, Agudelo C, Pisko E. Oral contraceptives and systemic lupus erythematosus. *Arthritis Rheum* 1980; **23**: 1396−8.

14 Furukawa F, Tachibana T, Imamura S, Tamura T. Oral contraceptive-induced lupus erythematosus in a Japanese woman. *J Dermatol (Tokyo)* 1991; **18**: 56−8.

15 Degos R, Touraine R, Kalis B, Delort J, Bonvalet D. Porphyrie cutanée tardive après prise prolongé de contraceptifs oraux. *Ann Dermatol Syphiligr (Paris)* 1969; **96**: 5−14.

16 Byrne JPH, Boss JM, Dawber RPR. Contraceptive pill-induced porphyria cutanea tarda presenting with onycholysis of the finger nails. *Postgrad Med J* 1976; **52**: 535−8.

17 Roberts DT, Brodie MJ, Moore MR, Thompson GG, Goldberg A, MacSween RNM. Hereditary coproporphyria presenting with photosensitivity induced by the contraceptive pill. *Br J Dermatol* 1977; **96**: 549−54.

18 Erickson LR, Peterka ES. Sunlight sensitivity from oral contraceptives. *JAMA* 1968; **203**: 980−1.

19 Baum JK, Holtz F, Bookstein JJ, Klein EW. Possible association between benign hepatomas and oral contraceptives. *Lancet* 1973; **ii**: 926−8.

Autoimmune progesterone dermatitis

A number of eruptions, including urticaria, eczema, pompholyx, and erythema multiforme have been reported to recur cyclically in the second, luteal phase of the menstrual cycle, with premenstrual peaking in severity [1−5]. It has been proposed that they result from sensitization to endogenous progesterone. There is frequently, but not always, a history of prior exposure to synthetic progesterones [1,3]. Two patients with recurrent premenstrual erythema multiforme and autoreactivity to 17α-hydroxyprogesterone have been described [4,5]; in one case the eruption spread in pregnancy, cleared after abortion, and was associated with a high affinity binding factor to 17α-hydroxyprogesterone in the serum [5]. A premenstrual urticarial reaction was exacerbated by oestrogen, rather than progesterone [6].

1 Hart R. Autoimmune progesterone dermatitis. *Arch Dermatol* 1977; **113**: 426−30.

2 Wojnarowska F, Greaves MW, Peachey RDG, *et al*. Progesterone-induced erythema multiforme. *J R Soc Med* 1985; **78**: 407−8.

3 Stephens CJM, Black MM. Perimenstrual eruptions: autoimmune progesterone dermatitis. *Semin Dermatol* 1989; **8**: 26–9.
4 Cheesman KL, Gaynor LV, Chatterton RT Jr, *et al.* Identification of a 17α-hydroxyprogesterone-binding immunoglobulin in the serum of a woman with periodic rashes. *J Clin Endocrinol Metab* 1982; **55**: 597–9.
5 Pinta JS, Sobrinho L, da Silva MB, *et al.* Erythema multiforme associated with autoreactivity to 17α-hydroxyprogesterone. *Dermatologica* 1990; **180**: 146–50.
6 Mayou SC, Charles-Holmes R, Kenney A, *et al.* A premenstrual urticarial eruption treated with bilateral oophorectomy and hysterectomy. *Clin Exp Dermatol* 1988; **13**: 114–16.

Tamoxifen

This oestrogen receptor antagonist used in the therapy of breast cancer in women has caused hirsutism, hair loss, dry skin and a variety of rashes.

13.3 Androgens

Anabolic steroids

Exacerbation of acne vulgaris with development of acne conglobata has been reported [1]. Both the size of sebaceous glands and the rate of sebum secretion is increased [2,3]. A lichenoid eruption was reported in a patient with aplastic anaemia treated with nandrolone furylpropionate (Cemelon) [4].

Danazol

This 17-ethinyltestosterone derivative, which is an inhibitor of pituitary gonadotrophin, is a very weak androgen. Acne, hirsutism, seborrhoea, rash, and generalized alopecia are documented [5–7]. Exacerbation of lupus erythematosus-like eruptions have been reported in patients receiving this drug for non-C1-esterase inhibitor-dependent angioedema [8] or for hereditary angioneurotic oedema [9].

Gestrinone

This derivative of 19-nortestosterone, like danazol, may cause weight gain, hirsutism, acne, voice change or irregular menstrual bleeding [10].

Testosterone

Severe acne (Fig. 13.9) or acne fulminans has followed therapy with testosterone, with [2,11] or without [12] anabolic steroids.

1 Merkle T, Landthaler M, Braun-Falco O. Acne-conglobata-artige Exazerbation einer Acne vulgaris nach Einnahme von Anabolika und Vitamin-B-Komplex-haltigen Präparaten. *Hautarzt* 1990; **41**: 280–2.
2 Kiraly CL, Collan Y, Alén M. Effect of testosterone and anabolic steroids on

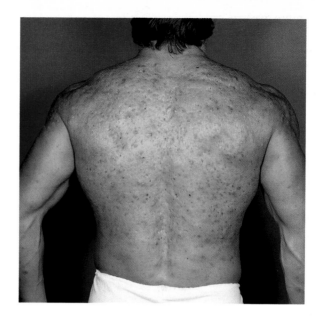

Figure 13.9 Extensive acneiform eruption in a professional sportsman who took testosterone. (Courtesy of Professor J. Zelger, Salzburg.)

the size of sebaceous glands in power athletes. *Am J Dermatopathol* 1987; **9**: 515–19.

3 Király CL, Alén M, Rahkila P, Horsmanheimo M. Effect of androgenic and anabolic steroids on the sebaceous gland in power athletes. *Acta Derm Venereol (Stockh)* 1987; **67**: 36–40.

4 Aihara M, Kitamura K, Ikezawa Z. Lichenoid drug eruption due to nandrolone furylpropionate (Cemelon). *J Dermatol (Tokyo)* 1989; **16**: 330–4.

5 Spooner JB. Classification of side-effects to danazol therapy. *J Int Med Res* 1977; **5** (Suppl 3): 15–17.

6 Greenberg RD. Acne vulgaris associated with antigonadotrophic (Danazol) therapy. *Cutis* 1979; **24**: 431–2.

7 Duff P, Mayer AR. Generalized alopecia: an unusual complication of danazol therapy. *Am J Obstet Gynecol* 1981; **141**: 349–50.

8 Fretwell MD, Altman LC. Exacerbation of a lupus-erythematosus-like syndrome during treatment of non-C1-esterase-inhibitor dependent angioedema with danazol. *J Allergy Clin Immunol* 1982; **69**: 306–10.

9 Sassolas B, Guillet G. Lupus, hereditary angioneurotic oedema and the risks of danazol treatment. *Br J Dermatol* 1991; **125**: 190–1.

10 Anonymous. Gestrinone (Dimetriose) — another option in endometriosis. *Drug Ther Bull* 1991; **29**: 45.

11 Heydenreich G. Testosterone and anabolic steroids and acne fulminans. *Arch Dermatol* 1989; **125**: 571–2.

12 Traupe H, von Mühlendahl KE, Brämswig J, Happle R. Acne of the fulminans type following testosterone therapy in three excessively tall boys. *Arch Dermatol* 1988; **124**: 414–17.

13.4 Insulin

Adverse reactions to insulin are relatively common [1–8]. Bovine insulin has most potential for production of allergic reactions, followed by porcine and human insulin [8]. Anaphylaxis may nevertheless occur with recombinant human insulin [9]. Local allergic reactions are often of immediate hypersensitivity type; they are more common in the first few months, and usually subside with continued therapy. Generalized pruritus and urticaria occur rarely. Typically, more severe anaphylactoid reactions follow re-introduction of insulin in patients who previously have received long-term therapy. Delayed reactions may also occur, and take the form of pruritic erythema and induration, sometimes with papulation, within 24 hours of injection [10]. Biphasic responses may be seen in the same individual, with initial immediate urticaria and a delayed reaction after 4−6 hours. Allergy may develop to the insulin itself (i.e. bovine or porcine protein), or to preservatives such as parabens, and zinc [11,12], or to surfen present in depot preparations [13]. Sterile furunculoid lesions at injection sites, which heal with scars, and which have a granulomatous histology, may result [11,12]. Lipo-atrophy at injection sites, or more rarely distally, perhaps the result of an immunological reaction [14], occurs especially with longer acting preparations; affected patients may have lesional immuno-globulin deposits and circulating anti-insulin antibodies. Exceptionally, hypertrophic lipodystrophy [15], or hyperkeratotic verrucous plaques at the site of repeated injections [16], may develop.

1 Hasche H, Haslbeck M, Bachmann W, Mehnert H. Verteilung allergischer Hautreaktionen bei Insulintherapie. *Dtsch Med Wochenschr* 1981; **106**: 1451−6.
2 Sibbald RG, Schachter RK. The skin and diabetes mellitus. *Int J Dermatol* 1984; **23**: 567−84.
3 Small P, Lerman S. Human insulin allergy. *Ann Allergy* 1984; **53**: 39−41.
4 Grammer L. Insulin allergy. *Clin Rev Allergy* 1986; **4**: 189−200.
5 Jegasothy BV. Cutaneous complications of insulin treatment. In Jelinek JE (ed) *The Skin and Diabetes*. Lea & Febiger, Philadelphia, 1986, pp 217−26.
6 De Shazo RD, Mather P, Grant W, *et al*. Evaluation of patients with local reactions to insulin with skin tests and *in vitro* techniques. *Diabetes Care* 1987; **10**: 330−6.
7 Plantin P, Sassolas B, Guillet M-H, *et al*. Accidents cutanés allergiques aux insulines. Aspects actuels a propos de 2 cas. *Ann Dermatol Vénéréol (Paris)* 1988; **115**: 813−17.
8 Sussman GL, Dolovich J. Prevention of anaphylaxis. *Semin Dermatol* 1989; **8**: 158−65.
9 Fineberg SE, Galloway JA, Fineberg NS, *et al*. Immunogenicity of recombinant human insulin. *Diabetologica* 1983; **25**: 465−9.
10 White WN, DeMartino SA, Yoshida T. Severe delayed inflammatory reactions from injected insulin. *Am J Med* 1983; **74**: 909−13.
11 Feinglos MN, Jegasothy BV. 'Insulin' allergy due to zinc. *Lancet* 1979; **i**: 122−4.
12 Jordaan HF, Sandler M. Zinc-induced granuloma − a unique complication of insulin therapy. *Clin Exp Dermatol* 1989; **14**: 227−9.
13 Goerz G, Ruzicka T, Hofmann N, *et al*. Granulomatöse allergische Reaktion vom verzögerten Typ auf Surfen. *Hautarzt* 1981; **32**: 187−90.
14 Reeves WG, Allen BR, Tattersall RB. Insulin-induced lipoatrophy: evidence for an immune pathogenesis. *Br Med J* 1980; **280**: 1500−3.
15 Johnson DA, Parlette HL. Insulin-induced hypertrophic lipodystrophy. *Cutis* 1983; **32**: 273−4.
16 Fleming MG, Simon SI. Cutaneous insulin reaction resembling acanthosis nigricans. *Arch Dermatol* 1986; **122**: 1054−6.

13.5 Thyroxine

Chronic urticaria and angioedema was reported in a patient, associated with exogenous thyrotoxicosis, related to thyroid replacement therapy [1].

1 Pandya AG, Beaudoing DL. Chronic urticaria associated with exogenous thyroid use. *Arch Dermatol* 1990; **126**: 1238—9.

13.6 Antithyroid drugs

Thiouracils

Hypersensitivity reactions include drug fever, pruritus, urticaria, angioedema, exanthemata, acneiform rashes, depigmentation of hair, and lupus erythematosus-like syndromes. Propylthiouracil has caused allergic vasculitis [1,2], and methylthiouracil has resulted in erythema multiforme. Thiouracils may cause excessive hair loss. These drugs may cause marrow failure [3].

1 Vasily DB, Tyler WB. Propylthiouracil-induced cutaneous vasculitis. *JAMA* 1980; **243**: 458—60.
2 Gammeltoft M, Kristensen JK. Propylthiouracil-induced cutaneous vasculitis. *Acta Derm Venereol (Stockh)* 1982; **62**: 171—3.
3 The International Agranulocytosis and Aplastic Anemia Study. Risk of agranulocytosis and aplastic anemia in relation to use of antithyroid drugs. *Br Med J* 1988; **287**: 262—5.

Chapter 14
Chemotherapeutic Agents

14.1 General side-effects

There have been a number of excellent reviews of the dermatological complications of these compounds [1−9], including histopathological reactions [10]. Bone marrow depression, with aplastic anaemia, agranulocytosis or thrombocytopenia, and gastrointestinal intolerance may occur with any of these drugs. Mucocutaneous surfaces are especially vulnerable to the toxic effects of this group of drugs on rapidly dividing cells. Common side-effects therefore include alopecia [8] and stomatitis [11]. Cytotoxic drugs may cause alopecia by either anagen or telogen effluvium. Severe alopecia of anagen type within 2 weeks of administration of the drug is frequently seen with cyclophosphamide, doxorubicin, and the nitroso-ureas; it is usually reversible with cessation of therapy. Other chemotherapeutic agents implicated in the production of alopecia include: amsacrine, bleomycin, cyclophosphamide, cytarabine, dactinomycin, daunorubicin, etoposide, fluorouracil, and methotrexate. Stomatitis occurs most frequently with acridinyl anisidide, dactinomycin, daunorubicin, doxorubicin, fluorouracil, and methotrexate (Fig. 14.1); it may respond to reduced dosage. Similarly, a number of drugs may cause pigmentation of the buccal mucosa [12] or of the nails [13−15].

Many of these agents have distinctive cutaneous side-effects, ranging from localized or diffuse hyperpigmentation to less usual ones, including radiation enhancement and recall phenomena, photosensitivity and hypersensitivity reactions, and phlebitis or chemical cellulitis.

Photosensitivity reactions occur with dacarbazine, fluorouracil, mitomycin and vinblastine. Hypersensitivity reactions such as urticaria and angioedema are common with some agents, such as asparaginase and cisplatin, but very rare with others, for example methotrexate. Radiation recall effects involve reactivation of an inflammatory response in areas irradiated months or years previously. Clinically, these range from erythema to vesiculation, with erosions and subsequent hyperpigmentation. They have most often been reported in association with dactinomycin and doxorubicin therapy [16]; bleomycin, fluorouracil, hydroxyurea, and methotrexate may also cause radiation enhancement.

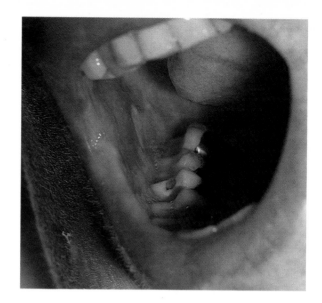

Figure 14.1 Erosive stomatitis due to methotrexate.

Rare complications such as diffuse sclerosis of the hands and feet, Raynaud's phenomenon [17], sterile folliculitis, and flushing reactions may also occur. Multiple drug regimes may pose special problems in trying to elucidate the cause of a specific reaction, such as white banded nails [18] or multiple Beau's lines [19]. A pityriasis lichenoides-like eruption occurred during therapy for myelogenous leukaemia with vincristine and mercaptopurine, antibiotics, and acyclovir [20].

Most cytotoxic drugs are teratogenic, and are contraindicated during pregnancy, especially during the first trimester. Alkylating drugs usually cause sterility in males, and may shorten reproductive life in women.

1 Weiss RB, Bruno S. Hypersensitivity reactions to cancer chemotherapeutic agents. *Ann Intern Med* 1981; **94**: 66–72.
2 Weiss RB. Hypersensitivity reactions to cancer chemotherapy. *Semin Oncol* 1982; **9**: 5–13.
3 Bronner AK, Hood AF. Cutaneous complications of chemotherapeutic agents. *J Am Acad Dermatol* 1983; **9**: 645–63.
4 McDonald CJ. Cytotoxic agents for use in dermatology. I. *J Am Acad Dermatol* 1985; **12**: 753–5.
5 McDonald CJ. Use of cytotoxic drugs in dermatologic diseases. II. *J Am Acad Dermatol* 1985; **12**: 965–75.
6 Hood AF. Cutaneous side effects of cancer chemotherapy. *Med Clin North Am* 1986; **70**: 187–209.
7 Delaunay M. Effets cutanés indésirables de la chimiothérapie antitumorale. *Ann Dermatol Vénéréol (Paris)* 1989; **116**: 347–61.
8 Kerker BJ, Hood AF. Chemotherapy-induced cutaneous reactions. *Semin Dermatol* 1989; **8**: 173–81.
9 Rapini RP. Cytotoxic drugs in the treatment of skin disease. *Int J Dermatol* 1991; **30**: 313–22.
10 Fitzpatrick JE, Hood AF. Histopathologic reactions to chemotherapeutic agents. *Adv Dermatol* 1988; **3**: 161–84.
11 Bottomley WK, Perlin E, Ross GR. Antineoplastic agents and their oral manifestations. *Oral Surg* 1977; **44**: 527–34.

12 Krutchik AN, Buzdar AU. Pigmentation of the tongue and mucous membranes associated with cancer chemotherapy. *South Med J* 1979; **72**: 1615–16.

13 Sulis E, Floris C. Nail pigmentation following cancer chemotherapy: a new genetic entity? *Eur J Cancer* 1980; **16**: 1517–19.

14 Daniel CR III, Scher RK. Nail changes secondary to systemic drugs or ingestants. *J Am Acad Dermatol* 1984; **10**: 250–8.

15 Daniel CR III, Scher RK. Nail changes secondary to systemic drugs or ingestants. In: Scher RK, Daniel CR III (eds) *Nails: Therapy, Diagnosis, Surgery.* W.B. Saunders, Philadelphia, 1990, pp 192–201.

16 Solberg LA Jr, Wick MR, Bruckman JE. Doxorubicin-enhanced skin reaction after whole-body electron beam irradiation for leukemia cutis. *Mayo Clinic Proc* 1980; **55**: 711–15.

17 Vogelzang NJ, Bosl GJ, Johnson D, *et al.* Raynaud's phenomenon: a common toxicity after combination chemotherapy for testicular cancer. *Ann Intern Med* 1981; **95**: 288–92.

18 James WD, Odom RB. Chemotherapy-induced transverse white lines in the fingernails. *Arch Dermatol* 1983; **119**: 334–5.

19 Singh M, Kaur S. Chemotherapy-induced multiple Beau's lines. *Int J Dermatol* 1986; **25**: 590–1.

20 Isoda M. Pityriasis lichenoides-like eruption occurring during therapy for myelogenous leukemia. *J Dermatol (Tokyo)* 1989; **16**: 73–5.

Extravasation

Extravasation, leading to skin necrosis with ulceration (Fig. 14.2), occurs with several agents [1–5]. Phlebitis typically results from amsacrine, dacarbazine, dactinomycin, daunorubicin, doxorubicin, mechlorethamine, mitomycin, mitoxantrone, and vinblastine. Chemical cellulitis is recorded with bleomycin, cisplatin, dacarbazine, dactinomycin, daunorubicin, doxorubicin, fluorouracil, mechlorethamine, methotrexate, mithramycin, mitomycin, mitoxantrone, streptozotocin, and the vinca alkaloids. Residual drug should be aspirated, and the limb elevated; plastic surgical advice should be sought as soon as possible. High dermal concentrations

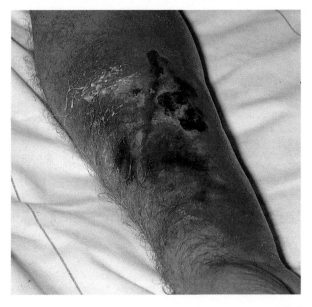

Figure 14.2 Skin necrosis and erythematous infiltration due to extravasation of cytotoxic agents (epirubicin, cyclophosphamide, and vincristine).

of doxorubicin have been documented as late as 28 days after accidental extravasation [6]. Histological examination of doxorubicin-related extravasation lesions demonstrated exaggerated interface-type dermatitis with thrombosis of venous tributaries [7].

1 Ignoffo RJ, Friedman MA. Therapy of local toxicities caused by extravasation of cancer chemotherapeutic drugs. *Cancer Treat Rev* 1980; **7**: 17−27.
2 Vansvloten Harwood K, Aisner J. Treatment of chemotherapeutic extravasation: Current status. *Cancer Treat Rep* 1984; **86**: 939−45.
3 Banerjee A, Brotherston TM, Lamberty BGH, *et al.* Cancer chemotherapy agent-induced perivenous extravasation injury. *J Postgrad Med* 1987; **63**: 5−9.
4 Rudolph R, Larson DL. Etiology and treatment of chemotherapeutic agent extravasation injuries. A review. *J Clin Oncol* 1987; **5**: 1116−26.
5 Dufresne RG Jr. Skin necrosis from intravenously infused materials. *Cutis* 1989; **39**: 197−8.
6 Sonneveld P, Wassenaar HA, Nooter K. Long persistence of doxorubicin in human skin after extravasation. *Cancer Treat Rep* 1984; **68**: 895−6.
7 Bhawan J, Petry J, Rybak ME. Histologic changes induced in skin by extravasation of doxorubicin (adriamycin). *J Cutan Pathol* 1989; **16**: 158−63.

Acral erythema

Several drugs (especially cytosine arabinoside, fluorouracil, and doxorubicin, and rarely cyclophosphamide, hydroxyurea, mercaptopurine, methotrexate, and mitotane) can cause dose-dependent acral erythema, either alone or in combination [1−9]. Bulla formation, desquamation, and subsequent re-epithelialization may occur. Reactions may occur sooner (from 24 hours to 3 weeks) and more severely with bolus or short-term chemotherapy than with low-dose continuous infusion [9], and are usually reproducible on challenge. Intravenous cyclosporin, given in bone marrow transplant patients, reportedly worsens the pain of the acral erythema [10]. The condition should be distinguished from graft-versus-host disease in patients who receive chemotherapy followed by bone marrow transplantation, and from chemotherapy-induced Raynaud's phenomenon.

1 Burgdorf WHC, Gilmore WA, Ganick RG. Peculiar acral erythema secondary to high-dose chemotherapy for acute myelogenous leukemia. *Ann Intern Med* 1982; **97**: 61−2.
2 Doyle LA, Berg C, Bottino G, Chabner E. Erythema and desquamation after high-dose methotrexate. *Ann Intern Med* 1983; **98**: 611−22.
3 Feldman LD, Jaffer A. Fluorouracil-associated palmar−plantar erythrodysesthesia syndrome. *JAMA* 1985; **254**: 3479.
4 Crider MK, Jansen J, Norins AL, McHale MS. Chemotherapy-induced acral erythema in patients receiving bone marrow transplantation. *Arch Dermatol* 1986; **122**: 1023−7.
5 Cox GJ, Robertson DB. Toxic erythema of palms and soles associated with high-dose mercaptopurine chemotherapy. *Arch Dermatol* 1986; **122**: 1413−14.
6 Guillaume J-C, Carp E, Rougier P, Charpentier P, André P, Carde P, Avril M-F. Effets secondaires cutanéo-muqueux des perfusions continues de 5-fluorouracile: 12 observations. *Ann Dermatol Vénéréol (Paris)* 1988; **115**: 1167−9.
7 Vukelja SJ, Lombardo RA, James WD, *et al.* Pyridoxine for the palmar−plantar erythrodysesthesia syndrome. *Ann Intern Med* 1989; **111**: 688−9.

8 Horwitz LJ, Dreizen S. Acral erythemas induced by chemotherapy and graft-versus-host disease in adults with hematogenous malignancies. *Cutis* 1990; **46**: 397–404.

9 Baack BR, Burgdorf WHC. Chemotherapy-induced acral erythema. *J Am Acad Dermatol* 1991; **24**: 457–61.

10 Kampmann KK, Graves T, Rogers SD. Acral erythema secondary to high-dose cytosine arabinoside with pain worsened by cyclosporin infusions. *Cancer* 1989; **63**: 2482–5.

Neutrophilic eccrine hidradenitis

Neutrophilic eccrine hidradenitis may represent a reaction pattern to a variety of chemotherapeutic agents [1–6], but particularly cytarabine and bleomycin. Clinically, erythematous papules or plaques or nodules are most frequent, although hyperpigmented plaques, pustules, purpura, and urticaria have been described. Lesions resolve spontaneously over the course of several days. The histology is characterized by infiltration of eccrine coils with neutrophils and necrosis of the secretory epithelium. Neutrophilic eccrine hidradenitas has also been described in a patient receiving haemodialysis without chemotherapy [7] and in a patient without a malignancy who was taking acetominophen [8].

A related but distinct entity termed syringosquamous metaplasia, which may be confused with well-differentiated squamous cell carcinoma histologically, has been described in patients receiving chemotherapy for leukaemia and other cancers [9,10]. Clinically, this may appear as an erythematous, blanching, papular crusted eruption [10].

1 Beutner KR, Packman CH, Markowitch W. Neutrophilic eccrine hidradenitis associated with Hodgkin's disease and chemotherapy. A case report. *Arch Dermatol* 1986; **122**: 809–11.

2 Fitzpatrick JE, Bennion SD, Reed OM, *et al.* Neutrophilic eccrine hidradenitis associated with induction chemotherapy. *J Cutan Pathol* 1987; **14**: 272–8.

3 Scallan PJ, Kettler AH, Levy ML, *et al.* Neutrophilic eccrine hidradenitis. *Cancer* 1988; **62**: 2532–6.

4 Fernández Cogolludo E, Ambrojo Antunez P, Aguilar Martínez A, *et al.* Neutrophil eccrine hidradenitis — a report of two additional cases. *Clin Exp Dermatol* 1989; **14**: 341–6.

5 Burg G, Bieber T, Langecker P. Lokalisierte neutrophile ekkrien Hidradenitis unter Mitoxantron: eine typische Zytostatikanebenwirkung. *Hautarzt* 1988; **39**: 233–6.

6 Allegue F, Soria C, Rocamora A, *et al.* Neutrophilic eccrine hidradenitis in two neutropenic patients. *J Am Acad Dermatol* 1990; **23**: 1110–13.

7 Moreno A, Barnadas MA, Ravella A, Moragas JM. Infectious eccrine hidradenitis in a patient undergoing hemodialysis. *Arch Dermatol* 1985; **121**: 1106–7.

8 Kuttner BJ, Kurban RS. Neutrophilic eccrine hidradenitis in the absence of an underlying malignancy. *Cutis* 1988; **41**: 403–5.

9 Bhawan J, Malhotra R. Syringosquamous metaplasia. A distinctive eruption in patients receiving chemotherapy. *Am J Dermatopathol* 1990; **12**: 1–6.

10 Hurt MA, Halvorson RD, Petr FC Jr, *et al.* Eccrine squamous syringometaplasia. A cutaneous sweat gland reaction in the histologic spectrum of 'chemotherapy-associated eccrine hidradenitis' and 'neutrophilic eccrine hidradenitis'. *Arch Dermatol* 1990; **126**: 73–7.

Side-effects related to immunosuppression

The cutaneous manifestations of immunosuppression have been reviewed [1–5]. Immunosuppressive therapy, as azathioprine and prednisone for renal transplant patients, may encourage skin infections of various types such as warts, herpes simplex, and herpes zoster [6], pityriasis versicolor and fungal infections [7]. Development of disseminated superficial actinic porokeratosis [8,9], porokeratosis of Mibelli [10–13], and increased numbers of benign [14,15] or eruptive dysplastic [16] melanocytic naevi may be promoted.

Internal malignancy

The frequency of cancers common in the general population is not increased in transplant patients. However, that of a variety of otherwise uncommon malignancies is increased [17–19], including non-Hodgkin's type lymphomas (mostly B cell, with 14% of T cell, and less than 1% of null cell, origin), which account for 21% of cancers in transplant recipients; Kaposi's sarcoma (Fig. 14.3); other sarcomas; carcinoma of the vulva and perineum; carcinoma of the kidney; and hepatobiliary tumours. Non-Hodgkin's lymphomas appear commoner and develop earlier where potent immunosuppressive agents such as cyclosporin and/or the monoclonal antibody OKT3 have been used; however, although cancer develops in 6% of all transplant recipients, only 1% of patients die from this complication [19]. Leukaemia may develop following chemotherapy [20], and bladder cancer has been associated with cyclophosphamide therapy [21].

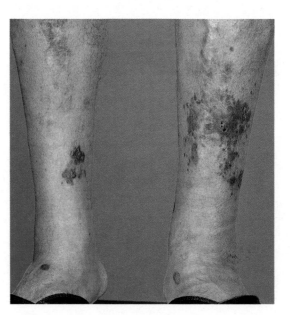

Figure 14.3 Kaposi's sarcoma following immunosuppression in a renal transplant patient.

Skin cancers

Actinic keratoses, squamous cell and basal cell cancer of the lip and skin [17–19,22–28], and malignant melanoma [29] have been reported to be more common, especially in immunosuppressed renal transplant patients. The majority of these patients have received azathioprine and corticosteroids. Interestingly, the immunosuppressed recipients of renal transplants have been reported to be at a high risk for skin cancer unless they express the HLA class I allele, A11 [30]. Furthermore, patients with longstanding renal grafts mismatched for HLA-B have a significantly higher incidence of squamous cell cancers than other mismatches, and patients who are homozygous for HLA-DR are at an increased risk for actinic keratoses and skin cancer [31]. These findings imply that major histocompatibility complex gene products participate in the pathogenesis of skin cancer in immunosuppressed patients, probably via influences on T cell recognition of neoantigens [32]. There was no difference from control levels in the number of $CD1^+HLA\text{-}DR^+$ antigen presenting Langerhans cells in the epidermis of immunosuppressed renal transplant recipients treated with either azathioprine/prednisone or cyclosporin/prednisone [33].

1 Koranda FC, Dehmel EM, Kahn G, Penn I. Cutaneous complications in immunosuppressed renal homograft recipients. *JAMA* 1974; **229**: 419–24.
2 Cohen EB, Komorowski RA, Clowry LJ. Cutaneous complications in renal transplant recipients. *Am J Clin Pathol* 1987; **88**: 32–7.
3 Abel EA. Cutaneous manifestations of immunosuppression in organ transplant recipients. *J Am Acad Dermatol* 1989; **21**: 167–79.
4 Boitard C, Nach J-F. Long-term complications of conventional immunosuppressive treatment. *Adv Nephrol* 1989; **18**: 335–54.
5 Paller AS, Mallory SB. Acquired forms of immunosuppression. *J Am Acad Dermatol* 1991; **24**: 482–8.
6 Spencer ES, Anderson HK. Viral infections in renal allograft recipients treated with long-term immunosuppression. *Br Med J* 1979; **2**: 829–30.
7 Shelley WB. Induction of tinea cruris by topical nitrogen mustard and systemic chemotherapy. *Acta Derm Venereol (Stockh)* 1981; **61**: 164–5.
8 Bencini PL, Crosti C, Sala F. Porokeratosis: immunosuppression and exposure to sunlight. *Br J Dermatol* 1987; **116**: 113–16.
9 Neumann RA, Knobler RM, Metze D, Jurecka W. Disseminated superficial porokeratosis and immunosuppression. *Br J Dermatol* 1988; **119**: 375–80.
10 Lederman JS, Sober AJ, Lederman GS. Immunosuppression: a cause of porokeratosis? *J Am Acad Dermatol* 1985; **13**: 75–9.
11 Grattan CEH, Christopher AP. Porokeratosis and immunosuppression. *J R Soc Med* 1987; **80**: 597–8.
12 Tatnall FM, Sarkany I. Porokeratosis of Mibelli in an immunosuppressed patient. *J R Soc Med* 1987; **80**: 180–1.
13 Wilkinson SM, Cartwright PH, English JSC. Porokeratosis of Mibelli and immunosuppression. *Clin Exp Dermatol* 1991; **16**: 61–2.
14 McGregor JM, Barker JNWN, MacDonald DM. The development of excess numbers of melanocytic naevi in an immunosuppressed identical twin. *Clin Exp Dermatol* 1991; **16**: 131–2.
15 Hughes BR, Cunliffe WJ, Bailey CC. Excess benign melanocytic naevi after chemotherapy for malignancy in childhood. *Br Med J* 1989; **299**: 88–91.
16 Barker JNWN, MacDonald DM. Eruptive dysplastic naevi following renal transplantation. *Clin Exp Dermatol* 1988; **13**: 123–5.
17 Penn I. Depressed immunity and the development of cancer. *Clin Exp Immunol* 1981; **146**: 459–74.

18 Penn I. Tumors of the immunocompromised patient. *Annu Rev Med* 1988; **39**: 63−73.

19 Penn I. Cancers complicating organ transplantation. *N Engl J Med* 1990; **323**: 1767−9.

20 Williams CJ. Leukaemia and cancer chemotherapy. The risk is acceptably small but may be reducible further. *Br Med J* 1990; **301**: 73−4.

21 Elliot RW, Essenhigh DM, Morley AR. Cyclophosphamide treatment of systemic lupus erythematosus: risk of bladder cancer exceeds benefit. *Blood* 1970; **35**: 543−8.

22 Walder BK, Robertson MR, Jeremy D. Skin cancer and immunosuppression. *Lancet* 1971; **ii**: 1282−3.

23 Lowney ED. Antimitotic drugs and aggressive squamous cell tumors. *Arch Dermatol* 1972; **105**: 924.

24 Kinlen LJ, Sheil AGR, Peto J, Doll R. Collaborative United Kingdom−Australasian study of cancer in patients treated with immunosuppressive drugs. *Br Med J* 1979; **ii**: 1461−6.

25 Boyle J, Briggs JD, MacKie RM, *et al*. Cancer, warts and sunshine in renal transplant patients. *Lancet* 1984; **i**: 702−5.

26 McLelland J, Rees A, Williams G, *et al*. The incidence of immunosuppression-related skin disease in long-term transplant patients. *Transplantation* 1988; **46**: 871−4.

27 Gupta AK, Cardella CJ, Haberman HF. Cutaneous malignant neoplasms in patients with renal transplants. *Arch Dermatol* 1986; **122**: 1288−93.

28 Hintner H, Fritsch P. Skin neoplasia in the immunodeficient host. *Curr Probl Dermatol* 1989; **18**: 210−17.

29 Greene MH, Young TI. Malignant melanoma in renal transplant recipients. *Lancet* 1981; **i**: 1196−9.

30 Bouwes Bavinck JN, Kootte AMM, van der Woude FJ, *et al*. HLA-A11−associated resistance to skin cancer in renal-transplant recipients. *N Engl J Med* 1990; **323**: 1350.

31 Bouwes Bavinck JM, Vermeer BJ, vans der Woude FJ, *et al*. Relation between skin cancer and HLA antigens in renal-transplant recipients. *N Engl J Med* 1991; **325**: 843−8.

32 Streilein JW. Immunogenetic factors in skin cancer. *N Engl J Med* 1991; **325**: 884−7.

33 Scheibner KG, Murray A, Sheil R, *et al*. T6$^+$ and HLA-DR$^+$ cell numbers in epidermis of immunosuppressed renal transplant recipients. *J Cutan Pathol* 1987; **14**: 202−6.

14.2 Alkylating agents

These drugs act by interfering with cell replication by damaging DNA. Gametogenesis is often severely affected, and their use is associated with a marked increase in non-lymphocytic leukaemia, especially when used in conjunction with radiotherapy.

Alkyl sulphonates

Busulphan

Reactions are rare, but have included urticaria, bullous erythema multiforme [1], Addisonian-like pigmentation [2,3] due to increased epidermal and dermal melanin, and drug-induced porphyria cutanea tarda [4]. Vasculitis has been reported. Keratinocyte nuclear abnormalities with abundant pale cytoplasm have been described [5]. Progressive pulmonary fibrosis may occur.

1 Dosik H, Hurewitz DJ, Rosner F, Schwartz JM. Bullous eruptions and elevated leukocyte alkaline phosphatase in the course of busulphan-treated chronic granulocytic leukaemia. *Blood* 1970; **35**: 543–8.
2 Harrold BP. Syndrome resembling Addison's disease following prolonged treatment with busulphan. *Br Med J* 1966; **1**: 463–4.
3 Burns WA, McFarland W, Matthews MJ. Toxic manifestations of busulfan therapy. *Med Ann DC* 1971; **40**: 567–9.
4 Kyle RA, Dameshek W. Porphyria cutanea tarda associated with chronic granulocytic leukemia treated with busulfan. *Blood* 1964; **23**: 776–85.
5 Hymes SR, Simonton SC, Farmer ER, *et al.* Cutaneous busulfan effect in patients receiving bone marrow transplantation. *J Cutan Pathol* 1985; **12**: 125–9.

Nitrogen mustard derivatives

Chlorambucil

Morbilliform rashes occur; urticarial plaques and periorbital oedema have been described rarely [1–3]. Alopecia is uncommon. Sterility with azoospermia and amenorrhoea is documented.

1 Knisely RE, Settipane GA, Albala MM. Unusual reaction to chlorambucil in a patient with chronic lymphocytic leukemia. *Arch Dermatol* 1971; **104**: 77–9.
2 Millard LG, Rajah SM. Cutaneous reaction to chlorambucil. *Arch Dermatol* 1977; **113**: 1298.
3 Peterman A, Braunstein B. Cutaneous reaction to chlorambucil therapy. *Arch Dermatol* 1986; **122**: 1358–60.

Cyclophosphamide and mesna

Alopecia is common and occurs in 5–30% of cases [1]. Pigmentation, which may be widespread or localized to the palms, soles or nails, is well documented and usually reversible [2,3]. Nail dystrophy may be seen (Fig. 14.4). Allergic exanthemata are rare, but anaphylactic and urticarial reactions are less so [4,5]; there may be cross-sensitivity to other alkylating agents, especially mechlorethamine and chlorambucil [6]. Sterility may supervene.

Haemorrhagic cystitis, the result of toxicity of the metabolite acrolein, is a complication in up to 40% of cases if cyclophosphamide is used alone. Introduction of the thiol compound, mesna (2-mercaptoethane sulphonate), has virtually eliminated this complication. There have been recent reports of urticaria, angioedema, allergic maculopapular pruritic rashes, and occasional more severe reactions with flushing, widespread erythema, and ulceration or blistering of mucous membranes related to mesna; patch tests may be positive [7–10].

1 Ahmed AR, Hombal SM. Cyclophosphamide (Cytoxan). *J Am Acad Dermatol* 1984; **11**: 1115–26.
2 Harrison BM, Wood CBS. Cyclophosphamide and pigmentation. *Br Med J* 1972; **1**: 352.
3 Shah PC, Rao KRP, Patel AR. Cyclophosphamide induced nail pigmentation. *Br J Dermatol* 1978; **98**: 675–80.

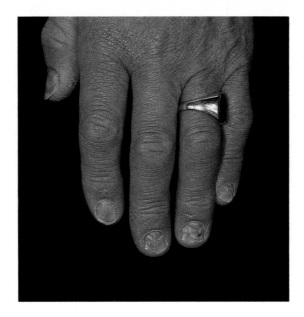

Figure 14.4 Dystrophic nails and hyperpigmentation of the hands due to cyclophosphamide.

4 Murti L, Horsman LR. Acute hypersensitivity reaction to cyclophosphamide. *J Pediatr* 1979; **94**: 844−5.
5 Lakin JD, Cahill RA. Generalized urticaria to cyclophosphamide: Type I hypersensitivity to an immunosuppressive agent. *J Allergy Clin Immunol* 1976; **58**: 160−71.
6 Kritharides L, Lawrie K, Varigos GA. Cyclophosphamide hypersensitivity and cross-reactivity with chlorambucil. *Cancer Treat Rep* 1987; **71**: 1323−4.
7 Pratt CB, Sandlund JT, Meyer WH, Cain AM. Mesna-induced urticaria. *Drug Intell Clin Pharm* 1988; **22**; 914.
8 Seidel A, Andrassy K, Ritz E, *et al*. Allergic reactions to mesna. *Lancet* 1991; **338**: 381.
9 Gross WL, Mohr J, Christophers E. Allergic reactions to mesna. *Lancet* 1991; **338**: 381.
10 D'Cruz D, Haga H-J, Hughes GRV. Allergic reactions to mesna. *Lancet* 1991; **338**: 705−6.

Lomustine

Flushing has been reported.

Mechlorethamine

Angioedema and pruritus have been recorded [1], but in view of the large number of patients receiving this drug as part of the MOPP regime (mechlorethamine, oncovin, procarbazine, prednisone) for lymphoma, it must be exceedingly rare. Topical mechlorethamine [2] used to treat psoriasis or mycosis fungoides may cause hyperpigmentation of involved and uninvolved skin [3], contact sensitization [4,5] and rarely immediate type hypersensitivity with urticaria or anaphylactoid reactions [6].

1 Wilson KS, Alexander S. Hypersensitivity to mechlorethamine. *Ann Intern Med* 1981; **94**: 823.

2 Price NM, Deneau DG, Hoppe RT. The treatment of mycosis fungoides with ointment-based mechlorethamine. *Arch Dermatol* 1982; **118**: 234−7.

3 Flaxman BA, Sosis AC, Van Scott EJ. Changes in melanosome distribution in Caucasoid skin following topical application of nitrogen mustard. *J Invest Dermatol* 1973; **60**: 321−6.

4 Van Scott EJ, Winters PL. Responses of mycosis fungoides to intensive external treatment with nitrogen mustard. *Arch Dermatol* 1970; **102**: 507−14.

5 Ramsay DL, Halperin PS, Zeleniuch-Jacquotte A. Topical mechlorethamine therapy for early stage mycosis fungoides. *J Am Acad Dermatol* 1988; **19**: 684−91.

6 Daughters D, Zackheim H, Maibach H. Urticaria and anaphylactoid reactions after topical application of mechlorethamine. *Arch Dermatol* 1973; **107**: 429−30.

Melphalan

Trivial morbilliform rashes are relatively common with this drug [1]. Severe anaphylactic reactions may occur after intravenous use, especially in patients with IgA κ myeloma [2]. Urticaria or angio-oedema after oral use is very rare [3]. Vasculitis has been documented, and melanonychia striata has been recorded [4]. Radiation recall is uncommon [5]. Sterility with azoospermia and amenorrhoea are reported to have occurred.

1 Costa GG, Engle RL Jr, Schilling A, *et al*. Melphalan and prednisone: an effective combination for the treatment of multiple myeloma. *Am J Med* 1973; **54**: 589−99.

2 Cornwell GG, Pajak TF, McIntyre OR. Hypersensitivity reactions to i.v. melphalan during the treatment of multiple myeloma: Cancer and leukemia group B experience. *Cancer Treat Rep* 1979; **63**: 399−403.

3 Lawrence BV, Harvey HA, Lipton A. Anaphylaxis due to oral melphalan. *Cancer Treat Rep* 1980; **64**: 731−2.

4 Malacarne P, Zavagli G. Melphalan-induced melanonychia striata. *Arch Dermatol Res* 1977; **258**: 81−3.

5 Kellie SJ, Plowman PN, Malpas JS. Radiation recall and radio-sensitization with alkylating agents. *Lancet* 1987; **i**: 1149−50.

Ethylenemine derivatives

Thiotepa (triethylenethiophosphoramide)

Intravesical installation caused pruritus, urticaria or angioedema in 5 of 164 patients with bladder carcinoma [1]. Intravenous administration resulted in patterned hyperpigmentation confined to skin occluded by adhesive bandages or electrocardiograph pads, probably due to secretion of the drug in sweat [2]. By contrast, topical thiotepa has produced periorbital leucoderma [3].

1 Veenema RJ, Dean AL, Uson AC, *et al*. Thiotepa bladder installations: Therapy and prophylaxis for superficial bladder tumors. *J Urol* 1969; **101**: 711−15.

2 Horn TD, Beveridge RA, Egorine MJ, *et al*. Observations and proposed mechanism of *N,N',N''*-triethylenethiophosphoramide (thiotepa)-induced hyperpigmentation. *Arch Dermatol* 1989; **125**: 524−7.

3 Harben DJ, Cooper PH, Rodman OG. Thiotepa-induced leukoderma. *Arch Dermatol* 1979; **115**: 973−4.

Nitrosoureas

Carmustine

Topical carmustine (BCNU) used for the treatment of cutaneous T cell lymphoma may result in erythema, skin tenderness, telangiectasia; contact sensitization may develop [1]. Mild marrow suppression is recorded.

1 Zackheim HS, Epstein EH Jr, Crain WR. Topical carmustine (BCNU) for cutaneous T cell lymphoma: A 15-year experience in 143 patients. *J Am Acad Dermatol* 1990; **22**: 802–10.

Dacarbazine (DTIC)

Photosensitivity [1,2] and a fixed eruption-like rash [3] have been reported. A patient with malignant melanoma treated with DTIC developed sudden fatal hepatic vein thrombosis (Budd–Chiari syndrome) following intravenous administration [4]. Increasing blood eosinophilia appears to be a sign of the imminent development of this DTIC complication. Chemical cellulitis occurs following extravasation.

1 Bolling R, Meyer-Hamme S, Schauder S. Lichtsensibilisierung unter DTIC-Therapie beim metastasierenden malignen Melanom. *Hautarzt* 1980; **31**: 602–5.
2 Yung CW, Winston EM, Lorincz AL. Dacarbazine-induced photosensitivity reaction. *J Am Acad Dermatol* 1981; **4**: 451–3.
3 Koehn GG, Balizet LR. Unusual local cutaneous reaction to dacarbazine. *Arch Dermatol* 1982; **118**: 1018–19.
4 Swensson-Beck H, Trettel WH. Budd–Chiari-Syndrom bei DTIC-Therapie. *Hautarzt* 1981; **33**: 30–1.

Procarbazine

Type I reactions are rare; recurrent angioedema, urticaria, and arthralgia with decreased serum complement have been reported [1,2].

1 Glovsky MM, Braunwald J, Opelz G, Alenty A. Hypersensitivity to procarbazine associated with angio-edema, urticaria and low serum complement activity. *J Allergy Clin Immunol* 1976; **57**: 134–40.
2 Andersen E, Videbaeck A. Procarbazine-induced skin reactions in Hodgkin's disease and other malignant lymphomas. *Scand J Haematol* 1980; **24**: 149–51.

14.3 Cytotoxic antibiotics

Bleomycin

Alopecia, glossitis and buccal ulceration occur, and drug fever is common, usually 1–4 hours after injection. Distinctive localized erythematous, tender, macules, nodules or infiltrated plaques on the hands, elbows, knees, and buttocks have been documented [1,2]. Their causation is uncertain, since the rash may resolve despite continued therapy [3]. Raynaud's phenomenon with and without ischaemic ulcerations, and systemic sclerosis-like changes in men, have been described [4–6]. Capillary microscopy has been advocated for the investigation of bleomycin acral vascular toxicity [7]. Intra-lesional therapy for warts may cause persistent Raynaud's phenomenon [8,9] and loss of nails [10].

Cutaneous erythema or hyperpigmentation, which may be diffuse [11], patchy or linear and prominent over pressure areas, especially the elbows, is seen in approximately 30% of patients [12]. 'Flagellate' streaked erythema [13] or pigmentation [14–18] on the trunk (Fig. 14.5) and proximal extremities is common. It has been proposed that trauma from scratching induces localized vasodilatation, with increased concentration of cutaneous bleomycin. In this regard, it is of interest that hyperpigmentation has been documented in a patient treated with bleomycin where a heating pad had been applied [19]. There may be darkening of the nail cuticle and palmar creases. The principal problem of systemic therapy is progressive pulmonary fibrosis.

1 Lincke-Plewig H. Bleomycin-Exanthem. *Hautarzt* 1980; **31**: 616–18.
2 Cohen IS, Mosher MB, O'Keefe EJ. Cutaneous toxicity of bleomycin therapy. *Arch Dermatol* 1973; **107**: 553–5.
3 Bennett JP, Burns CP. Absence of progression of recurrent bleomycin skin toxicity without postponement or attenuation of therapy. *Am J Med* 1988; **85**: 585–6.
4 Finch WR, Rodnan GP, Buckingham RB, *et al*. Bleomycin-induced scleroderma. *J Rheumatol* 1980; **7**: 651–9.
5 Bork K, Korting GW. Symptomatische Sklerodermie durch Bleomyzin. *Hautarzt* 1983; **34**: 10–12.
6 Snauwaert J, Degreef H. Bleomycin-induced Raynaud's phenomenon and acral sclerosis. *Dermatologica* 1984; **169**: 172–4.
7 Bellmunt J, Navarro M, Morales S, *et al*. Capillary microscopy is a potentially useful method for detecting bleomycin vascular toxicity. *Cancer* 1990; **65**: 303–9.
8 Epstein E, O'Keefe EJ, Hayes M, Bovenmyer DA. Persisting Raynaud's

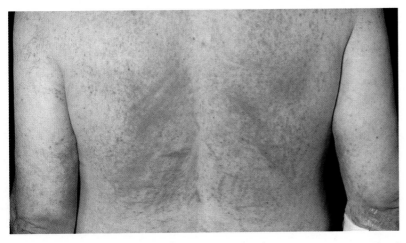

Figure 14.5 Flagellate streaked erythema caused by bleomycin.

phenomenon following intralesional bleomycin treatment of finger warts. *J Am Acad Dermatol* 1985; **13**: 468−71.

9 Epstein E. Intralesional bleomycin and Raynaud's phenomenon. *J Am Acad Dermatol* 1991; **24**: 785−6.

10 Gonzalez FU, Gil MCC, Martinez AA, *et al.* Cutaneous toxicity of intralesional bleomycin in the treatment of periungual warts. *Arch Dermatol* 1986; **122**: 974−5.

11 Wright AL, Bleehen SS, Champion AE. Reticulate pigmentation due to bleomycin: light- and electron-microscopic studies. *Dermatologica* 1990; **181**: 255−7.

12 Ohnuma T, Selawry OS, Holland JF, *et al.* Clinical study with bleomycin: Tolerance to twice weekly dosage. *Cancer* 1972; **30**: 914−22.

13 Cortina P, Garrido JA, Tomas JF, *et al.* 'Flagellate' erythema from bleomycin. With histopathological findings suggestive of inflammatory oncotaxis. *Dermatologica* 1990; **180**: 106−9.

14 Schuler G, Auböck J, Huber H. Bleomycininduzierte lineare Hyperpigmentierungen. *Hautarzt* 1984; **35**: 383−6.

15 Fernandez-Obregon AC, Hogan KP, Bibro MK. Flagellate pigmentation from intrapleural bleomycin. A light and electron microscopic study. *J Am Acad Dermatol* 1985; **13**: 464−8.

16 Guillet G, Guillet M-H, de Meaux H, *et al.* Cutaneous pigmented stripes and bleomycin treatment. *Arch Dermatol* 1986; **122**: 381−2.

17 Polla BS, Saurat JG, Merot Y, Slosman D. Flagellate pigmentation from bleomycin. *J Am Acad Dermatol* 1986; **14**: 690.

18 Rademaker M, Meyrick Thomas RH, Lowe DG, Munro DD. Linear streaking due to bleomycin. *Clin Exp Dermatol* 1987; **12**: 457−9.

19 Kukla LJ, McGuire WP. Heat-induced recall of bleomycin skin changes. *Cancer* 1982; **50**: 2283−4.

Dactinomycin (actinomycin D)

A papulo-pustular acneiform sterile folliculitis, spreading from the face to the trunk and buttocks, and which may mimic septic cutaneous emboli, is common [1].

1 Epstein EH, Lutzner MA. Folliculitis induced by actinomycin D. *N Engl J Med* 1969; **281**: 1094−6.

Daunorubicin

Angioedema with generalized urticaria [1], and hyperpigmentation [2] have been described.

1 Freeman AI. Clinical note. Allergic reaction to daunomycin (NSC-82151). *Cancer Chemother Rep* 1970; **54**: 475−6.

2 Kelly TM, Fishman LM, Lessner HE. Hyperpigmentation with Daunorubicin therapy. *Arch Dermatol* 1984; **120**: 262−3.

Doxorubicin (Adriamycin)

Short-lived localized erythema or urticaria with pruritus along the vein proximal to the injection site may occur in up to 3% of patients [1]. Angioedema, generalized urticaria with or without anaphylaxis, and chronic urticaria have been reported rarely [2]. Cutaneous and nail pigmentation are well recognized [3,4]. Erythema and desquamation of palmar and plantar skin, with or without onycholysis, occurs frequently in patients receiving doxorubicin [5−7]. Allergic cross-reaction occurs with daunorubicin. Toxic epidermal injury after intra-arterial injection [8], phlebitis, and chemical cellulitis with extensive tissue necrosis and ulceration following extravasation [9] are well documented.

1 Vogelzang NJ. 'Adriamycin flare': A skin reaction resembling extravasation. *Cancer Treat Rep* 1979; **63**: 2067−9.
2 Hatfield AK, Harder L, Abderhalden RT. Chronic urticarial reactions caused by doxorubicin-containing regimens. *Cancer Chemother Rep* 1981; **65**: 353−4.
3 Kew CM, Mzamane D, Smith AG, Shuster S. Melanocyte stimulating-hormone levels in doxorubicin-induced hyperpigmentation. *Lancet* 1977; **ii**: 811.
4 Giacobetti R, Estely NB, Morgan ER. Nail hyperpigmentation secondary to therapy with doxorubicin. *Am J Dis Child* 1981; **135**: 317−18.
5 Vogelzang NJ, Ratain MJ. Cancer chemotherapy and skin changes. *Ann Intern Med* 1985; **103**: 303−4.
6 Jones AP, Crawford SM. Anthracycline-induced toxicity affecting palmar and plantar skin. *Br J Cancer* 1989; **59**: 814.
7 Curran CF. Onycholysis in doxorubicin-treated patients. *Arch Dermatol* 1990; **126**: 1244.
8 Von Eyben FE, Bruze M, Eksborg S, *et al.* Toxic epidermal injury following intraarterial Adriamycin treatment. *Cancer* 1981; **48**: 1535−8.
9 Reilly JJ, Neifeld JP, Rosenberg SA. Clinical course and management of accidental Adriamycin extravasation. *Cancer* 1977; **40**: 2053−6.

Mitomycin

Urticaria, and dermatitis [1−3], particularly on the face, palms and soles, have been reported after intravesical therapy. Sunlight-induced recall of ulceration following extravasation has been recorded [4].

1 Neild VS, Sanderson KV. Dermatitis due to mitomycin bladder instillations. *J R Soc Med* 1984; **77**: 610−11.
2 Colver GB, Inglis JA, McVittie E, *et al.* Dermatitis due to intravesical mitomycin C: a delayed-type hypersensitivity reaction? *Br J Dermatol* 1990; **122**: 217−24.
3 De Groot AC, Conemans JMH. Systemic allergic contact dermatitis from intravesical instillation of the antitumor antibiotic mitomycin C. *Contact Dermatitis* 1991; **24**: 201−9.
4 Fuller B, Lind M, Bonomi P. Mitomycin C extravasation exacerbated by sunlight. *Ann Intern Med* 1981; **94**: 542.

14.4 Antimetabolites

Aminoglutethimide

This inhibitor of adrenal steroid synthesis has been reported to induce systemic lupus erythematosus [1].

1 McCraken M, Benson EA, Hickling P. Systemic lupus erythematosus induced by aminoglutethimide. *Br Med J* 1980; **281**: 1254.

Azathioprine

Dermatological aspects of this derivative of the antimetabolite mercaptopurine have been reviewed [1–4]. Bone marrow suppression is the main problem; blood counts should be performed weekly for the first month, then monthly thereafter. Gastrointestinal upset is common and may necessitate discontinuation of therapy. Hypersensitivity reactions [5], including cholestatic jaundice, hepatitis, liver necrosis, fever, maculopapular rashes, interstitial pneumonitis, polyneuropathy, pancreatitis, and shock are well recognized. An association with atrial fibrillation has been postulated [6]. An acneiform exanthem has been described, confirmed on challenge [7]. Multiple large resistant warts are common on the hands of renal transplant recipients maintained on long-term azathioprine and prednisolone therapy; herpes simplex and herpes zoster infection may occur [8], and Norwegian scabies may be promoted [9].

Disseminated superficial actinic porokeratosis [10] and porokeratosis of Mibelli [11] have been documented. Kerato-acanthomas and squamous cell carcinomata may develop [12–14]. Long-term therapy may predispose to the development of malignancy, especially of non-Hodgkin's lymphoma [15,16]. Azathioprine crosses the placenta, but there is little evidence that azathioprine is teratogenic in humans, and detailed analysis of successful pregnancies notified to the European Dialysis and Transplant Association did not suggest an excessive congenital abnormality rate [17]. However, depressed fetal haemopoiesis and resultant neonatal thrombocytopenia and leucopenia have been documented [18]. Pregnancy is therefore best avoided in patients receiving this drug [19]. Allopurinol may potentiate the effect of azathioprine by inhibiting its metabolism; the dose of azathioprine should therefore be reduced to one-quarter of the regular dose.

1 Ahmed AR, Mox R. Azathioprine. *Int J Dermatol* 1981; **20**: 461–7.
2 Speerstra F, Boerbooms AM, van de Putte LB, *et al.* Side effects of azathioprine treatment in rheumatoid arthritis: analysis of ten years of experience. *Ann Rheum Dis* 1982; **41** (Suppl): 37–9.
3 Gendler E. Azathioprine for use in dermatology. *J Dermatol Surg Oncol* 1984; **10**: 462–4.
4 Younger IR, Harris DWS, Colver GB. Azathioprine in dermatology. *J Am Acad Dermatol* 1991; **25**: 281–6.
5 Saway PA, Heck LW, Bonner JR, *et al.* Azathioprine hypersensitivity: case report and review of the literature. *Am J Med* 1988; **84**: 960–4.
6 Dodd HJ, Tatnall FM, Sarkany I. Fast atrial fibrillation induced by treatment of psoriasis with azathioprine. *Br Med J* 1985; **291**: 706.
7 Schmoeckel C, von Liebe V. Akneiformes Exanthem durch Azathioprin. *Hautarzt* 1983; **34**: 413–15.
8 Spencer ES, Anderson HK. Viral infections in renal allograft recipients treated with long-term immunosuppression. *Br Med J* 1979; **2**: 829–30.
9 Paterson WD, Allen BR, Beveridge GW. Norwegian scabies during immunosuppressive therapy. *Br Med J* 1973; **4**: 211–12.
10 Neumann RA, Knobler RM, Metze D, *et al.* Disseminated superficial porokeratosis and immunosuppression. *Br J Dermatol* 1988; **119**: 375–80.
11 Tatnell FM, Sarkany I. Porokeratosis of Mibelli in an immunosuppressed patient. *J R Soc Med* 1987; **80**: 180–1.

12 Walder BK, Robertson MR, Jeremy D. Skin cancer and immunosuppression. *Lancet* 1971; **ii**: 1282−3.

13 Lowney ED. Antimitotic drugs and aggressive squamous cell tumors. *Arch Dermatol* 1972; **105**: 924.

14 McLelland J, Rees A, Williams G, *et al*. The incidence of immunosuppression-related skin disease in long-term transplant patients. *Transplantation* 1988; **46**: 871−4.

15 Phillips LT, Salisbury J, Leigh I, Baker H. Non-Hodgkin's lymphoma associated with long-term azathioprine therapy. *Clin Exp Dermatol* 1987; **12**: 444−5.

16 Kinlen LJ, Sheil AGR, Peto J, *et al*. Collaborative United-Kingdom−Australasian study of cancer in patients treated with immunosuppressive drugs. *Br Med J* 1979; **2**: 1461−6.

17 The Registration Committee of the European Dialysis and Transplant Association. Successful pregnancies in women treated by dialysis and kidney transplantation. *Br J Obstet Gynaecol* 1980; **87**: 839−45.

18 Davison JM, Dellagrammatikas H, Parkin JM. Maternal azathioprine therapy and depressed haemopoiesis in the babies of renal allograft patients. *Br J Obstet Gynaecol* 1985; **92**: 233−9.

19 Gebhart DOE. Azathioprine teratogenicity: review of the literature and case report. *Obstet Gynecol* 1983; **61**: 270.

Cytosine arabinoside

This drug interferes with pyrimidine synthesis. A self-limited palmar−plantar erythema, occasionally with bullae, may occur [1−3]. Neutrophilic eccrine hidradenitis has been reported [4]. A syndrome with fever, malaise, arthralgia, conjunctivitis and diffuse erythematous maculopapular rash is documented [5].

1 Walker IR, Wilson WEC, Sauder DN, *et al*. Cytarabine-induced palmar−plantar erythema. *Arch Dermatol* 1985; **121**: 1240−1.

2 Shall L, Lucas GS, Whittaker JA, Holt PJA. Painful red hands: a side-effect of leukaemia therapy. *Br J Dermatol* 1988; **119**: 249−53.

3 Brown J, Burck K, Black D, Collins C. Treatment of cytarabine acral erythema with corticosteroids. *J Am Acad Dermatol* 1991; **24**: 1023−5.

4 Flynn TC, Harrist TJ, Murphy GF, *et al*. Neutrophilic eccrine hidradenitis: A distinctive type of neutrophilic dermatosis associated with cytarabine therapy and acute leukemia. *J Am Acad Dermatol* 1984; **11**: 584−90.

5 Shah SS, Rybak ME, Griffin TW. The cytarabine syndrome in an adult. *Cancer Treat Rep* 1983; **67**: 405−6.

Fluorouracil

Anaphylaxis is rare; alopecia and radiation recall may be seen. Erythema followed by hyperpigmentation of sun-exposed areas occurs in up to 5% of patients [1]. Photosensitivity is recorded; pellagra may be caused by direct inhibition of the transformation of tryptophan into nicotinamide. Rarely, hyperpigmented streaks, 'serpentine supravenous hyperpigmentation', develop over arm veins used for injection [1,2]. Continuous infusion may be followed by the development of erythema, oedema and desquamation of the hands [3−5]. Pyridoxine may decrease the intensity and pain of fluorouracil-induced acral erythema [5]. Oral adminstration resulted in painful erythema multiforme-like erosions and blisters on the soles and arms in one case [6]. Fluorouracil may result in marked

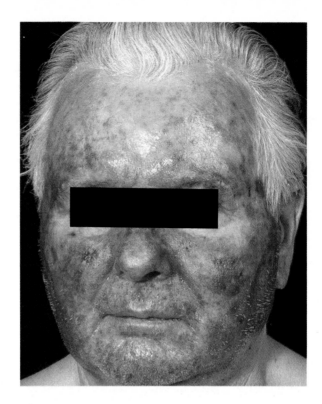

Figure 14.6 Irritant contact dermatitis caused by topical 5-fluorouracil.

inflammation of metastatic skin lesions [7]. Topical application may lead to hyperpigmentation with or without a preceding irritant (Fig. 14.6) or allergic contact dermatitis [8].

1 Hrushesky WJ. Unusual pigmentary changes associated with 5-fluorouracil therapy. *Cutis* 1980; **26**: 181–2.
2 Hrushesky WJ. Serpentine supravenous 5-fluorouracil (NSC-19893) hyperpigmentation. *Cancer Treat Rep* 1976; **60**: 639.
3 Feldman LD, Jaffer A. Fluorouracil-associated palmar–plantar erythrodysesthesia syndrome. *JAMA* 1985; **254**: 3479.
4 Guillaume J-C, Carp E, Rougier P, *et al*. Effets secondaires cutanéo-muqueux des perfusions continues de 5-fluorouracile: 12 observations. *Ann Dermatol Vénéréol (Paris)* 1988; **115**: 1167–9.
5 Vukelja SJ, Lombardo RA, James WD, *et al*. Pyridoxine for the palmar–plantar erythrodysesthesia syndrome. *Ann Intern Med* 1989; **111**: 688–9.
6 Ueki H, Namba M. Arznelmittelexanthem durch ein neues 5-Fluorourazil-derivat. *Hautarzt* 1980; **31**: 207–8.
7 Schlang HA. Inflammation of malignant skin involvement with fluorouracil. *JAMA* 1977; **238**: 1722.
8 Goette DK, Odom RB. Allergic contact dermatitis to topical fluorouracil. *Arch Dermatol* 1977; **113**: 1058–61.

Methotrexate

Dermatological aspects of methotrexate have been reviewed [1–3]. This drug is a folic acid analogue and antagonist, which inactivates dihydrofolate reductase. There is marked individual variation in absorption from the gastrointestinal tract, and hence in expression of toxic effects.

Alopecia occurs in 6% of patients receiving low dose therapy for psoriasis, and in 8% of patients on high dose regimes for malignancy, and is usually the result of telogen effluvium. Intermittent high dosage has resulted in horizontal pigmented banding of hair (the 'flag sign' of chemotherapy) [4]. Urticaria develops in about 4% of patients on low dose oral or parenteral therapy for psoriasis [5]. Photosensitivity occurs in up to 5% of cases. Methotrexate use has been associated with severe reactivation of sunburn [6,7]; in one case, there was sparing of chronically sun-exposed skin [7]. Chronic viral wart and molluscum infections may result from immunosuppression. Cutaneous toxicity with epidermal necrosis may occasionally occur [8,9]. A macular erythema occurring in 15% of patients, and biopsy-proven capillaritis, have been reported with high dose therapy [3]. Anaphylactic reactions [10], and pain, burning, erythema and desquamation of the palms and soles [11], are seen with high dose intravenous methotrexate, but are extremely rare. Vasculitis has been very rarely documented with both intermediate dosage therapy for leukaemia [12] and high dose therapy [13].

Systemic side-effects

Since folic acid is an essential cofactor for DNA synthesis and cell division, bone marrow suppression may occur even on low dose therapy [14−16]. Severe marrow suppression with the dosage used in the therapy of psoriasis is fortunately not that common. Stomatitis may be a warning sign of overdosage. The risk of myelosuppression is much greater in the presence of renal impairment. Gastrointestinal upset is common. Abnormalities of taste sensation occur rarely [17].

The main hazard is hepatotoxicity with long-term use [18]. The risk of developing severe hepatotoxicity is related to the daily dose, the dose frequency, and the cumulative dose [19]. Alcohol consumption, underlying liver disease, and obesity, especially in the presence of diabetes, are aggravating factors. Recommendations include obtaining baseline haematological, renal and hepatic function tests and a liver biopsy before or within 4 months of starting therapy, and repeating this after every 1.5 g [20]. Liver function tests may be unreliable indicators of fibrosis of cirrhosis. These guidelines appear prudent but have never been rigorously tested, and are variously applied in clinical practice [20]. Radionucleotide liver scans are thought to be of little value in the detection of methotrexate-induced liver disease [20], but liver ultrasound may be of some assistance [21]. Abnormal liver biopsy may improve after cessation of therapy [22]. Acute renal failure may follow high-dose methotrexate therapy, but renal damage is rare in patients treated for psoriasis. Pulmonary complications, such as pneumonitis or fibrosis, are rare [23,24]. There do not appear to be adverse effects on humoral or cellular immunity from low weekly doses as given for rheumatoid arthritis or psoriasis [25].

Methotrexate is a known teratogen, and may cause oligospermia [26,27]. It is recommended that patients avoid pregnancy or impregnation during and for 12 weeks after cessation of methotrexate therapy.

Drug interactions

Care must be taken with regard to potential drug interactions with methotrexate [28,29]. Drugs that also interfere with folate metabolism, such as trimethoprim—sulphamethoxazole [30–34], may cause pancytopenia; both trimethoprim and sulphamethoxazole bind to dihydrofolate reductase. Drugs that displace methotrexate from plasma protein-binding sites, such as salicylates, sulphonamides, and diphenylhydantoin, as well as drugs which impair the renal clearance of methotrexate, such as non-steroidal anti-inflammatory agents and sulphonamides, may also cause pancytopenia.

1 Plantin P, Saraux A, Guillet G. Méthotrexate en dermatologie: aspects actuels. *Ann Dermatol Vénéréol (Paris)* 1989; **116**: 109–15.
2 Zachariae H. Methotrexate side-effects. *Br J Dermatol* 1990; **122** (Suppl 36): 127–33.
3 Olsen EA. The pharmacology of methotrexate. *J Am Acad Dermatol* 1991; **25**: 306–18.
4 Wheeland RG, Burgdorf WH, Humphrey GB. The flag sign of chemotherapy. *Cancer* 1983; **51**: 1356–8.
5 Weinstein GD, Frost P. Methotrexate for psoriasis. A new therapeutic schedule. *Arch Dermatol* 1971; **103**: 33–8.
6 Mallory SB, Berry DH. Severe reactivation of sunburn following methotrexate use. *Pediatrics* 1986; **78**: 514–15.
7 Westwick TJ, Sherertz EF, McCarley D, Flowers FP. Delayed reactivation of sunburn by methotrexate: sparing of chronically sun-exposed skin. *Cutis* 1987; **39**: 49–51.
8 Harrison PV. Methotrexate-induced epidermal necrosis. *Br J Dermatol* 1987; **116**: 867–9.
9 Kaplan DL, Olsen EA. Erosion of psoriatic plaques after chronic methotrexate administration. *Int J Dermatol* 1988; **27**: 59–62.
10 Klimo P, Ibrahim E. Anaphylactic reaction to methotrexate used in high doses as an adjuvant treatment of osteogenic sarcoma. *Cancer Treat Rep* 1981; **65**: 725.
11 Doyle LA, Berg C, Bottino G, *et al.* Erythema and desquamation after high-dose methotrexate. *Ann Intern Med* 1983; **98**: 611–12.
12 Fondevila CG, Milone GA, Pavlovsky S. Cutaneous vasculitis after intermediate dose of methotrexate (IDMTX). *Br J Haematol* 1989; **72**: 591–2.
13 Navarro M, Pedragosa R, Lafuerza A, *et al.* Leukocytoclastic vasculitis after high-dose methotrexate. *Ann Intern Med* 1986; **105**: 471–2.
14 MacKinnon SK, Starkebaum G, Wilkens RF. Pancytopenia associated with low-dose pulse methotrexate in the treatment of rheumatoid arthritis. *Semin Arthritis Rheum* 1985; **15**: 119–26.
15 Shupack JL, Webster GF. Pancytopenia following low-dose oral methotrexate therapy for psoriasis. *JAMA* 1988; **259**: 3594–6.
16 Abel EA, Farber EM. Pancytopenia following low-dose methotrexate therapy. *JAMA* 1988; **259**: 3612.
17 Duhra P, Foulds IS. Methotrexate-induced impairment of taste acuity. *Clin Exp Dermatol* 1988; **13**: 126–7.
18 Zachariae H, Kragballe K, Søgaard H. Methotrexate induced liver cirrhosis: studies including serial liver biopsies during continued treatment. *Br J Dermatol* 1980; **102**: 407–12.

19 Lewis JH, Schiff E. ACG Committee on FDA-Related Matters. Methotrexate-induced chronic liver injury: guidelines for detection and prevention. *Am J Gastroenterol* 1988; **88**: 1337−45.

20 Roenigk HH Jr, Auerbach R, Maibach HI, Weinstein GD. Methotrexate in psoriasis: revised guidelines. *J Am Acad Dermatol* 1988; **19**: 145−56.

21 Coulson IH, McKenzie J, Neild VS, *et al*. A comparison of liver ultrasound with liver biopsy histology in psoriatics receiving long-term methotrexate therapy. *Br J Dermatol* 1987; **116**: 491−5.

22 Newman M, Auerbach R, Feiner H, *et al*. The role of liver biopsies in psoriatic patients receiving long-term methotrexate treatment. Improvement in liver abnormalities after cessation of therapy. *Arch Dermatol* 1989; **125**: 1218−24.

23 Phillips TJ, Jones DH, Baker H. Pulmonary complications following methotrexate therapy. *J Am Acad Dermatol* 1987; **16**: 373−5.

24 Carson CW, Cannon GW, Egger MJ, *et al*. Pulmonary disease during the treatment of rheumatoid arthritis with low dose pulse methotrexate. *Semin Arthritis Rheum* 1987; **16**: 186−95.

25 Andersen PA, West SG, O'Dell JR, *et al*. Weekly pulse methotrexate in rheumatoid arthritis: clinical and immunologic effects in a randomized, double-blind study. *Ann Intern Med* 1985; **103**: 489−96.

26 Sussman A, Leonard JM. Psoriasis, methotrexate, and oligospermia. *Arch Dermatol* 1980; **116**: 215−17.

27 Shamberger RC, Rosenberg SA, Seipp CA, *et al*. Effects of high-dose methotrexate and vincristine on ovarian and testicular functions in patients undergoing postoperative adjuvant treatment of osteosarcoma. *Cancer Treat Rep* 1981; **65**: 739−46.

28 Evans WE, Christensen ML. Drug interactions with methotrexate. *J Rheumatol* 1985; **12** (Suppl 12): 15−20.

29 Liddle BJ, Marsden JR. Drug interactions with methotrexate. *Br J Dermatol* 1989; **120**: 582−3.

30 Maricic M, Davis M, Gall EP. Megaloblastic pancytopenia in a patient receiving concurrent methotrexate and trimethoprim−sulfamethoxazole treatment. *Arthritis Rheum* 1986; **29**: 133−5.

31 Thomas MH, Gutterman LA. Methotrexate toxicity in a patient receiving trimethoprim−sulfamethoxazole. *J Rheumatol* 1986; **13**: 440−1.

32 Thomas DR, Dover JS, Camp RDR. Pancytopenia induced by the interaction between methotrexate and trimethoprim−sulfamethoxazole. *J Am Acad Dermatol* 1987; **17**: 1055−6.

33 Ferrazzini G, Klein J, Sulh H, *et al*. Interaction between trimethoprim−sulfamethoxazole and methotrexate in children with leukemia. *J Pediatr* 1990; **117**: 823−6.

34 Groenendal H, Rampen FHJ. Methotrexate and trimethoprim−sulphamethoxazole − a potentially hazardous combination. *Clin Exp Dermatol* 1990; **15**: 358−60.

14.5 Vinca alkaloids and etoposide

These drugs cause metaphase arrest by interfering with microtubule assembly.

Etoposide (VP-16)

This semisynthetic podophyllotoxin derivative has caused Stevens−Johnson syndrome and radiation recall. Four cases of a diffuse erythematous maculopapular rash occurring 5−9 days after initiation of therapy, with spontaneous resolution within 3 weeks, have been reported [1]. Histologically, scattered markedly enlarged individual keratinocytes with a 'starburst' nuclear chromatin pattern were seen. Hypersensitivity reactions are rare.

Vincristine

Peripheral neuropathy is well recognized with long-term therapy [2].

Vinblastine

Photosensitivity is common [3]. Acute alopecia and radiation recall are documented.

1 Yokel BK, Friedman KJ, Farmer ER, Hood AF. Cutaneous pathology following etoposide therapy. *J Cutan Pathol* 1987; **14**: 326–30.
2 Watkins SM, Griffin JP. High incidence of vincristine-induced neuropathy in lymphomas. *Br Med J* 1978; **i**: 610–12.
3 Breza TS, Halprin KM, Taylor JR. Photosensitivity reaction to vinblastine. *Arch Dermatol* 1975; **111**: 1168–70.

14.6 Enzymes

L-Asparaginase

Dose-dependent IgE-mediated hypersensitivity reactions, including urticaria and anaphylaxis, are frequent, especially when the drug is used alone [1].

1 Ertel IJ, Nesbit ME, Hammond D, *et al*. Effective dose of L-asparaginase for induction of remission in previously treated children with acute lymphocytic leukemia: A report from Childrens Cancer Study Group. *Cancer Res* 1979; **39**: 3893–6.

14.7 Miscellaneous chemotherapeutic agents

Acridinyl anisidide (AMSA)

Skin reactions are rare, but widespread erythema has been reported [1].

1 Rosenfelt FP, Rosenbloom BE, Weinstein IM. Allergic reaction following administration of AMSA. *Cancer Treat Rep* 1982; **66**: 549–5.

Bromodeoxyuridine

A distinctive eruption comprising linear supravenous papules and erythroderma has been described with bromodeoxyuridine given in combination with radiotherapy for central nervous system tumours [1]. Ipsilateral facial dermatitis with epilation of eyebrows and eyelashes, ocular irritation, bilateral nail dystrophy, oral ulceration, exanthem or erythema multiforme have also been described [2].

1 Fine J-D, Breathnach SM. Distinctive eruption characterized by linear supra-venous papules and erythroderma following broxuridine (Bromodeoxyuridine) therapy and radiotherapy. *Arch Dermatol* 1986; **122**: 199–200.
2 McCuaig CM, Ellis CN, Greenberg HS, *et al*. Mucocutaneous complications of intraarterial 5-bromodeoxyuridine and radiation. *J Am Acad Dermatol* 1989; **21**: 1235–40.

Cisplatin

Severe hypersensitivity reactions, including flushing, erythema, maculopapular eruptions, urticaria, and anaphylaxis occur in about 5% of cases when this drug is used as a single agent, and in up to 20% when given with other chemotherapeutic agents [1]. Atopic subjects are especially at risk. Local reactions follow extravasation [2].

1 Vogl SE, Zaravinos T, Kaplan BH. Toxicity of *cis*-diamminedichloro-platinum II given in a two-hour outpatient regimen of diuresis and hydration. *Cancer* 1980; **45**: 11–15.
2 Fields S, Koeller J, Topper RL, *et al*. Local soft tissue toxicity following cisplatin extravasation. *J Natl Cancer Inst* 1990; **82**: 1649–50.

Colchicine

Alopecia is recorded [1].

1 Haarms M. Haarausfall und Haarveränderungen nach Kolchizintherapie. *Hautarzt* 1980; **31**: 161–3.

Hydroxyurea

Dermatological aspects of this drug have been reviewed [1–3]. A modest fall in haemoglobin and development of macrocytosis is almost constant. Fixed drug eruption has been reported [3]. Stomatitis occurs, but alopecia is rare. Morbilliform erythema occurs, and hyperpigmentation, generalized or localized to pressure areas is recorded in up to 4.7% of cases [2]. Nail changes such as multiple pigmented nail bands [4], or onycholysis with nail dystrophy occur. Dermatomyositis-like acral erythema, scaling, and atrophy especially on the dorsum of the hands with lesser involvement of the feet [1,5,6], and palmar and plantar keratoderma have been rarely described with long-term therapy for leukaemia. The dermatomyositis-like lesions have been seen only in patients with chronic myeloid leukaemia. Photosensitivity is documented, and vasculitis has been reported. An ulcerative lichen planus-like dermatitis has been recorded [7]. Radiation recall occurs [8]. Leg ulcers which improved following cessation of therapy have been described in patients treated for chronic myeloid leukaemia [9]. Impaired renal function has been reported in some, but not other, studies [3].

1 Kennedy BJ, Smith LR, Goltz RW. Skin changes secondary to hydroxyurea therapy. *Arch Dermatol* 1975; **111**: 183–7.

2 Layton AM, Sheehan-Dare RA, Goodfield MJD, Cotterill JA. Hydroxyurea in the management of therapy resistant psoriasis. *Br J Dermatol* 1989; **121**: 647−53.

3 Boyd AS, Neldner KH. Hydroxyurea therapy. *J Am Acad Dermatol* 1991; **25**: 518−24.

4 Vomvoura S, Pakula AS, Shaw JM. Multiple pigmented nail bands during hydroxyurea therapy: an uncommon finding. *J Am Acad Dermatol* 1991; **24**: 1016−17.

5 Richard M, Truchetet F, Friedel J, *et al.* Skin lesions simulating chronic dermatomyositis during long-term hydroxyurea therapy. *J Am Acad Dermatol* 1989; **21**: 797−9.

6 Sigal M, Crickx B, Blanchet P, *et al.* Lésion cutanées induites par l'utilisation au long cours de l'hydroxyurée. *Ann Dermatol Véneréol (Paris)* 1984; **111**: 895−900.

7 Renfro L, Kamino H, Raphael B, *et al.* Ulcerative lichen planus-like dermatitis associated with hydroxyurea. *J Am Acad Dermatol* 1991; **24**: 143−5.

8 Sears ME. Erythema in areas of previous irradiation in patients treated with hydroxyurea (NSC-32065). *Cancer Chemother Rep* 1964; **40**: 31−2.

9 Montefusco E, Alimena G, Gastaldi R, *et al.* Unusual dermatologic toxicity of long-term therapy with hydroxyurea in chronic myelogenous leukemia. *Tumori* 1986; **72**: 317−21.

OKT 3

Orthoclone OKT3, a murine monoclonal antibody directed against the CD3 subset of T lymphocytes, has been used as an immunosuppressive agent in renal transplant recipients, and has been anecdotally associated with anaphylaxis [1].

1 Werier J, Cheung AHS, Matas AJ. Anaphylactic hypersensitivity reaction after repeat OKT3 treatment. *Lancet* 1991; **337**: 1351.

Triazinate

Acanthosis nigricans-like hyperpigmentation has been recorded [1].

1 Greenspan AH, Shupack JL, Foo S-H. Acanthosis nigricans-like hyperpigmentation secondary to triazinate therapy. *Arch Dermatol* 1985; **121**: 232−5.

Chapter 15
Drugs Affecting the Immune Response

15.1 Cyclosporin A and FK506

Cyclosporin A

Cyclosporin A is a ligand for the immunophilin cyclophilin A, and, like FK506, is thought to block early events in T cell gene activation, by interfering with the intracellular translocation of a substance known as nuclear factor of activated T cells [1,2]. It selectively inhibits antigen-induced activation of, and interleukin 2 production by, CD4[+] helper T lymphocytes, thereby blocking T cell proliferation [3,4]. It inhibits transcription of genes encoding for interleukin 2 and γ-interferon [5], and blocks expression of interleukin 2 receptors. Cyclosporin also inhibits Langerhans cell antigen-presenting function [6−8], and suppresses intercellular adhesion molecule 1 (ICAM-1) expression by papillary endothelium in inflamed skin, thus reducing T cell recruitment [9]. Much of the information on side-effects is derived from patients who have undergone organ transplants, and in diseases such as rheumatoid arthritis [10]. However, this drug is now being used by dermatologists [11−18], especially in the management of difficult psoriasis [13−16], but also in refractory atopic eczema [17] and a number of other conditions [16].

Dermatological complications

Hypertrichosis develops in a high proportion of patients; it affects especially the face and eyebrows (Fig. 15.1), the upper back along the spinal column, and the lateral upper arms [18−23]. The hypertrichosis is reversible, and children and adolescents seem to be at a greater risk of developing this complication [23]. Other cutaneous complications include gum hypertrophy [21,24] and angioedema [25]. Anaphylaxis may occur in response to intravenous cyclosporin [11], probably due to the solvent. A mild capillary leak syndrome has resulted in purpuric lesions in the flexures and at pressure points [26].

There have been isolated reports of the development of benign lymphocytic infiltrates in patients with psoriasis or alopecia areata [27,28], of pseudolymphoma after therapy of actinic reticuloid [29], and of an aggressive T cell lymphoma after cyclosporin therapy for

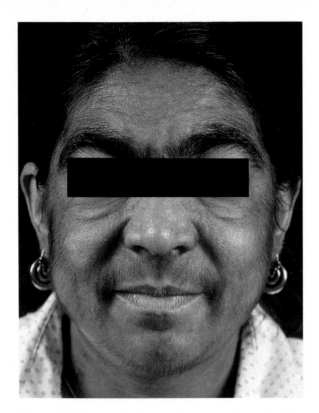

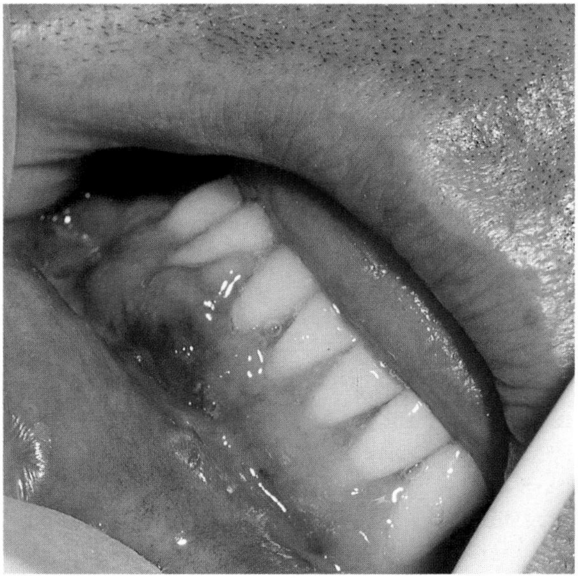

Figure 15.2 Gingival Kaposi's sarcoma in a renal transplant patient treated with oral corticosteroids and cyclosporin.

Figure 15.1 Hypertrichosis in a renal transplant patient treated with cyclosporin and minoxidil.

Sézary syndrome [30]. Squamous cell skin cancer may develop [31–33], and could potentially be predisposed to by previous psoralens with UV-A (PUVA) therapy [32]. A recent study showed no difference in the incidence of cutaneous malignancy between renal allograft recipients treated either with cyclosporin or with azathioprine [33]. Kaposi's sarcoma may occur (Fig. 15.2); a renal transplant patient treated with cyclosporin and methylprednisolone developed a Kaposi's sarcoma which completely regressed on reducing the dosage of both drugs [34]. There have been isolated reports of development of malignant melanoma in cyclosporin-treated patients, but the incidence of this complication does not seem to be increased above the risk in the general population [35,36].

Systemic side-effects

Headache, gastrointestinal and musculoskeletal symptoms are well recognized. There is an increased risk of nephrotoxicity [37,38], which appears to be caused by arteriolar vasoconstriction due to local thromboxane A_2 release [39], and consequent hypertension [40]. Impaired renal function may develop after short- as well as long-term treatment for psoriasis [41]. Both renal dysfunction and hypertension are reversible, and lymphoma development is unlikely,

[306]

in patients on short-term low dose (less than 5 mg/kg) therapy [11]. Adverse effects on renal function and systolic blood pressure appear greater in psoriasis patients receiving higher doses [15]. Rarely, a serious capillary leak syndrome which may be fatal occurs, with marked fluid retention and periorbital oedema; there may be associated gastrointestinal bleeding, pneumonitis, uraemia and urinary sodium loss followed by hypertension and convulsions [21]. Hepatotoxicity is a complication [42], and hypercholesterolaemia is recorded [43]. Cyclosporin may be associated with myopathy without rhabdomyolysis, or with rhabdomyolysis; the latter occurs in the setting of concomitant lovastatin or colchicine therapy [44]. Lymphoma and other cancers have developed on high dosage as for organ grafting [19,45]. Transplant patients treated with cyclosporin have not been shown to have a higher incidence of neoplasms than those receiving other immunosuppressive agents [12].

A successful pregnancy occurred in a patient receiving cyclosporin for psoriasis [46]. Although pregnancy remains a major exclusion criteria for treatment with cyclosporin, there is no conclusive evidence of a teratogenic effect in man, based on the experience of 107 transplant recipients [47].

Interactions with cyclosporin and other drugs have been reviewed [48]. Cyclosporin blood levels may be increased by concomitant therapy with erythromycin or ketoconazole, as a result of inhibition of the hepatic microsomal cytochrome P450 enzyme system [49], as well as by danazol and norethindrone, oral contraceptives, and calcium channel antagonists. Decreased blood levels may be caused by drugs which induce hepatic enzymes, including phenytoin, phenobarbital, and tuberculostatic therapy with rifampicin and isoniazid. Aminoglycoside antibiotics, melphalan, amphotericin B, and trimethoprim alone or in combination with sulphamethoxazole, interact with cyclosporin by altering renal function.

1 Gallagher RB, Cambier JC. Signal transmission pathways and lymphocyte function. *Immunol Today* 1990; **11**: 187–9.
2 Anon. Unmasking immunosuppression. *Lancet* 1991; **338**: 789.
3 Ryffel B. Pharmacology of cyclosporine. 6. Cellular activation: regulation of intracellular events by cyclosporine. *Pharmacol Rev* 1989; **41**: 407–22.
4 Borel JF. Pharmacology of cyclosporin (Sandimmune). 4. Pharmacological properties *in vivo*. *Pharmacol Rev* 1989; **41**: 259–371.
5 Granelli-Piperno A. Lymphokine gene expression *in vivo* is inhibited by cyclosporin A. *J Exp Med* 1990; **171**: 533–44.
6 Furue M, Katz SI. The effects of cyclosporin on epidermal cells. I. Cyclosporin inhibits accessory cell functions of epidermal Langerhans cells *in vitro*. *J Immunol* 1988; **140**: 4139–43.
7 Demidem A, Taylor JR, Grammer SF, Streilein JW. Comparison of effects of transforming growth factor-beta and cyclosporin A on antigen-presenting cells of blood and epidermis. *J Invest Dermatol* 1991; **96**: 401–7.
8 Dupuy P, Bagot M, Michel L, *et al*. Cyclosporin A inhibits the antigen-presenting functions of freshly isolated human Langerhans cells *in vitro*. *J Invest Dermatol* 1991; **96**: 408–13.
9 Petzelbauer P, Stingl G, Wolff K, Volc-Platzer B. Cyclosporin A suppresses ICAM-1 expression by papillary endothelium in healing psoriatic plaques. *J Invest Dermatol* 1991; **96**: 362–9.

10 Dougados M, Awada H, Amor B. Cyclosporin in rheumatoid arthritis: a double blind placebo controlled study in 52 patients. *Ann Rheum Dis* 1988; **47**: 127–33.

11 Gupta AK, Brown MD, Ellis CN, *et al*. Cyclosporine in dermatology. *J Am Acad Dermatol* 1989; **21**: 1245–56.

12 Fradin MS, Ellis CN, Voorhees JJ. Management of patients and side effects during cyclosporine therapy for cutaneous disorders. *J Am Acad Dermatol* 1990; **23**: 1265–74.

13 De Rie MA, Meinardi MMHM, Bos JD. Analysis of side-effects of medium- and low-dose cyclosporin maintenance therapy in psoriasis. *Br J Dermatol* 1990; **123**: 347–53.

14 Mihatsch MJ, Wolff K (eds) Risk/benefit ratio of cyclosporin A (Sandimmun) in psoriasis. *Br J Dermatol* 1990; **122** (Suppl 36): 1–115.

15 Ellis CN, Fradin MS, Messana JM, *et al*. Cyclosporine for plaque-type psoriasis. Results of a multidose, double-blind trial. *N Engl J Med* 1991; **324**: 277–84.

16 Ellis CN (ed.) Cyclosporine in dermatology. Proceedings of a symposium. *J Am Acad Dermatol* 1991; **23**: 1231–4.

17 Sowden JM, Berth-Jones J, Ross JS, *et al*. Double-blind, controlled, crossover study of cyclosporin in adults with severe refractory atopic dermatitis. *Lancet* 1991; **338**: 137–40.

18 Fradin MS, Ellis CN, Voorhees JJ. Management of patients and side effects during cyclosporine therapy for cutaneous disorders. *J Am Acad Dermatol* 1990; **23**: 1265–75.

19 European Multicentre Trial. Cyclosporin A as sole immunosuppressive agent in recipients of kidney allografts from cadaver donors. Preliminary results. *Lancet* 1982; **ii**: 57–60.

20 Mortimer PS, Thompson JF, Dawber RP, *et al*. Hypertrichosis and multiple cutaneous squamous cell carcinomas in association with cyclosporin A therapy. *J R Soc Med* 1983; **76**: 786–7.

21 Harper JI, Kendra JR, Desai S, *et al*. Dermatological aspects of the use of Cyclosporin A for prophylaxis of graft-versus-host disease. *Br J Dermatol* 1984; **110**: 469–74.

22 Bencini PL, Montagnino G, Sala F, *et al*. Cutaneous lesions in 67 cyclosporin-treated renal transplant recipients. *Dermatologica* 1986; **172**: 24–30.

23 Wysocki GP, Daley TD. Hypertrichosis in patients receiving cyclosporine therapy. *Clin Exp Dermatol* 1987; **12**: 191–6.

24 Frosch PJ, Ruder H, Stiefel A, *et al*. Gingivahyperplasie und Seropapeln unter Cyclosporinbehandlung. *Hautarzt* 1988; **39**: 611–16.

25 Isenberg DA, Snaith ML, Al-Khader AA, *et al*. Cyclosporin relieves arthralgia, causes angiodema. *N Engl J Med* 1980; **303**: 754.

26 Ramon D, Bettloch E, Jimenez A, *et al*. Remission of Sézary's syndrome with cyclosporin A. Mild capillary leak syndrome as an unusual side effect. *Acta Derm Venereol (Stockh)* 1986; **66**: 80–2.

27 Brown MD, Ellis CN, Billings J, *et al*. Rapid occurrence of nodular cutaneous T-lymphocyte infiltrates with cyclosporine therapy. *Arch Dermatol* 1988; **124**: 1097–100.

28 Gupta AK, Cooper KD, Ellis CN, *et al*. Lymphocytic infiltrates of the skin in association with cyclosporine therapy. *J Am Acad Dermatol* 1990; **23**: 1137–41.

29 Thestrup-Pedersen K, Zachariae C, Kaltoft K, *et al*. Development of cutaneous pseudolymphoma following cyclosporin therapy of actinic reticuloid. *Dermatologica* 1988; **177**: 376–81.

30 Catterall MD, Addis BJ, Smith JL, Coode PE. Sézary syndrome: transformation to a high grade T-cell lymphoma after treatment with Cyclosporin A. *Clin Exp Dermatol* 1983; **8**: 159–69.

31 Thompson JF, Allen R, Morris PJ, Wood R. Skin cancer in renal transplant patients treated with cyclosporin. *Lancet* 1985; **i**: 158–9.

32 Stern RS. Risk assessment of PUVA and cyclosporine. Lessons from the past; challenges for the future. *Arch Dermatol* 1989; **125**: 545–7.

33 Bunney MH, Benton EC, Barr BB, *et al*. The prevalence of skin disorders in

renal allograft recipients receiving cyclosporin A compared with those receiving azathioprine. *Nephrol Dial Transplant* 1990; **5**: 379–82.

34 Pilgrim M. Spontane Manifestation und Regression eines Kaposi-Sarkoms unter Cyclosporin A. *Hautarzt* 1988; **39**: 368–70.

35 Mérot Y, Miescher PA, Balsiger F, *et al*. Cutaneous malignant melanomas occurring under cyclosporin A therapy: a report of two cases. *Br J Dermatol* 1990; **123**: 237–9.

36 Arellano F, Krupp PF. Cutaneous malignant melanoma occurring after cyclosporin A therapy. *Br J Dermatol* 1991; **124**: 611.

37 Myers BD, Ross J, Newton L, *et al*. Cyclosporine-associated chronic nephropathy. *N Engl J Med* 1984; **311**: 699–705.

38 Myers BD, Sibley R, Newton L, *et al*. The long-term course of cyclosporine-associated chronic nephropathy. *Kidney Int* 1988; **33**: 590–600.

39 Coffman TM, Carr DR, Yarger WE, Klotman PE. Evidence that renal prostaglandin and thromboxane production is stimulated in chronic cyclosporine nephrotoxicity. *Transplantation* 1987; **43**: 282–5.

40 Porter GAM, Bennett WM, Sheps SG. Cyclosporine-associated hypertension. *Arch Intern Med* 1990; **150**: 280–3.

41 Powles AV, Carmichael D, Julme B, *et al*. Renal function after long-term low-dose cyclosporin for psoriasis. *Br J Dermatol* 1990; **122**: 665–9.

42 Lorber MI, Van Buren CT, Flechner SM, *et al*. Hepatobiliary and pancreatic complications of cyclosporine therapy in 466 renal transplant recipients. *Transplantation* 1987; **43**: 35–40.

43 Ballantyne CM, Podet EJ, Patsch WP, *et al*. Effects of cyclosporine therapy on plasma lipoprotein levels. *JAMA* 1989; **262**: 53–6.

44 Arellano F, Krupp P. Muscular disorders associated with cyclosporin. *Lancet* 1991; **337**: 915.

45 Penn I, First MR. Development and incidence of cancer following cyclosporin therapy. *Transplant Proc* 1986; **18** (Suppl 1): 210–13.

46 Wright S, Glover M, Baker H. Psoriasis, cyclosporine, and pregnancy. *Arch Dermatol* 1991; **127**: 426.

47 Cockburn I, Krupp P, Monka C. Present experience of Sandimmune in pregnancy. *Transplant Proc* 1989; **21**: 3730–2.

48 Yee GC, McGuire TR. Pharmacokinetic drug interactions with cyclosporin (Part I). *Clin Pharmacokinet* 1990; **19**: 319–32.

49 Abel EA. Isotretinoin treatment of severe cystic acne in a heart transplant patient receiving cyclosporine: Consideration of drug interactions. *J Am Acad Dermatol* 1991; **24**: 511.

FK 506

This novel macrolide immunosuppressant has a similar mode of action to cyclosporin as a powerful and selective anti-T cell agent. The side-effects of both drugs are similar in man, although hirsutism, gingival hyperplasia, and coarsening of facial features have not yet been reported, whereas neurological side-effects do occur [1].

1 Macleod AM, Thomson AW. FK506: an immunosuppressant for the 1990s? *Lancet* 1991; **337**: 25–7.

15.2 PUVA therapy

The side-effects of psoralen plus long-wave ultraviolet light A (PUVA) therapy have been reviewed [1–8]. Acute side-effects of PUVA include nausea, worse with 8-methoxypsoralen than with 5-methoxypsoralen, dose-related erythema followed by tanning, and pruritus; there may be a painful burning sensation towards the end of a treatment course [9]. Severe erythema and burning (Fig. 15.3) or phototoxic blistering (Fig. 15.4) may develop as a result of overdosage. Care must be exercised in eliminating the possibility that a patient is taking phototoxic drugs simultaneously with PUVA therapy [10]. Phototoxic reactions may occur from handling tablets of psoralen [11]. Spontaneous non-haemorrhagic blistering, associated with granular C_3 deposition at the dermo-epidermal junction and/or round upper blood vessels, occurs on clinically normal skin of the limbs in 10% of patients on PUVA [12]. This blistering is related to impaired dermo-epidermal adhesion on friction or minor trauma, which is present in all treated patients. There have been reports of bullous pemphigoid precipitated by PUVA therapy [13]. Antinuclear antibodies, at low titre and usually of homogeneous pattern, appear during PUVA therapy [14]. Photo-onycholysis [15], and subungual haemorrhage induced by a phototoxic mechanism, are well recognized (Fig. 15.5). Nail pigmentation has also been described [16]. Acneiform rashes, eruptions simulating polymorphous light eruption and transient facial hypertrichosis are recorded. Drug fever is documented [17]. PUVA therapy using topical 8-methoxypsoralen is associated with a low (0.8%) incidence of allergic contact and photocontact dermatitis; the incidence is higher with monofunctional psoralens such as 3-carbethoxypsoralen, 4,6,4'-trimethylangelicin and 7-methyl pyridopsoralen [18].

Chronic PUVA therapy is associated with premature ageing of

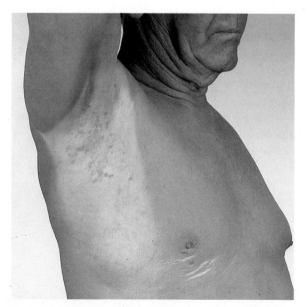

Figure 15.3 Marked erythema in exposed areas following PUVA therapy.

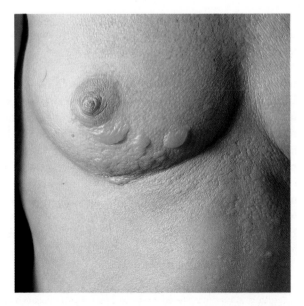

Figure 15.4 Phototoxic bullae after self-medication with methoxypsoralen prior to sun-bed UV light exposure.

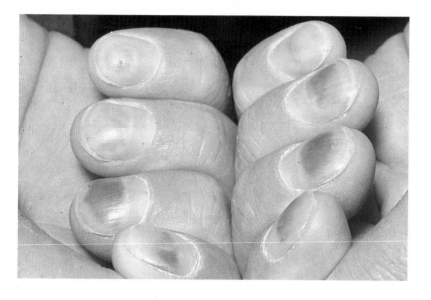

Figure 15.5 Photo-onycholysis with subungual haemorrhage resulting from PUVA therapy.

the skin [19]. Dermal colloid-amyloid bodies have been reported following PUVA therapy [20]. Other histological changes include eosinophilic homogenization of the dermo-epidermal junction, a reduction in, and fragmentation of, elastic fibres, and accumulation of amorphous eosinophilic material around blood vessels [21,22]. PUVA induces clustering and increased size of melanocytes, with heavy melanization of melanocytes [23] and accumulation of lipid [24]. Patients on long-term PUVA may develop pigmented PUVA lentigos [25–30], with large atypical melanocytes containing larger or giant melanosomes (Fig. 15.6). The palms and soles may be involved [29]. Mottled hypopigmentation which occurs in a minority of patients may be related to areas of overdosage. There is a potential for premature cataract formation in animal studies [31]. However, there is no evidence that cataracts are significantly more frequent in patients treated with PUVA [5]. Nevertheless, it is recommended that protective UV-A-opaque goggles or spectacles be worn during the period of increased photosensitivity following psoralen ingestion. A study showed no evidence to suggest that PUVA is a potent teratogen or substantially increased the risk of major malformations or stillbirth, although the power of the study to detect an increase in the risk of specific defects was limited [32]. However, the recommendation remains that PUVA should be avoided during pregnancy where practical.

1 Wolff K, Fitzpatrick TB, Parrish JA, *et al*. Photochemotherapy for psoriasis with orally administered methoxsalen. *Arch Dermatol* 1976; **112**: 943–50.
2 Farber EM, Abel EA, Cox AJ. Long-term risks of psoralen and UVA therapy for psoriasis. *Arch Dermatol* 1983; **119**: 426–31.

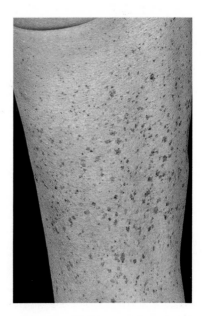

Figure 15.6 PUVA-induced lentigines.

3 Nater JP, de Groot AC. Side effects of photochemotherapy. In *Unwanted Effects of Cosmetics and Drugs Used in Dermatology*, 2nd edn. Amsterdam, Elsevier, Amsterdam, 1985, pp 221–44.

4 Gupta AK, Anderson TF. Psoralen photochemotherapy. *J Am Acad Dermatol* 1987; **17**: 703–34.

5 Cox NH, Jones SK, Downey DJ, *et al*. Cutaneous and ocular side-effects of oral photochemotherapy: results of an 8-year follow-up study. *Br J Dermatol* 1987; **116**: 145–52.

6 Abdullah AN, Keczkes K. Cutaneous and ocular side-effects of PUVA photochemotherapy — a 10-year follow-up study. *Clin Exp Dermatol* 1989; **14**: 421–4.

7 Morison WL. *Phototherapy and Photochemotherapy of Skin Disease*, 2nd edn. Raven Press, New York, 1990.

8 Wolff K. Side-effects of psoralen photochemotherapy (PUVA). *Br J Dermatol* 1990; **122** (Suppl 36): 117–25.

9 Norris PG, Maurice PDL, Schott GD, Greaves MW. Persistent pain after PUVA. *Clin Exp Dermatol* 1987; **12**: 403–5.

10 Stern RS, Kleinerman RA, Parrish JA, *et al*. Phototoxic reactions to photoactive drugs in patients treated with PUVA. *Arch Dermatol* 1980: **116**: 1269–71.

11 Morison WL. Topical phototoxicity from oral methoxsalen. *Arch Dermatol* 1989; **125**: 433.

12 Friedmann PS, Coburn P, Dahl MGC, *et al*. PUVA-induced blisters, complement deposition, and damage to the dermoepidermal junction. *Arch Dermatol* 1987; **123**: 1471–7.

13 Abel EA, Bennett A. Bullous pemphigoid. Occurrence in psoriasis treated with psoralens plus long-wave ultraviolet radiation. *Arch Dermatol* 1979; **115**: 988–9.

14 Bruze M, Ljunggren B. Antinuclear antibodies appearing during PUVA therapy. *Acta Derm Venereol (Stockh)* 1985; **65**: 31–6.

15 Warin AP. Photo-onycholysis secondary to psoralen use. *Arch Dermatol* 1979; **115**: 235–6.

16 Weiss E, Sayegh-Carreno R. PUVA-induced pigmented nails. *Int J Dermatol* 1989; **28**: 188–9.

17 Tóth Kása I, Dobozy A. Drug fever caused by PUVA treatment. *Acta Derm Venereol (Stockh)* 1985; **65**: 557–8.

18 Takashima A, Yamamoto K, Kumura S, *et al*. Allergic contact and photocontact dermatitis due to psoralens in patients with psoriasis treated with topical PUVA. *Br J Dermatol* 1991; **124**: 37–42.

19 Oikarinen A, Karvonen J, Uitto J, Hannuksela M. Connective tissue alterations in skin exposed to natural and therapeutic UV-radiation. *Photodermatology* 1985; **2**: 15–26.

20 Hashimoto K, Kumakiri M. Colloid–amyloid bodies in PUVA-treated human psoriatic patients. *J Invest Dermatol* 1979; **72**: 70–80.

21 Gschnait F, Wolff K, Hönigsmann H, *et al*. Long-term photochemotherapy: histopathological and immunofluorescence observations in 243 patients. *Br J Dermatol* 1980; **103**: 11–22.

22 Zelickson AS, Mottaz JH, Zelickson BD, *et al*. Elastic tissue changes in skin following PUVA therapy. *J Am Acad Dermatol* 1980; **3**: 186–92.

23 Zaynoun S, Konrad K, Gschnait F, *et al*. The pigmentary response to photochemotherapy. *Acta Derm Venereol (Stockh)* 1977; **57**: 431–40.

24 Schuler G, Hönigsmann H, Jaschke E, *et al*. Selective accumulation of lipid within melanocytes during photochemotherapy (PUVA) of psoriasis. *Br J Dermatol* 1982; **107**: 173–81.

25 Szekeres E, Török L, Szücs M. Auftreten disseminierter hyperpigmentierter Flecke unter PUVA-Behandlung. *Hautarzt* 1981; **32**: 33–5.

26 Rhodes AR, Harrist TJ, Momtaz TK. The PUVA-induced pigmented macule: a lentiginous proliferation of large, sometimes cytologically atypical, melanocytes. *J Am Acad Dermatol* 1983; **9**: 47–58.

27 Rhodes AR, Stern RS, Melski JW. The PUVA lentigo: an analysis of predisposing factors. *J Invest Dermatol* 1983; **81**: 459–63.

28 Swart R, Kenter I, Suurmond D. The incidence of PUVA-induced freckles. *Dermatologica* 1984; **168**: 304—5.

29 Bruce DR, Berger TG. PUVA-induced pigmented macules: A case involving palmoplantar skin. *J Am Acad Dermatol* 1987; **16**: 1087—90.

30 Senff H, Reinel D, Schaeg G. PUVA-induced disseminated lentigenes. *Cutis* 1988; **41**: 199—202.

31 Lerman S, Megaw J, Willis I. Potential ocular complications from PUVA therapy and their prevention. *J Invest Dermatol* 1980; **74**: 197—9.

32 Stern RS, Lange R, Members of The Photochemotherapy Follow-up Study. Outcomes of pregnancies among women and partners of men with a history of exposure to methoxsalen photochemotherapy (PUVA) for the treatment of psoriasis. *Arch Dermatol* 1991; **127**: 347—50.

PUVA, immunosuppression and carcinogenesis

Psoralen plus long-wave ultraviolet light A causes a reversible inhibition of contact sensitization, which appears to be mediated by antigen-specific suppressor T cells [1—4]. PUVA also inhibits the elicitation phase of allergic contact dermatitis, but this effect is antigen-non-specific since irritant reactions are also inhibited [4]. PUVA-induced immunosuppression is thought to involve, at least in part, effects on the skin immune system [5]. Reported effects of PUVA on lymphocytes have included a variable decrease in the numbers of the different subsets of circulating T cells, and inhibition of *in vitro* alloantigen-stimulated and mitogen-induced lymphocyte proliferation in some but not all studies, perhaps as a result of impaired interleukin 2 production (reviewed in [5,6]). PUVA also suppresses T lymphocyte migration [7]. In addition to effects on lymphocytes, PUVA results in a dose- and time-dependent reversible decrease in the number and function of antigen-presenting epidermal Langerhans cells [5]. Despite the immunosuppressive actions of PUVA, five human immunodeficiency virus (HIV)-infected patients without serum HIV antigenaemia remained well 1 year after PUVA therapy [8]. PUVA therapy has been implicated in the development of lymphomatoid papulosis in a patient treated for mycosis fungoides [9].

PUVA induces focal histological evidence ot epidermal dystrophic change, which is however reversible in the short term [10,11], and predisposes to development of disseminated superficial actinic porokeratosis [12] and actinic keratoses [11]. A number of groups, amongst them large cooperative ones, have reported the results of long-term studies for the detection of non-melanoma skin cancer [13—23].

Initial reports of an increase in squamous cell carcinoma came from the US [13]. A substantial dose-related increase in the incidence of squamous cell carcinoma was confirmed in the update of the 16-centre US prospective cohort study [14]; the percentage with squamous cell carcinoma was greater in those exposed to more than 1500 J/cm^2. In a retrospective case-control study of 551 psoriasis patients on PUVA for up to 10 years, there was a significant increase in basal cell carcinoma at 2.4% and in squamous cell carcinoma at 1.6% of patients [15]. The increase in basal cell carcinoma, but not that in squamous cell carcinoma, occurred only in patients with exposure to other carcinogenic agents. Some studies from Europe reported either no increase in squamous cell carcinoma or only in relation to previous exposure to other carcinogens [16,18]. It has been proposed that this is accounted for by the fact that in Europe, PUVA schedules usually involve fewer but higher single-dose treatments than in the US. However, a recent Swedish study reported that male patients who had received more than 200 treatments had a more than 30 times increase in the incidence of squamous cell cancer of the skin [21]; a possible link with internal malignancy was also postulated. In addition, a recent Dutch study reported that the incidence of both squamous and basal cell carcinomas, as well as actinic keratoses, was increased [22]. The use of monofunctional psoralens such as 3-carbethoxypsoralen in PUVA therapy may be associated with a lower risk of skin cancer [24]. Relatively low PUVA exposures have at most small effects on skin cancer risk, and so far PUVA-associated squamous cell cancers are unlikely to metastasize [25]. There does not seem to be an increased risk of melanoma so far [26,27].

1 Strauss GH, Greaves M, Price M, *et al*. Inhibition of delayed hypersensitivity reaction in skin (DNCB test) by 8-methoxypsoralen photochemotherapy. *Lancet* 1980; **ii**: 556–9.

2 Moss C, Friedmann PS, Shuster S. Impaired contact hypersensitivity in untreated psoriasis and the effects of photochemotherapy and dithranol/UV-B. *Br J Dermatol* 1981; **105**: 503–8.

3 Kripke ML, Morison WL, Parrish JA. Systemic suppression of contact hypersensitivity in mice by psoralen plus UVA radiation (PUVA). *J Invest Dermatol* 1983; **81**: 87–92.

4 Thorvaldsen J, Volden G. PUVA-induced diminution of contact allergic and irritant skin reactions. *Clin Exp Dermatol* 1980; **5**: 43–6.

5 Ashworth J, Kahan MC, Breathnach SM. PUVA therapy decreases HLA-DR⁺CD1a⁺ Langerhans cells and epidermal cell antigen-presenting capacity in human skin, but flow cytometrically-sorted residual HLA-DR⁺CD1a⁺ Langerhans cells exhibit normal alloantigen-presenting function. *Br J Dermatol* 1989; **120**: 329–39.

6 Okamoto H, Horio T, Maeda M. Alteration of lymphocyte functions by 8-methoxypsoralen and long-wave ultraviolet radiation. II. The effect of *in vivo* PUVA on IL-2 production. *J Invest Dermatol* 1987; **89**: 24–6.

7 Okamoto H, Takigawa M, Horio T. Alteration of lymphocyte functions by 8-methoxypsoralen and long-wave ultraviolet radiation. I. Suppressive effects of PUVA on T lymphocyte migration *in vitro*. *J Invest Dermatol* 1985; **84**: 203–5.

8 Ranki A, Puska P, Mattinen S, *et al*. Effect of PUVA on immunologic and virologic findings in HIV-infected patients. *J Am Acad Dermatol* 1991; **24**: 404–10.

9 Wolf P, Cerroni L, Smolle J, Kerl H. PUVA-induced lymphomatoid papulosis in a patient with mycosis fungoides. *J Am Acad Dermatol* 1991; **25**: 422–6.

10 Cox AJ, Abel EA. Epidermal dystrophy. Occurrence after psoriasis therapy with psoralen and long-wave ultraviolet light. *Arch Dermatol* 1979; **115**: 567–70.

11 Abel EA, Cox AJ, Farber EM, *et al*. Epidermal dystrophy and actinic keratoses in patients following oral psoralen photochemotherapy (PUVA). *J Am Acad Dermatol* 1982; **7**: 333–40.

12 Hazen PG. Carney JF, Walker AE, *et al*. Disseminated superficial actinic

porokeratosis: Appearance with photochemotherapy for psoriasis. *J Am Acad Dermatol* 1985; **12**: 1077-8.

13 Stern RS, Laird N, Melski J, *et al.* Cutaneous squamous cell carcinoma in patients treated with PUVA. *N Engl J Med* 1984; **310**: 1156-61.

14 Stern RS, Lange R, and Members of the Photochemotherapy Follow-Up Study. Non-melanoma skin cancer occurring in patients treated with PUVA five to ten years after first treatment. *J Invest Dermatol* 1988; **91**: 120-4.

15 Forman AB, Roenigk HH, Caro WA, Magid ML. Long-term follow-up of skin cancer in the PUVA-48 cooperative study. *Arch Dermatol* 1989; **125**: 515-19.

16 Tanew A, Hönigsmann H, Ortel B, *et al.* Non-melanoma skin tumors in long-term photochemotherapy treatment of psoriasis. *J Am Acad Dermatol* 1986; **15**: 960-5.

17 Cox NH, Jones SK, Downey DJ, *et al.* Cutaneous and ocular side-effects of oral photochemotherapy: results of an 8-year follow-up study. *Br J Dermatol* 1987; **116**: 145-52.

18 Henseler T, Christopher E, Hönigsmann H, Wolff K. Skin tumors in the European PUVA study. *J Am Acad Dermatol* 1987; **16**: 108-16.

19 Barth J, Meffert H, Schiller F, Sönnichsen N. Zehn Jahre PUVA-Therapie in der DDR — Analyse Zum Langzeitrisiko. *Z Klin Med* 1987; **42**: 889-92.

20 Torinuki W, Tagami H. Incidence of skin cancer in Japanese psoriatic patients treated with either PUVA, Goeckerman regimen or both therapies. *J Am Acad Dermatol* 1988; **18**: 1278-81.

21 Lindelöf B, Sigurgeirsson B, Tegner E, *et al.* PUVA and cancer: a large-scale epidemiological study. *Lancet* 1991; **338**: 91-3.

22 Bruynzeel I, Bergman W, Hartevelt HM, *et al.* 'High single-dose' European PUVA regimen also causes an excess of non-melanoma skin cancer. *Br J Dermatol* 1991; **124**: 49-55.

23 Thomas P, Pannequin C. Puvathérapie et carcinogenese. *Ann Dermatol Vénéréol (Paris)* 1991; **118**: 503-6.

24 Dubertret L, Averbeck D, Zajdela F, *et al.* Photochemotherapy (PUVA) of psoriasis using 3-carbethoxypsoralen, a non-carcinogenic compound in mice. *Br J Dermatol* 1979; **101**: 379-89.

25 Stern RS. Risk Assessment of PUVA and cyclosporine. Lessons from the past; challenges for the future. *Arch Dermatol* 1989; **125**: 545-7.

26 Stern RS, Lange R. Cardiovascular disease, cancer, and cause of death in patients with psoriasis: 10 years prospective experience in a cohort of 1380 patients. *J Invest Dermatol* 1988; **91**: 197-201.

27 Gupta AK, Stern RS, Swanson NA, *et al.* Cutaneous melanomas in patients treated with psoralens plus ultraviolet A. *J Am Acad Dermatol* 1988; **19**: 67-76.

15.3 Immunotherapy

Sera

Animal immune sera can produce any type of early or late hypersensitivity reactions from urticaria, asthma, or fatal anaphylaxis to serum sickness. Clinical manifestations of serum sickness include fever, arthritis, nephritis, neuritis, myocarditis, uveitis, oedema, and an urticarial or papular rash. A characteristic serpiginous, erythematous and purpuric eruption developed on the hands and feet, at the borders of palmar and plantar skin, in patients treated with equine antithymocyte globulin [1,2]. Low serum C4 and C3 levels, elevated plasma C3a anaphylatoxin levels, and circulating immune complexes were found. Immunoreactants including IgM, C3, IgE, and IgA were deposited in the walls of dermal blood vessels on direct immunofluorescence [1,2]. Patients with autoimmune disease may have a particular liability to react to antilymphocyte globulin.

1 Lawley TJ, Bielory L, Gascon P, *et al.* A prospective clinical and immunologic analysis of patients with serum sickness. *N Engl J Med* 1984; **311**: 1407–13.
2 Bielory L, Yancey KB, Young NS, *et al.* Cutaneous manifestations of serum sickness in patients receiving antithymocyte globulin. *J Am Acad Dermatol* 1985; **13**: 411–17.

Vaccines

Local reactions include erythema, swelling and tenderness, which may result from an Arthus reaction (Fig. 15.7) [1,2]. Keloid scarring may develop. Local inflammatory reactions, fever, lymphadenopathy, urticaria, and lichenoid rashes have been observed following vaccination in patients sensitive to the preservative merthiolate; patch testing and intradermal testing may be positive [3]. Inflammatory nodular reactions may occur as a result of aluminium sensitization, as with hepatitis B, diphtheria and tetanus vaccination [4,5]; patch testing to aluminium may be positive [4]. Itching, eczema and circumscribed hypertrichosis developed over nodules following immunization with vaccines adsorbed on aluminium hydroxide in three children [5]. Transient subcutaneous nodule formation at the injection site, and increased regional adenopathy, have been rarely noted in patients with HIV infection treated with gp160 vaccination [6]. Urticaria, angioedema or anaphylaxis may occur in patients vaccinated with live measles vaccine, who are allergic to egg protein. Urticaria and systemic symptoms including malaise and fever, or

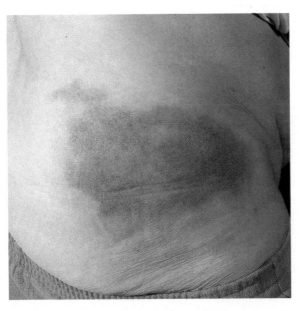

Figure 15.7 Arthus reaction with local erythema and induration following a booster injection of tetanus toxoid.

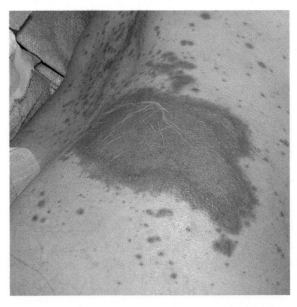

Figure 15.8 Blistering at injection site in a patient with Stevens–Johnson syndrome following vaccination with tetanus toxoid.

Stevens—Johnson syndrome (Fig. 15.8) may follow tetanus toxoid vaccination [7,8]. Vaccination may result in development of an autoimmune state; dermatomyositis has been provoked. Fatalities have rarely occurred following vaccination as a result of anaphylaxis [9,10]. Influenza vaccination in the elderly is, however, reported to cause no more systemic side-effects than placebo [11]. Recent reports have implicated vaccination against Japanese encephalitis in the development of serious adverse reactions, including urticaria, angioedema, hypotension and collapse [12].

Vaccination with vaccinia virus, formerly used as prophylaxis against smallpox, was associated with local reactions including keloid formation (Fig. 15.9), dissemination to other sites (e.g. eczema vaccinatum in atopic patients), and toxic erythema (Fig. 15.10) [13]. These reactions are now mainly of historical interest.

1 Jacobs RL, Lowe RS, Lanier BQ. Adverse reactions to tetanus toxoid. *JAMA* 1982; **247**: 40—2.
2 Marrinan LM, Andrews G, Alsop-Shields L, Dugdale AE. Side effects of rubella immunisation in teenage girls. *Med J Aust* 1990; **153**: 631—2.
3 Lindemayr H, Drobil M, Ebner H. Impfreaktionen nach Tetanus- und Frühsommermeningoenzephalitis-Schutzimpfungen durch Merthiolat (Thiomersal). *Hautarzt* 1984; **35**: 192—6.

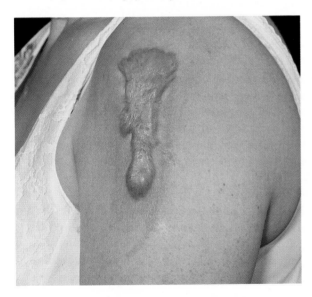

Figure 15.9 Keloid scarring at site of vaccination with vaccinia.

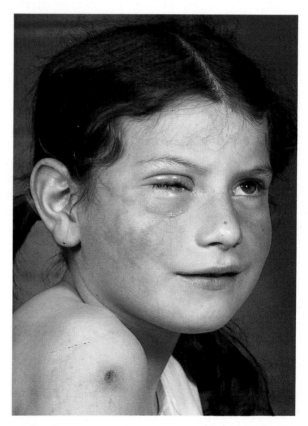

Figure 15.10 Toxic erythema and oedema of the face following smallpox vaccination with vaccinia at the right deltoid area.

[317]

4 Cosnes A, Flechet M-L, Revuz J. Inflammatory nodular reactions after hepatitis B vaccination due to aluminium sensitization. *Contact Dermatitis* 1990; **23**: 65–7.

5 Pembroke AC, Marten RH. Unusual cutaneous reactions following diphtheria and tetanus immunization. *Clin Exp Dermatol* 1979; **4**: 345–8.

6 Redfield RR, Birx DL, Ketter N, *et al*. A phase I evaluation of the safety and immunogenicity of vaccination with recombinant gp160 in patients with early human immunodeficiency virus infection. *N Engl J Med* 1991; **324**: 1677–84.

7 Kuhlwein A, Bleyl A. Tetanusantitoxintiter und Reaktionen nach Tetanusimpfungen. *Hautarzt* 1985; **36**: 462–4.

8 Weisse ME, Bass JW. Tetanus toxoid allergy. *JAMA* 1990; **264**: 2448.

9 Boston Collaborative Drug Surveillance Program. Drug-induced anaphylaxis. A cooperative study. *JAMA* 1973; **224**: 613–15.

10 Lockey RF, Benedict LM, Turkeltaub PC, Bukantz SC. Fatalities from immunotherapy (IT) and skin testing (ST). *J Allergy Clin Immunol* 1987; **79**: 660–77.

11 Margolis KL, Nichol KL, Poland GA, Pluhar RE. Frequency of adverse reactions to influenza vaccine in the elderly. A randomized, placebo-controlled trial. *JAMA* 1990; **264**: 1139–41.

12 Ruff TA, Eisen D, Fuller A, Kass R. Adverse reactions to Japanese encephalitis vaccine. *Lancet* 1991; **338**: 881–2.

13 Landthaler M, Strasser S, Schmoeckel C. Vaccinia inoculata. *Hautarzt* 1988; **39**: 322–3.

Hyposensitization immunotherapy

Hyposensitization immunotherapy is a standard therapy for recalcitrant hay fever and bee or wasp stings in many countries in the world, including the US, Scandinavia, and the continent of Europe [1]. However, in the UK, allergen injection immunotherapy for IgE-mediated diseases has been largely discontinued, following the recommendations of the Committee on Safety of Medicines in 1986 [2], because of concern about deaths related to bronchospasm and anaphylaxis. The Committee recommended that immunotherapy be given only where full facilities for cardiopulmonary resuscitation are available, and that patients be kept under medical observation for at least 2 hours. The necessity for the latter recommendation has been questioned recently, since serious reactions occur within minutes [1]. Fatalities from allergen immunotherapy are reportedly extremely rare [3]. β-Blocker drugs did not increase the frequency of systemic reactions in patients receiving allergen immunotherapy in one series, but patients developed more severe systemic reactions which were more refractory to therapy [4].

Local urticarial reactions are by contrast common (Fig. 15.11) [1]. Desensitization injections for hay fever have resulted in occasional tender nodules lasting for several months or years [5,6]; these are thought to develop as a result of allergy to aluminium, since it is present in the lesions and patch tests may be positive [6]. Inflammatory nodules at injection sites first developing several years later have also been described [7]. Vasculitis [8–10] and serum sickness [11] have been described following hyposensitization therapy as for pollen and house dust mite allergy. Cold urticaria developed during the course of hyposensitization to wasp venom [12].

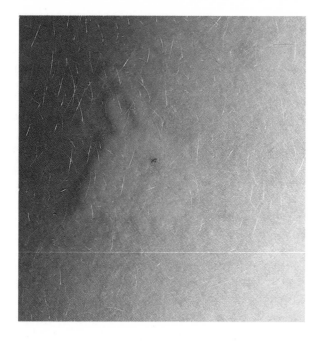

Figure 15.11 Local immediate
whealing after injection of purified
bee venom.

1 Varney VA, Gaga M, Frew AJ, *et al.* Usefulness of immunotherapy in patients
   with severe summer hay fever uncontrolled by antiallergic drugs. *Br Med J*
   1991; **302**: 265−9.
2 Anonymous. CSM update. Desensitising vaccines. *Br Med J* 1986; **293**: 948.
3 Lockey RF, Benedict LM, Turkeltaub PC, Bukantz SC. Fatalities from
   immunotherapy and skin testing. *J Allergy Clin Immunol* 1987; **79**: 660−77.
4 Hepner MJ, Ownby DR, Anderson JA, *et al.* Risk of systemic reactions in
   patients taking beta-blocker drugs receiving allergen immunotherapy injections. *J Allergy Clin Immunol* 1990; **86**: 407−11.
5 Osterballe O. Side effects during immunotherapy with purified grass pollen
   extracts. *Allergy* 1982; **37**: 553−62.
6 Frost L, Johansen S, Pedersen S, *et al.* Persistent subcutaneous nodules in
   children hypo-sensitised with aluminium-containing allergen extracts. *Allergy*
   1985; **40**: 368−72.
7 Jones SK, Lovell CR, Peachey RDG. Delayed onset of inflammatory nodules
   following hay fever desensitization injections. *Clin Exp Dermatol* 1988; **13**:
   376−8.
8 Phanuphak P, Kohler PF. Onset of polyarteritis nodosa during allergic hyposensitisation treatment. *Am J Med* 1980; **68**: 479−85.
9 Merk H, Kober ML. Vasculitis nach spezifischer Hyposensibilisierung. *Z
   Hautkr* 1982; **57**: 1682−5.
10 Berbis P, Carena MC, Auffranc JC, Privat Y. Vascularite nécrosante cutanéo-
   systémique survenue en cours de désensibilisation. *Ann Dermatol Vénéréol
   (Paris)* 1986; **113**: 805−9.
11 Umetsu DT, Hahn JS, Perez-Atayde AR, Geha RS. Serum sickness triggered
   by anaphylaxis: a complication of immunotherapy. *J Allergy Clin Immunol*
   1985; **76**: 713−16.
12 Anfosso-Capra F, Philip-Joet F, Reynaud-Gaubert M, Arnaud A. Occurrence
   of cold urticaria during venom desensitization. *Dermatologica* 1990; **181**:
   276−7.

Bacille Calmette−Guérin (BCG) vaccination

Vaccination with BCG causes a benign self-limiting lesion consisting
of a small papule, pustule or ulcer which heals to leave a small scar

within weeks. Occasionally local abscess formation may follow vaccination of strongly tuberculin positive individuals, administration of too much vaccine, or injecting it too deeply [1,2]. BCG abscesses may also rarely arise following needlestick injury in health care professionals [3]. In Austria, where the Ministry of Health's recommendation is for all neonates to be vaccinated, the normal complication rate is between 0.3 and 0.6%, with suppurative lymphadenitis, generalized lymphadenopathy, and osteitis [4]. This rate temporarily increased substantially, with 5.3% of 659 children vaccinated at the University Hospital, Innsbruck, requiring surgical excision of suppurating lymph nodes, following a change to use of a more virulent strain [4]. Anaphylactoid reactions to BCG vaccine, probably as a result of immune complex reactions mediated by antibodies to dextran in the vaccine, have been reported [5]. A papulonecrotic type of vasculitis has been documented [6]. Dermatomyositis may occasionally be a complication [7].

BCG immunotherapy for malignant melanoma has been associated with [8]: local ulceration [9], local recurrent erysipelas, keloid formation, influenza-like symptoms, lymphadenopathy, urticaria and angioedema, granulomatous hepatitis, arthritis [10], and reactivation of pulmonary tuberculosis. Widespread miliary granulomas were present in a patient with fatal disseminated bacillus Calmette–Guérin infection following intralesional immunotherapy of cutaneous malignant melanoma [11].

1 Lotte A, Wasz-Hockert O, Poisson N, *et al.* BCG complications. *Adv Tuberculosis Res* 1984; **21**: 107–93, 194–245.
2 de Souza GRM, Sant'anna CC, Lapa e Silva JR, *et al.* Intradermal BCG complications — analysis of 51 cases. *Tubercle* 1983; **64**: 23–7.
3 Warren JP, Nairn DS, Robertson MH. Cold abscess after accidental BCG inoculation. *Lancet* 1984; **ii**: 289.
4 Hengster P, Fille M, Menardi G. Suppurative lymphadenitis in newborn babies after change of BCG vaccine. *Lancet* 1991; **337**: 1168–9.
5 Rudin C, Amacher A, Berglund A. Anaphylactoid reactions to BCG vaccination. *Lancet* 1991; **337**: 377.
6 Lübbe D. Vasculitis allergica vom papulonekrotischen Typ nach BCG-Impfung. *Dermatol Monatsschr* 1982; **168**: 186–92.
7 Kass E, Staume S, Mellbye OJ, *et al.* Dermatomyositis associated with BCG vaccination. *Scand J Rheumatol* 1979; **8**: 187–91.
8 Schult C. Nebenwirkungen der BCG-Immuntherapie bei 511 Patienten mit malignem Melanom. *Hautarzt* 1984; **35**: 78–83.
9 Korting HC, Strasser S, Konz B. Multiple BCG-Ulzera nach subkutaner Impfstoffapplikation im Rahmen der Immunochemotherapie des malignen Melanoms. *Hautarzt* 1988; **39**: 170–3.
10 Torisu M, Miyahara T, Shinohara A, *et al.* A new side effect of BCG immunotherapy: BCG-induced arthritis in man. *Cancer Immunol Immunother* 1978; **5**: 77–83.
11 de la Monte SM, Hutchins GM. Fatal disseminated bacillus Calmette–Guérin infection and arrested growth of cutaneous malignant melanoma following intralesional immunotherapy. *Am J Dermatopathol* 1986; **8**: 331–5.

Cyotokines

Cytokines are being increasingly used in the management of neoplastic and haematological disorders and acquired immuno-deficiency syndrome (AIDS), and in addition are starting to be used for the therapy of specific dermatological disorders; side-effects have been reviewed [1].

1 Luger TA, Schwarz T. Therapeutic use of cytokines in dermatology. *J Am Acad Dermatol* 1991; **24**: 915–26.

Colony-stimulating factors

Recombinant haematopoietic colony-stimulating factors used in the treatment of haematological disorders are usually well tolerated, but may induce itching and erythema at the site of subcutaneous injection, thrombophlebitis with intravenous infusion, facial flushing and a transient maculopapular eruption, transient leucopenia and bone pain [1].

Granulocyte-macrophage colony-stimulating factor (GM-CSF) plays a primary role in the haematopoietic maturation of cells of granulocyte and monocyte lineage, and has been used in aplastic anaemia, myelodysplastic syndrome, for neutropenia secondary to chemotherapy, during bone marrow transplantation, and in AIDS. The commonest side-effects are bone pain, fever, chills, myalgias, arthralgias, decreased appetite, and nausea, mild elevation of transaminase levels, and a local skin eruption. A capillary leak syndrome with pleural and pericardial effusions, ascites and large vessel thrombosis has been noted only with high dose GM-CSF therapy [2]. Intravenous recombinant GM-CSF therapy for leukaemia resulted in a widespread confluent maculopapular eruption in three patients, associated with a dermal lymphocyte, macrophage and granulocyte infiltration, exocytosis, and keratinocyte ICAM-1 expression [3]. Nine of 23 patients with advanced malignancy treated with GM-CSF had a cutaneous eruption characterized by local erythema and pruritus at the injection site, recall erythema at previous injection sites, or a generalized maculopapular rash [4]. Necrotizing vasculitis developed at GM-CSF injection sites in one patient with white cell aplasia, but not in over 150 other neutropenic patients who received the drug [5].

1 Wakefield PE, James WD, Samlaska CP, Meltzer MS. Colony-stimulating factors. *J Am Acad Dermatol* 1990; **23**: 903–12.
2 Antman KS, Griffin JD, Elias A, *et al*. Effect of recombinant human granulocyte-macrophage colony-stimulating factor on chemotherapy-induced myelo-suppression. *N Engl J Med* 1988; **319**: 593–8.
3 Horn TD, Burke PJ, Karp JE, Hood AF. Intravenous administration of recombinant human granulocyte-macrophage colony-stimulating factor causes a cutaneous eruption. *Arch Dermatol* 1991; **127**: 49–52.
4 Lieschke GJ, Maher D, Cebon J, *et al*. Effects of bacterially synthesized recombinant human granulocyte-macrophage colony-stimulating factor in patients with advanced malignancy. *Ann Intern Med* 1989; **110**: 357–64.
5 Farmer KL, Kurzrock R, Duvic M. Necrotizing vasculitis at granulocyte-macrophage-colony-stimulating factor injection sites. *Arch Dermatol* 1990; **126**: 1243–4.

Interferon

Cutaneous reactions to recombinant interferon given to patients with cancer or AIDS are frequent (5−10%) but usually of moderate degree. Most patients experience flu-like symptoms following systemic therapy; reversible leucopenia and thrombocytopenia are recorded with higher dosage. Exacerbation of underlying auto-immune disease is documented with α-interferon [1]. Neutralizing antibodies to recombinant α-interferon may be produced [2].

Local reactions consist of erythema or induration at injection sites or urticaria [3−5]. Of 63 patients treated with γ-interferon for prophylaxis of infection in chronic granulomatous disease one had a severe cutaneous reaction (unspecified), and rashes or injection-site erythema or tenderness occurred in 17 and 14% of cases respectively [3]. Side-effects of intralesional injection of a sustained release formulation of α2b-interferon for the treatment of basal cell carcinomas in 33 patients included, in addition to various influenza-like systemic complaints, a rash in 6%, as well as local inflammation in 85% and local pruritus in 22% of cases [6]. Patch testing to interferon was positive in one case [5]. Local skin necrosis has also occurred [7]. Reactivation of oral herpes simplex, and enhanced radiation toxicity have been recorded [4]. α2a-Interferon for the treatment of cutaneous T cell lymphoma has induced temporary alopecia [8]. By contrast, α-interferon therapy has caused increased growth of eyelashes [9]. No adverse cutaneous side-effects resulted from intralesional injection of γ-interferon in 10 patients treated for keloid scarring [10].

α-Interferon used in the treatment of disseminated carcinoma [11,12], or intralesionally for viral warts [13], has been reported to exacerbate or trigger onset of psoriasis; psoriatic arthritis was also triggered in one case [14]. Psoriasis appeared at the site of sub-cutaneous injection of recombinant γ-interferon in patients with psoriatic arthritis [15], and at the site of intralesional injection in a patient receiving recombinant β-interferon for a basal cell carcinoma [16].

1 Conlon KC, Urba WJ, Smith JW II, *et al*. Exacerbation of symptoms of autoimmune disease in patients receiving alpha-interferon therapy. *Cancer* 1990; **65**: 2237−42.
2 Steis RG, Smith JW, Urba WJ. Resistance to recombinant interferon alfa-2a in hairy-cell leukemia associated with neutralizing anti-interferon antibodies. *N Engl J Med* 1988; **318**; 1409−13.
3 The International Chronic Granulomatous Disease Cooperative Study Group. A controlled trial of interferon gamma to prevent infection in chronic granulomatous disease. *N Engl J Med* 1991; **324**: 509−16.
4 Kerker BJ, Hood AF. Chemotherapy-induced cutaneous reactions. *Semin Dermatol* 1989; **8**: 173−81.
5 Detmar U, Agathos M, Nerl C. Allergy of delayed type to recombinant interferon α 2c. *Contact Dermatitis* 1989; **20**: 149−50.
6 Edwards L, Tucker SB, Perednia D, *et al*. The effect of an intralesional sustained-release formulation of interferon alfa-2b on basal cell carcinomas. *Arch Dermatol* 1990; **126**: 1029−32.
7 Cnudde F, Gharakhanian S, Luboinski J, *et al*. Cutaneous local necrosis

following interferon injections. *Int J Dermatol* 1991; **30**: 147.

8 Olsen EA, Rosen ST, Vollmer RT, *et al*. Interferon alfa-2a in the treatment of cutaneous T cell lymphoma. *J Am Acad Dermatol* 1989; **20**: 395–407.

9 Foon KA, Dougher G. Increased growth of eyelashes in a patient given leukocyte A Interferon. *N Engl J Med* 1984; **311**: 1259.

10 Granstein RD, Rook A, Flotte RJ, *et al*. A controlled trial of intralesional recombinant interferon-γ in the treatment of keloidal scarring. *Arch Dermatol* 1990; **126**: 1295–302.

11 Quesada JR, Gutterman JU. Psoriasis and alpha-interferon. *Lancet* 1986; **i**: 1466–8.

12 Hartmann F, von Wussow P, Deicher H. Psoriasis — exacerbation bei therapie mit alpha-Interferon. *Dtsch Med Wochenschr* 1989; **114**: 96–8.

13 Shiohara T, Kobayashi M, Abe K, Nagashima M. Psoriasis occurring predominantly on warts. Possible involvement of interferon alpha. *Arch Dermatol* 1988; **124**: 1816–21.

14 Jucgla A, Marcoval J, Curco N, Servitje O. Psoriasis with articular involvement induced by interferon alfa. *Arch Dermatol* 1991; **127**: 910–11.

15 Fierlbeck G, Rassner G, Müller C. Psoriasis induced at the injection site of recombinant interferon gamma. *Arch Dermatol* 1990; **126**: 351–5.

16 Kowalzick L, Weyer U. Psoriasis induced at the injection site of recombinant interferons. *Arch Dermatol* 1990; **126**: 1515–16.

Interleukin 2

Immunotherapy with interleukin 2 either alone, or in conjunction with lymphokine-activated killer cells, is used in the treatment of metastatic cancer. Cutaneous complications [1–5] include macular erythema (principally restricted to the head, neck and upper chest), burning and pruritus, which resolves with mild desquamation, erythroderma, petechiae, and a generalized capillary leak syndrome, with non-pitting oedema and diffuse pulmonary infiltrate on chest X-ray. Exacerbation of psoriasis (including erythroderma) has been described [2–5]. Additional associated events in patients being treated with interleukin 2 with or without lymphokine-activated killer cells include mucositis, glossitis, telogen effluvium, punctate superficial ulcers, erosions in scars, and jaundice. Erythema nodosum has been documented [6]. It is of interest that lymphocytes activated by interleukin 2 can non-specifically destroy keratinocytes *in vitro* [7].

1 Lotze MT, Matory YL, Rayner AA, *et al*. Clinical effects and toxicity of interleukin-2 in patients with cancer. *Cancer* 1986; **58**: 2764–72.

2 Rosenberg SA, Lotze MT, Muul LM, *et al*. Clinical experience with the treatment of 157 patients with advanced cancer using lymphokine-activated killer cells and interleukin-2 or high dose interleukin 2 alone. *N Engl J Med* 1987; **316**: 889–97.

3 Gaspari AA, Lotze MT, Rosenberg SA, *et al*. Dermatologic changes associated with interleukin-2 administration. *JAMA* 1987; **258**: 1624–9.

4 Rosenberg SA. Immunotherapy of cancer using interleukin 2: current status and future prospects. *Immunol Today* 1988; **9**: 58–62.

5 Lee RE, Gaspari AA, Lotze MT, *et al*. Interleukin 2 and psoriasis. *Arch Dermatol* 1988; **124**: 1811–15.

6 Weinstein A, Bujak D, Mittelman A, *et al*. Erythema nodosum in a patient with renal cell carcinoma treated with Interleukin 2 and lymphokine-activated killer cells. *JAMA* 1987; **258**: 3120–1.

7 Kalish RS. Non-specifically activated human peripheral blood mononuclear

cells are cytotoxic for human keratinocytes *in vitro*. *J Immunol* 1989; **142**: 74–80.

Interleukin 3

The authors have seen erythema and purpura at the site of injection of interleukin 3 in a patient with bone marrow hypoplasia (Fig. 15.12).

Tumour necrosis factor

Subcutaneous or intramuscular administration of tumour necrosis factor for advanced malignancy is limited by local pain, erythema and swelling or frank ulceration, while intravenous infusion may cause hypotension [1].

1 Wakefield PE, James WD, Samlaska CP, Meltzer MS. Tumor necrosis factor. *J Am Acad Dermatol* 1991; **24**: 675–85.

15.4 Miscellaneous

Diphencyprone

Diphencyprone used for alopecia areata has resulted in urticaria [1] and erythema multiforme [2], and it has been linked to development of vitiligo [3,4]. Severe contact dermatitis reactions may be induced (Fig. 15.13).

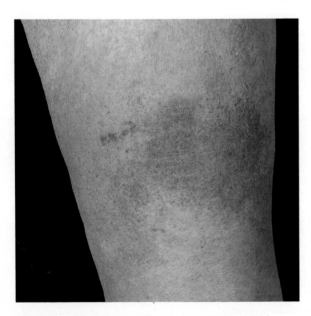

Figure 15.12 Purpuric erythematous eruption at the injection site of interleukin 3 in a patient with bone marrow hypoplasia.

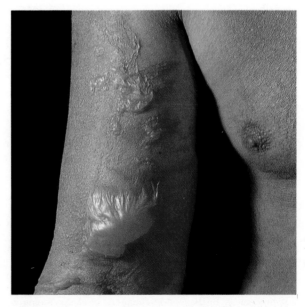

Figure 15.13 Severe bullous contact dermatitis reaction to diphencyprone.

1 van der Steen PHM, van Baar HMJ, Perret CM, Happle R. Treatment of alopecia areata with diphenylcyclopropenone. *J Am Acad Dermatol* 1991; **24**: 253−7.

2 Perret CM, Steijlen PM, Zaun H, Happle R. Erythema multiforme-like eruptions: a rare side effect of topical immunotherapy with diphenylcyclopropenone. *Dermatologica* 1990; **180**: 5−7

3 Hatzis J, Gourgiotou K, Tosca A, *et al*. Vitiligo as a reaction to topical treatment with diphencyprone. *Dermatologica* 1988; **177**: 146−8.

4 Duhra P, Foulds IS. Persistent vitiligo induced by diphencyprone. *Br J Dermatol* 1990; **123**: 415−16.

15.5 Antihistamines

H_1 Antihistamines

All traditional H_1 antagonists cause side-effects [1−4], especially sedation, most marked with the amino alkyl ether and phenothiazine groups. Dizziness, poor coordination, blurred vision and diplopia, as well as nervousness, insomnia and tremor may occur. In addition, atropine-like anticholinergic effects including dryness of mucous membranes, urinary retention, palpitations, agitation, increased intra-ocular pressure, and gastrointestinal upset are seen. Phenothiazine-derived drugs may cause photosensitivity or cholestatic jaundice. The effects of central nervous system depressants such as alcohol, hypnotics, sedatives, analgesics and anxiolytics may be potentiated. Decreased efficacy of drugs metabolized by the liver microsomal enzyme system, including oral anticoagulants, phenytoin and griseofulvin, may occur as a result of liver enzyme induction by antihistamines. The newer antihistamine drugs (e.g. terfenadine, astemizole, loratadine, cetirizine) are much less likely to cause sedation [1−4].

True hypersensitivity reactions are rare. Fixed eruptions have been caused by thonzylamine and cyclizine [5]. Skin eruptions have been documented with terfenadine [6], including possible exacerbation of psoriasis [7]; alopecia has been reported rarely [8]. Ventricular arrhythmia with prolonged QT interval on electrocardiography (torsade de pointes) has occurred rarely with excessive dosage of both terfenadine [9,10] and astemizole [11]. Torsade de pointes has also been documented in a single patient taking conventional dosage of terfenadine; there may have been pharmacological interactions with concomitantly administered ketoconazole [12].

H_2 Antihistamines

Severe adverse reactions are rare with cimetidine, ranitidine, nizatidine, and famotidine [13]. Gastrointestinal upset, headache, drowsiness, fatigue, or muscular pain occur in less than 3% of patients. Confusion, dizziness, somnolence, gynaecomastia or galactorrhoea with increased prolactin levels (cimetidine and ranitidine only), impotence and loss of libido (with cimetidine), marrow depression, hepatitis, abnormal renal function or nephritis, arthralgia, myalgia, cardiac abnormalities, and minor or severe skin reactions occur in less than 1% of patients.

Cimetidine

Mucocutaneous reactions are rare in relation to the enormous world-wide use of this drug. Reported reactions include a seborrhoeic dermatitis-like rash [14] and asteatotic dermatitis [15], erythema annulare centrifugum (Fig. 15.14) [16], erythrosis [17], giant urticaria [18], transitory alopecia [19], erythema multiforme [20], and exfoliative dermatitis [21]. Other effects have included thrombocytopenia [22] and a leucocytoclastic vasculitis [23]. Exacerbation of cutaneous lupus erythematosus [24] and systemic lupus erythematosus with granulocytopenia [25] are documented. Cimetidine binds to, and therefore blocks the binding of dihydrotestosterone to, androgen receptors, and gynaecomastia and hypogonadism are now well known [26]. The drug augments cell-mediated immunity *in vitro*, by blockade of H_2 receptors on T lymphocytes [27].

Ranitidine

This drug has a less marked effect on androgen receptors. Cross-sensitivity with cimetidine does not necessarily occur [16].

1 Woodward JK. Pharmacology and toxicology of nonclassical antihistamines. *Cutis* 1988; **42**: 5−9.
2 Lichtenstein LM, Simons FER (eds) Advancements in antiallergic therapy: beyond conventional antihistamines. *J Allergy Clin Immunol* 1990; **86** (Suppl): 995−1046.
3 Kennard CD, Ellis CN. Pharmacologic therapy for urticaria. *J Am Acad Dermatol* 1991: **25**: 176−89.
4 Soter NA. Treatment of urticaria and angioedema: low-sedating H_1-type antihistamines. *J Am Acad Dermatol* 1991; **24**: 1084−7.
5 Griffiths WAD, Peachey RDG. Fixed drug eruption due to cyclizine. *Br J Dermatol* 1970; **82**: 616−17.

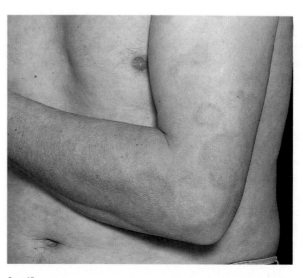

Figure 15.14 Erythema annulare centrifugum-like eruption due to cimetidine.

6 Stricker BHCH, Van Dijke CHP, Isaacs AJ, Lindquist M. Skin reactions to terfenadine. *Br Med J* 1986; **293**: 536.

7 Harrison PV, Stones RN. Severe exacerbation of psoriasis due to terfenadine. *Clin Exp Dermatol* 1988; **13**: 275.

8 Jones S, Morley W. Terfenadine causing hair loss (unreviewed report). *Br Med J* 1985; **291**: 940.

9 MacConnell TJ, Stanners AJ. Torsades de pointes complicating treatment with terfenadine. *Br Med J* 1991; **302**: 1469.

10 Warin RP. Torsades de pointes complicating treatment with terfenadine. *Br Med J* 1991; **303**: 58.

11 Simons FER, Kesselman MS, Giddins NG, *et al*. Astemizole induced torsade de pointes. *Lancet* 1988; **ii**: 624.

12 Monahan BP, Ferguson CL, Killeavy ES, *et al*. Torsades de pointes occurring in association with terfenadine use. *JAMA* 1990; **264**: 2788−90.

13 Feldman M, Burton ME. Histamine$_2$-receptor antagonists. Standard therapy for acid-peptide diseases (First of two parts). *N Engl J Med* 1990; **323**: 1672−80.

14 Kanwar A, Majid A, Garg MP, Singh G. Seborrheic dermatitis-like eruption caused by cimetidine. *Arch Dermatol* 1981; **117**: 65−6.

15 Greist MC, Epinette WW. Cimetidine-induced xerosis and asteatotic dermatitis. *Arch Dermatol* 1982; **118**: 253−4.

16 Merrett AC, Marks R, Dudley FJ. Cimetidine-induced erythema annulare centrifugum: no cross-sensitivity with ranitidine. *Br Med J* 1981; **283**: 698.

17 Angelini G, Bovo P, Vaona B, Cavallini G. Cimetidine and erythrosis-like lesions. *Br Med J* 1979; **i**: 1147−8.

18 Hadfield WA Jr. Cimetidine and giant urticaria. *Ann Intern Med* 1979; **91**: 128−9.

19 Vircburger MI, Prelevic GM, Brkic S, *et al*. Transitory alopecia and hypergonadotrophic hypogonadism during cimetidine treatment. *Lancet* 1981; **i**: 1160−1.

20 Ahmed AH, McLarty DG, Sharma SK, Masawe AEJ. Stevens−Johnson syndrome during treatment with cimetidine. *Lancet* 1978; **ii**: 433.

21 Yantis PL, Bridges ME, Pittman FE. Cimetidine-induced exfoliative dermatitis. *Dig Dis Sci* 1980; **25**: 73−4.

22 Rate R, Bonnell M, Chervenak C, Pavinich G. Cimetidine and hematologic effects. *Ann Intern Med* 1979; **91**: 795.

23 Dernbach WK, Taylor G. Leukocytoclastic vasculitis from cimetidine. *JAMA* 1981; **246**: 331.

24 Davidson BL, Gilliam JN, Lipsky PE. Cimetidine-associated exacerbation of cutaneous lupus erythematosus. *Arch Intern Med* 1982; **142**: 166−7.

25 Littlejohn GO, Urowitz MB. Cimetidine, lupus erythematosus, and granulocytopenia. *Ann Intern Med* 1979; **91**: 317−18.

26 Jensen RT, Collen MJ, Pandol SJ, *et al*. Cimetidine-induced impotence and breast changes in patients with gastric hypersecretory states. *N Engl J Med* 1983; **308**: 883−7.

27 Mavligit GM. Immunologic effects of cimetidine: potential uses. *Pharmacotherapy* 1987; **7** (Suppl 2): 120S−124S.

Chapter 16
Injections, Infusions, and Procedures

16.1 Radiographic contrast media and radiopharmaceuticals

Radiographic contrast media

Reactions to radiographic contrast media were previously reported to occur in about 4–8% of cases; severe reactions occur in 1 in 1000 administrations, and occasionally fatal anaphylactoid reactions (1 in 3000 for intravenous cholangiograms and between 1 in 10 000 and 1 in 100 000 for intravenous urography) develop [1–5]. The vast majority are not due to iodine allergy, but rather to non-immunological release of mast cell mediators or to direct complement activation [6,7]. The risk of severe reactions is increased in atopics, asthmatics and with higher doses; 40% of patients with a previous reaction may develop a recurrence [8].

Newer lower osmolality radiocontrast media are associated with fewer reactions [9,10], e.g. administration of iohexol in 50 660 patients undergoing excretory urography resulted in a frequency of adverse reactions of any type of 2.1% [9]. Lower osmolality radiocontrast media (e.g. iohexol or iopamidol) should be the contrast media of choice for patients with a prior immediate generalized reaction to conventional contrast media, and in addition patients should receive prednisone–diphenhydramine–ephedrine (adrenaline) or prednisone–diphenhydramine prophylaxis therapy [10].

Isolated cases of bullous lichen planus [11] and vasculitis [12] have been recorded. There has been a single case report of fatal toxic epidermal necrolysis following the second exposure to diatrizoate solution for excretory pyelography [13].

1 Coleman WP, Ochsner SF, Watson BE. Allergic reactions in 10 000 consecutive intravenous urographies. *South Med J* 1964; **57**: 1401–4.
2 Greenberg PA. Contrast media reactions. *J Allergy Clin Immunol* 1984; **74**: 600–5.
3 Lieberman P, Siegle RL, Treadwell G. Radiocontrast reactions. *Clin Rev Allergy* 1986; **4**: 229–45.
4 Grammer LC, Patterson R. Adverse reactions to radiographic contrast material. *Clin Dermatol* 1986; **4**: 149–54.
5 Katayama H, Tanaka T. Clinical survey of adverse reactions to contrast media. *Invest Radiol* 1988; **23** (Suppl): S88–S89.
6 Arroyave CM, Bhatt KN, Crown NR. Activation of the alternative pathway of

the complement system by radiocontrast media. *J Immunol* 1976; **117**: 1866–9.

7 Rice MC, Lieberman P, Siegle RL, Mason J. *In vitro* histamine release induced by radiocontrast media and various chemical analogs in reactor and control subjects. *J Allergy Clin Immunol* 1983; **72**: 180–6.
8 Enright T, Chua-Lim A, Duda E, Lim DT. The role of a documented allergic profile as a risk factor for radiographic contrast media reaction. *Ann Allergy* 1989; **62**: 302–5.
9 Schrott KM, Behrends B, Clauss W, *et al.* Iohexol in excretory urography: results of the drug monitoring programs. *Fortschr Med* 1986; **104**: 153–6.
10 Greenberger PA, Patterson R. The prevention of immediate generalized reactions to contrast media in high-risk patients. *J Allergy Clin Immunol* 1991; **87**: 867–71.
11 Grunwald MH, Halevy S, Livni E, Feuerman EJ. Bullous lichen planus after intravenous pyelography. *J Am Acad Dermatol* 1985; **13**: 512–13.
12 Kerdel FA, Fraker DL, Haynes HA. Necrotizing vasculitis from radiographic contrast media. *J Am Acad Dermatol* 1984; **10**: 25–9.
13 Kaftori JK, Abraham Z, Gilhar A. Toxic epidermal necrolysis after excretory pyelography. Immunologic-mediated contrast medium reaction? *Int J Dermatol* 1988; **27**: 346–7.

Radiopharmaceuticals

The reported incidence of reactions to agents used in nuclear medicine is low; these usually take the form of immediate urticaria or angioedema [1–3]. Urticarial or anaphylactic reactions to technetium-99m (^{99m}Tc) sulphur colloid and ^{99m}Tc human albumin microspheres together accounted for 50% of reported reactions [2]. The bone scanning agent ^{99m}Tc methylene diphosphonate produces a delayed-onset erythematous pruritic eruption within 4–24 hours [4].

1 Rhodes BA, Cordova MA. Adverse reactions to radio-pharmaceuticals: Incidence in 1978, and associated symptoms. *J Nucl Med* 1980; **2**: 1107.
2 Cordova MA, Hladik WB III, Rhodes BA. Validation and characterization of adverse reactions to radiopharmaceuticals. *Noninv Med Imag* 1984; **1**: 17–24.
3 Keeling D, Sampson CB. Adverse reactions to radiopharmaceuticals: incidence, reporting, symptoms, treatment. *Nuklearmedizin* 1986; **23** (Suppl): 478–82.
4 Collins MRL, James WD, Rodman OG. Adverse cutaneous reaction to technetium Tc 99m methylene diphosphonate. *Arch Dermatol* 1988; **124**: 180–1.

16.2 Halides

Bromides

Bromides have a long half-life and are excreted slowly by the kidney; bromism may develop in patients with impaired renal function, and eruptions may not develop until as much as 2 months after the drug has been discontinued. Acneiform and vegetating lesions occur more often, and bullae less frequently, than with iodism [1,2]. Vegetating bromoderma presents as single or multiple papillomatous nodules or plaques, studded with small pustules, on the face or limbs (Fig. 16.1). Bromism is also characterized by weakness, restlessness, headache, ataxia and personality changes [2].

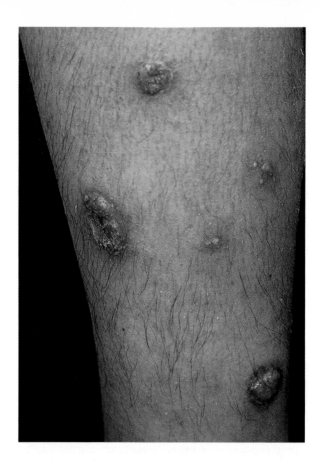

Figure 16.1 Vegetating bromoderma.

Iodides

Serious and even fatal reactions of anaphylactic type have been caused by radiographic contrast media containing organic iodine [3,4]. In iodism, nasal congestion and conjunctivitis, often accompanied by an exanthematic eruption, may be associated with a wide variety of systemic symptoms [5,6]. Prolonged administration of small doses of iodide, as in many cough mixtures, may provoke eruptions with or without mucosal or systemic symptoms. Lesions may first develop some days after the drug is discontinued. The following may occur: urticaria, an acneiform rash, papulopustular lesions, nodules, anthracoid or carbuncular lesions, or clear or haemorrhagic bullae on the face, forearms, neck and flexures, or buccal mucosa [6]. If the iodine is continued, the bullae may be replaced by vegetating masses which simulate pemphigus vegetans or a granulomatous infection [7]. Iododerma has developed after administration of oral [8] and intravenous [9,10] radiographic contrast media, and during thyroid protection treatment [11]. Iododerma seems more frequent in patients with renal failure, and may be accompanied by leucocytoclastic vasculitis [12]. The eruption recurs within days of readministration in a sensitized individual [12]. Cell mediated [5] and 'hyperinflammatory' [13] mechanisms have been postulated. Vegetating iododerma may be an idiosyncratic response which is commoner in patients with polyarteritis nodosa or para-proteinaemia [14]. Fixed eruptions occur rarely [15]. Generalized pustular psoriasis has been reportedly provoked by potassium iodide [16].

Histology of bromoderma and iododerma

In bromoderma, verrucous pseudo-epitheliomatous hyperplasia is associated with abscesses containing neutrophils and eosinophils in the epidermis, a dense dermal infiltrate initially consisting mainly of neutrophils and eosinophils, and later containing many lympho-cytes, plasma cells and histiocytes. The abundant dilated blood vessels may show endothelial proliferation. In iododermas, ulcer-ation is more marked, but there is usually less epithelial hyperplasia. Both conditions must be differentiated from blastomycosis and coccidiomycosis, and from pemphigus vegetans [17].

1 Blasik LG, Spencer SK. Fluoroderma. *Arch Dermatol* 1979; **115**: 1334−5.
2 Carney MWP. Five cases of bromism. *Lancet* 1971; **ii**: 523−4.
3 Sparrow GP. Iododerma due to radiographic contrast medium. *J R Soc Med* 1979; **72**: 60−1.
4 Vaillant L, Pengloan J, Blanchier D, De Muret A, Lorette G. Iododerma and acute respiratory distress with leucocytoclastic vasculitis following the intravenous injection of contrast medium. *Clin Exp Dermatol* 1990; **15**: 232−33.
5 Kincaid MC, Green WR, Hoover RE, Farmer ER. Iododerma of the conjunctiva and skin. *Ophthalmology (Rochester)* 1981; **88**: 1216−20.
6 O'Brien TJ. Iodic eruptions. *Australas J Dermatol* 1987; **28**: 119−22.
7 Rosenberg FR, Einbinder J, Walzer RA, Nelson CT. Vegetating iododerma. An immunologic mechanism. *Arch Dermatol* 1972; **105**: 900−5.
8 Boudoulas O, Siegle RJ, Grinwood RE. Iododerma occurring after orally administered iopanoic acid. *Arch Dermatol* 1987; **123**: 387−8.
9 Heydenreich G, Larsen PO. Iododerma after high dose urography in an oliguric patient. *Br J Dermatol* 1977; **97**: 567−9.
10 Lauret P, Godin M, Bravard P. Vegetating iodides after an intravenous pyelogram. *Dermatologica* 1985; **71**: 463−8.
11 Wilkin JK, Strobel D. Iododerma during thyroid protection treatment. *Cutis* 1985; **36**: 335−7.
12 Jones LE, Pariser H, Murray PF. Recurrent iododerma. *Arch Dermatol* 1958; **28**: 353−8.
13 Stone OJ. Proliferative iododerma: a possible mechanism. *Int J Dermatol* 1985; **24**: 565−6.
14 Soria C, Allegue F, España A, *et al*. Vegetating iododerma with underlying systemic diseases: Report of three cases. *J Am Acad Dermatol* 1990; **22**: 418−22.
15 Baker H. Fixed drug eruption due to iodide and antipyrine. *Br J Dermatol* 1962; **74**: 310−16.
16 Shelley WB. Generalized pustular psoriasis induced by potassium iodide. *JAMA* 1967; **201**: 1009−14.
17 Lever WF, Schaumburg-Lever G. *Histopathology of the Skin*, 7th edn. JB Lippincott, Philadelphia, 1990.

16.3 Agents used in general anaesthesia

Neuromuscular blocking agents, skeletal muscle relaxants and general anaesthetics

The incidence of life-threatening anaphylactic or anaphylactoid reactions during anaesthesia has been variously reported to occur in 1 in 1000 to 1 in 20000, and minor reactions probably occur in more than 1% of cases; neuromuscular blocking agents are the triggering agents in about 50% of these reactions [1−11]. The mortality rate in anaphylactic reactions to drugs used in general anaesthesia is between 4 and 6% [11].

Reactions appear most likely with suxamethonium and gallamine, then *d*-tubocurarine and alcuronium, and least likely with pancuronium and vecuronium [3,6]. Mucocutaneous manifestations including erythema, urticaria, and angioneurotic oedema, are reported in up to 80% of reactions, but may only be recognized after the acute phase has passed. Reactions are more frequent in women and in atopic patients. Proposed mechanisms for anaphylactic reactions include type I (IgE antibody-mediated) hypersensitivity to quaternary or tertiary ammonium ion determinants [7], and direct histamine release. Environmental contact with other quaternary or tertiary ammonium compounds in drugs, cosmetics and disinfectants, with resultant prior sensitization and generation of IgE antibodies, has been invoked as an explanation of cross-reactivity with different relaxants. Cross-reactivity is widespread with most of the drugs but is least with pancuronium. It has been suggested that pancuronium should be used where muscle relaxation during anaesthesia is essential but sensitivity to another relaxant exists [3], although others have questioned the safety of this procedure [10]. Intradermal [1−3] or prick [4,10] testing may be helpful in identifying the causative drug, and is essential in confirming lack of sensitivity to pancuronium before use in documented sensitivity to other relaxants [3]. IgE-dependent sensitivity to thiopental may result in anaphylactic reactions [5]. In one recent series [11] of patients with a history of anaphylaxis during induction of general anaesthesia, skin testing was performed by the prick and intracutaneous methods with dilutions of thiobarbiturates, muscle relaxants or β-lactam antibiotics, where administered. No patient experienced a recurrence of anaphylaxis during subsequent general anaesthesia, for which agents producing positive skin tests were avoided, provided a premedication regime of prednisone and diphenhydramine was given [11].

1 Fisher M McD. Intradermal testing in the diagnosis of acute anaphylaxis during anaesthesia — results of five years experience. *Anaesth Intensive Care* 1979; **7**: 58−61.
2 Fisher M McD. The diagnosis of acute anaphylactoid reactions to neuromuscular blocking agents: a commonly undiagnosed condition. *Anaesth Intensive Care* 1981; **9**: 235−41.
3 Galletly DC, Treuren BC. Anaphylactoid reactions during anaesthesia. Seven

years' experience of intradermal testing. *Anaesthesia* 1985; **40**: 329–33.

4 Leynadier F, Sansarricq M, Didier JM, Dry J. Prick tests in the diagnosis of anaphylaxis to general anaesthetics. *Br J Anaesth* 1987; **59**: 683–9.

5 Cheema AL, Sussman GL, Jancelewicz Z, *et al.* Update: Pentothal-induced anaphylaxis. *J Allergy Clin Immunol* 1988; **81**: 220.

6 Richardson FJ, Agoston S. Neuromuscular blocking agents and skeletal muscle relaxants. In: Dukes MNG, (ed.) *Meyler's Side Effects of Drugs,* 11th edn. Elsevier Science Publishers, Amsterdam, 1988.

7 Assem ESK, Ling YB. Fatal anaphylactic reaction to suxamethonium: new screening test suggests possible prevention. *Anaesthesia* 1988; **43**: 958–61.

8 Fisher M McD. Anaphylaxis. *Anaesthesia* 1989; **44**: 516–17.

9 Noble DW, Yap PL. Screening for antibodies to anaesthetics. No case for doing it yet. *Br Med J* 1989; **299**: 2.

10 Moneret-Vautrin DA, Laxenaire MC. Anaphylaxis to muscle relaxants: predictive tests. *Anaesthesia* 1990; **45**: 246–7.

11 Moscicki RA, Sockin SM, Corsello BF, *et al.* Anaphylaxis during induction of general anaesthesia: Subsequent evaluation and management. *J Allergy Clin Immunol* 1990; **86**: 325–32.

16.4 Local anaesthetic agents

Local anaesthetics may cause both immediate anaphylactic reactions and contact dermatitis [1–6]. Acute anaphylactic reactions are uncommon, but are probably less likely to occur when amide linkage agents are used [5,6]. Necrosis of the fingertip has followed local injection for nail extraction [7].

EMLA cream

EMLA cream, a eutectic mixture of prilocaine and lignocaine in a cream base, has been associated with methaemoglobinaemia [8–10]; two metabolites of prilocaine, namely 4-hydroxy-2-methylaniline and 2-methylaniline (*o*-toluidine), have been incriminated. A 3-month-old infant became cyanosed after application of 5 g, but this may have been contributed to by concomitant sulphonamide therapy [8]. Small but significant increases in methaemoglobin levels have been reported in children 1–6 years old following routine administration of 5 g before surgery, and may persist for at least 24 hours [9], so that it is recommended that the minimum effective dose be used in children requiring daily application. Blanching following application of EMLA is common [11]. Severe lidocaine intoxication with progressive neurological and psychiatric abnormalities and cardiorespiratory arrest occurred following topical application to painful ulcerated areas in a patient with cutaneous T cell lymphoma [12].

1 Schatz M. Skin testing and incremental challenge in the evaluation of adverse reactions of local anesthetics. *J Allergy Clin Immunol* 1984; **74**: 606–16.

2 Fisher MMcD, Graham R. Adverse responses to local anaesthetics. *Anaesth Intensive Care* 1984; **12**: 325–7.

3 Ruzicka T, Gerstmeier M, Przybilla B, Ring J. Allergy to local anesthetics: Comparison of patch test with prick and intradermal test results. *J Am Acad Dermatol* 1987; **16**: 1202–8.

4 Berlin J, Erdmann W, Cartellieri S. Lokalanästhetika. Unerwünschte

Wirkungen und ihre Behandlung. *Fortschr Med* 1989; **107**: 288—90.

5 Christie JL. Fatal consequences of local anesthesia: report of five cases and a review of the literature. *J Forensic Sci* 1975; **21**: 671—9.

6 Kennedy KS, Cave RH. Anaphylyactic reaction to lidocaine. *Arch Otolaryngol Head Neck Surg* 1986; **112**: 671—3.

7 Roser-Maaß E. Nekrosen an Fingerendgliedern nach Lokalanästhesie bei Nagelextraktion. *Hautarzt* 1981; **32**: 39—41.

8 Jakobson B, Nilsson A. Methaemoglobinaemia associated with a prilocaine— lidocaine cream and trimethoprim—sulphamethoxazole. A case report. *Acta Anaesthesiol Scand* 1985; **29**: 453—5.

9 Frayling IM, Addison GM, Chattergee K, Meakin G. Methaemoglobinaemia in children treated with prilocaine—lignocaine cream. *Br Med J* 1990; **301**: 153—4.

10 Nilsson A, Engberg G, Henneberg S, Danielson K, DeVerdier C-H. Inverse relationship between age-dependent erythrocyte activity of methaemoglobin reductase and prilocaine-induced methaemoglobinaemia during infancy. *Br J Anaesth* 1990; **64**: 72—6.

11 Villada G, Zetlaoui J, Revuz J. Local blanching after epicutaneous application of EMLA cream. *Dermatologica* 1990; **181**: 38—40.

12 Lie RL, Vermeer BJ, Edelbroek PM. Severe lidocaine intoxication by cutaneous absorption. *J Am Acad Dermatol* 1990; **23**: 1026—8.

16.5 Infusions and injections

Intravenous infusion

Pain, oedema, induration, and thrombophlebitis are well-recognized complications. Localized bullous eruptions following infusion of commonly used non-vesicant fluids, such as saline, have been described [1]. Extravasation was reported to occur in 11% of 16 380 administrations to children monitored over a 6-month period [2]. Skin necrosis following intravenous infusion [2—8], including after administration of chemotherapeutic agents (Section 14.1, Fig. 14.2, p. 283) [2,3,5—8] occurs in up to 6% of patients [1].

1 Robijns BJL, de Wit WM, Bosma NJ, van Vloten WA. Localized bullous eruptions caused by extravasation of commonly used intravenous infusion fluids. *Dermatologica* 1991; **182**: 39—42.

2 Brown AS, Hoelzer DJ, Piercy SA. Skin necrosis from extravasation of intravenous fluids in children. *Plast Reconstr Surg* 1979; **64**: 145—50.

3 Dufresne RG. Skin necrosis from intravenously infused materials. *Cutis* 1987; **39**: 197—8.

4 MacCara E. Extravasation: A hazard of intravenous therapy. *Drug Intell Clin Pharm* 1987; **17**: 713—17.

5 Ignoffo RJ, Friedman MA. Therapy of local toxicities caused by extravasation of cancer chemotherapeutic drugs. *Cancer Treat Rev* 1980; **7**: 17—27.

6 Harwood KV, Aisner J. Treatment of chemotherapeutic extravasation: current status. *Cancer Treat Rep* 1984; **68**: 939—45.

7 Banerjee A, Brotherston TM, Lamberty BGH, *et al.* Cancer chemotherapy agent-induced perivenous extravasation injury. *J Postgrad Med* 1987; **63**: 5—9.

8 Rudolph R, Larson DL. Etiology and treatment of chemotherapeutic agent extravasation injuries. A review. *J Clin Oncol* 1987; **5**: 1116—26.

Blood transfusion and leucopheresis

Urticaria occurs in about 1% of transfusions [1], and may be the result of allergy to soluble proteins in donor plasma. Post-transfusion purpura may rarely occur as a result of profound thrombocytopenia about 1 week after transfusion, and is associated with antiplatelet alloantibodies. Other potential side-effects include transmission of infectious diseases, including syphilis, hepatitis B, and human immunodeficiency virus-related syndromes (AIDS).

Graft-versus-host disease may develop following transfusion of unirradiated blood in immunosuppressed patients [2–8], including those with malignancies [2], and infants with severe congenital immunodeficiency [3]. Isolated reports of fatal transfusion-associated graft-versus-host disease in presumed immunocompetent hosts receiving fresh unirradiated blood have been reported [9–11]. This paradoxical situation may be in part explained by situations in which recipients heterozygous for a given major histocompatibility complex haplotype receive a transfusion from a donor homozygous for this haplotype, since the recipient would not react to the donor haplotype, but the donor lymphocytes would react to the non-identical recipient haplotype [8]. Thus some recipients of non-irradiated blood from their offspring may be at risk of developing graft-versus-host disease. An acute fatal illness, characterized by fever, diffuse erythematous rash, and progressive leucopenia, has been described in Japanese patients 10 days after surgical operation, under the name 'post-operative erythroderma' [12]. Histologically, scattered single cell epidermal cell eosinophilic necrosis, satellite cell necrosis, basal cell liquefaction degeneration, and a scanty dermal infiltrate may be seen; the reaction is compatible with an acute graft-versus-host reaction following blood transfusion [12].

Hydroxyethylstarch (hetastarch), used as a sedimenting agent to increase the yield of granulocytes during leucopheresis, has been implicated in the development of lichen planus [13], and severe generalized pruritus beginning 2 weeks after exposure and taking months to settle [14].

1 Shulman IA. Adverse reactions to blood transfusion. *Texas Med* 1990; **85**: 35–42.
2 Decoste SD, Boudreaux C, Dover JS. Transfusion-associated graft-vs-host disease in patients with malignancies. Report of two cases and review of the literature. *Arch Dermatol* 1990; **126**: 1324–9.
3 Hathaway WE, Githens JH, Blackburn WR, *et al*. Aplastic anemia, histiocytosis and erythrodermia in immunologically deficient children. *N Engl J Med* 1965; **273**: 953–8.
4 Brubaker DB. Human posttransfusion graft-versus-host disease. *Vox Sang* 1983; **45**: 401–20.
5 Leitman SF, Holland PV. Irradiation of blood products: indications and guidelines. *Transfusion* 1985; **25**: 292–300.
6 Anderson KC, Weinstein HJ. Transfusion-associated graft-versus-host disease. *N Engl J Med* 1990; **323**: 315–21.
7 Ray TL. Blood transfusions and graft-vs-host disease. *Arch Dermatol* 1990; **126**: 1347–50.
8 Ferrara JLM, Deeg HJ. Graft-versus-host disease. *N Engl J Med* 1991; **324**: 667–74.
9 Arsura EL, Bertelle A, Minkowitz S, *et al*. Transfusion-associated graft-vs-host disease in a presumed immunocompetent patient. *Arch Intern Med* 1988; **148**: 1941–4.

10 Capond SM, DePond WD, Tyan DB, *et al*. Transfusion-associated graft-versus-host disease in an immunocompetent patient. *Ann Intern Med* 1991; **114**: 1025−6.

11 Juji T, Takahashi K, Shibata Y, *et al*. Post-transfusion graft-versus-host disease in immunocompetent patients after cardiac surgery in Japan. *N Engl J Med* 1989; **321**: 56.

12 Hidano A, Yamashita N, Mizuguchi M, Toyoda H. Clinical, histological, and immunohistological studies of postoperative erythroderma. *J Dermatol (Tokyo)* 1989; **16**: 20−30.

13 Bode U, Deisseroth AB. Donor toxicity in granulocyte collections: association of lichen planus with the use of hydroxyethyl starch leukapheresis. *Transfusion* 1981; **21**: 83−5.

14 Parker NE, Porter JB, Williams HJM, Leftley N. Pruritus after administration of hetastarch. *Br Med J* 1982; **284**: 385−6.

16.6 Renal dialysis

Dermatological complications of renal dialysis have been reviewed [1,2]. These include marked premature ageing, hyperpigmentation, xeroderma, decreased sebaceous and sweat gland secretion, Raynaud's syndrome, generalized pruritus, and carpal tunnel syndrome due to β-amyloid deposition [1]. Extravasation, phlebitis, and bacterial infection of the cannula, with resulting septicaemia, may occur related to the site of insertion of the cannula into the arteriovenous fistula. A bullous dermatosis of haemodialysis has been described [2,3]. This resembles porphyria clinically (Fig. 16.2) and histologically, and porphyrins may be elevated [3], although cases with pseudo-porphyria in which there are no abnormalities of porphyrin metabolism have also been documented [2]. Two-thirds of patients with dialysis-associated anaphylaxis have IgE antibodies to ethylene oxide−human serum albumin [4]. Allergic contact dermatitis due to rubber chemicals in the haemodialysis equipment may be seen around the arteriovenous shunt [5]. Porokeratosis localized to the access region for haemodialysis has also been reported [6].

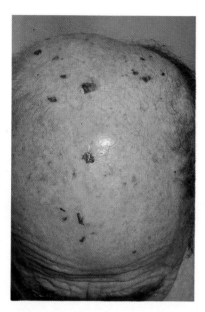

Figure 16.2 Porphyria cutanea tarda-like lesions of the scalp in a patient with renal failure treated with haemodialysis.

1 Altmeyer P, Kachel H-G, Jünger M, *et al*. Hautveränderungen bei Langzeit-dialysepatienten. *Hautarzt* 1982; **33**: 303−9.

2 Gupta AK, Gupta MA, Cardella CJ, Haberman HF. Cutaneous complications of chronic renal failure and dialysis. *Int J Dermatol* 1986; **25**: 498−504.

3 Poh-Fitzpatrick MB, Bellet N, DeLeo VA, *et al*. Porphyria cutanea tarda in two patients treated with hemodialysis for chronic renal failure. *N Engl J Med* 1978; **299**: 292−4.

4 Grammer LC, Roberts M, Wiggins CA, *et al*. A comparison of cutaneous testing and ELISA testing for assessing reactivity to ethylene oxide−human serum albumin in hemodialysis patients with anaphylactic reactions. *J Allergy Clin Immunol* 1991; **87**: 674−6.

5 Kruis-De Vries MH, Coenraads PJ, Nater JP. Allergic contact dermatitis due to rubber chemicals in haemodialysis equipment. *Contact Dermatitis* 1987; **17**: 303−5.

6 Nakazawa A, Matsuo I, Ohkido M. Porokeratosis localized to the access region for hemodialysis. *J Am Acad Dermatol* 1991; **25**: 338−40.

16.7 Necrosis from intramuscular injections

Aseptic necrosis (embolia cutis medicamentosa) may follow intramuscular therapeutic injections, particularly of preparations containing corticosteroids, local anaesthetics, or phenylbutazone; more rarely, chlorpromazine, penicillin, phenobarbitone, and sulphonamides have been implicated [1]. Clinically, stellate erythema and infiltration (Fig. 16.3) are followed by central deep necrosis (Fig. 16.4) which heals with scarring.

1 Bork K. *Cutaneous Side Effects of Drugs*. WB Saunders, Philadelphia, 1988.

16.8 Polyvinylpyrrolidone

High-molecular weight polyvinylpyrrolidone used in depot preparations of subcutaneously or intramuscularly administered medi-

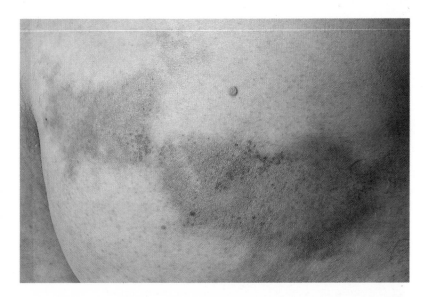

Figure 16.3 Stellate erythema following intramuscular injection of a preparation containing phenylbutazone.

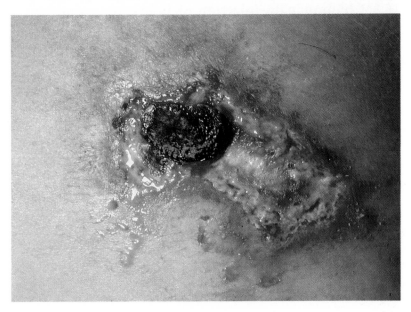

Figure 16.4 Embolia cutis medicamentosa resulting in central necrosis.

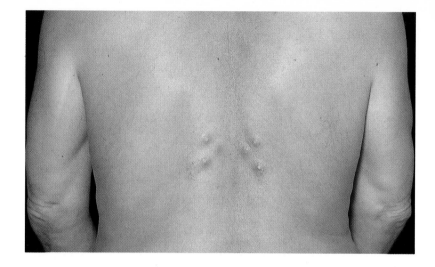

Figure 16.5 Granulomatous nodules
at sites of injection of procaine—
polyvinylpyrrolidone.

cations may induce local granulomatous lesions (Fig. 16.5) [1,2] and
pseudotumours distant from the site of injection [3,4].

1 Bode U, Ring J, Schmoeckel C. Granulombildung nach intrakutaner Applikation
von Procain-Polyvinylpyrrolidon (PVP). *Hautarzt* 1984; **35**: 447—7.
2 Fartasch M, Anton-Lamprecht I, Frosch PJ, Petzoldt D. Polyvinylpyrrolidon-
Dermatose. Klinik und ultrastrukturelle Morphologie. *Hautarzt* 1988; **39**:
569—75.
3 Oehlschlaegel G, Marquart K-H, Steuer G, Burg G. Iatrogener, durch Polyvinylpyrrolidon (PVP) induzierter 'Pseudotumor' der Haut. *Hautarzt* 1983; **34**:
555—60.
4 Bork K. Multiple Lymphozytome an den Einstichstellen als Komplikation
einer Akupunkturbehandlung. Zur traumatischen Entstehung des Lymphozytoms. *Hautarzt* 1983; **34**: 496—9.

16.9 Chymopapain injection of intervertebral discs

Intradisc injection for chemonucleosis has caused anaphylaxis,
which occurs in about 1% of previously untreated patients [1].

1 Grammer LC, Patterson R. Proteins: Chymopapain and insulin. *J Allergy Clin
Immunol* 1984; **74**: 635—40.

16.10 Dermal implants

Collagen implants

Zyderm I and Zyderm II consist of sterile suspensions of purified
bovine dermal collagen in phosphate buffered saline with lidocaine
at concentrations of 35 mg/ml and 65 mg/ml respectively [1,2]; the
preparations contain 95% type I collagen, and 5% type III collagen
[1]. Zyplast Implant is a similar product in which the bovine collagen
has been cross-linked by addition of glutaraldehyde [2]. More than
4 million collagen injections in more than 350 000 patients had been

safely administered from 1981, when Zyderm I was introduced, up to 1989 [2]. Adverse reactions to these medications have been extensively reviewed [1–6].

Virtually all treated patients develop transient erythema related to trauma to the site. Intradermal skin testing in the volar forearm is mandatory before definitive use in patients. Up to 5% of patients will develop a test site reaction consisting of local erythema, pain, itching and induration, or urticaria; 70% occur within 72 hours, a further 10% within 7 days [2–5]. Absent symptoms or signs one month after injection is taken as a negative reaction, although exceptional cases with reactions initially evident at 6 weeks have been described. Adverse treatment site reactions similar to the skin test site reactions may develop in up to 4% of patients with negative skin tests from 1 week to 2 months after injection, and are in general self-limited, resolving spontaneously within weeks to months [2–5]. Short-lived purpura, and rarely superficial necrosis, presumably due to mechanical obstruction of superficial blood vessels, occurs. Zyplast Implant may be associated with fewer hypersensitivity reactions [7]. A recent update on the 470 000 patients treated with collagen implants from 1981 to 1989 reported that abscess formation occurs in 0.04% of cases, and localized necrosis in 0.09% of cases; more than half the cases involved the skin of the glabella [6]. Rarely, recurrent intermittent swelling, erythema and induration at treatment sites develops, and may last up to 3 years [5]. Histological analysis of treatment site reactions shows foreign body or necrobiotic granuloma formation in two-thirds of cases [2,5,8–10]. Zyplast Implant may induce a much more intense lymphohistiocytic reaction than Zyderm I at injection sites [11]. A single case of an embolus entering the ophthalmic artery, with consequent partial blindness, followed attempted correction of glabellar frown lines [5]. No statistically significant systemic complications have been reported, although arthralgia, malaise and headache are recorded. It is thought that the isolated cases of rheumatoid arthritis, dermatomyositis and of polymyositis recorded in association with collagen implants in the more than 350 000 patients treated up to 1989 reflect the general population prevalence of these disorders [2,12].

Immunological aspects

Of patients with localized test-site hypersensitivity reactions 90% will have circulating species-specific IgG antibodies to bovine collagen [7,12–17], which react with multiple antigenic sites on Zyderm I [16,17]. These also occur with use of Zyplast Implant [7]. The prevalence of anti-bovine collagen antibodies, presumed to be the result of dietary exposure, in patients before treatment has been reported as 8.4%, as measured by an enzyme-linked immunosorbent assay (ELISA) [17]. Patients with significant pretreatment anti-collagen antibody levels may be about six times more likely to develop an adverse treatment reaction [17]. Anti-collagen antibodies may develop in a small number of patients with an initially negative skin test [17,18]. However, these antibodies may also be present in some patients who do not develop reactions to bovine collagen [19]. Abscesses related to collagen implants are also thought to represent a hypersensitivity reaction; anti-bovine collagen antibodies are present in 86% of cases, and immunoglobulin is deposited within the implant material [6].

1 Zeide DA. Adverse reactions to collagen implants. *Clin Dermatol* 1986; **4**: 176−82.
2 Clark DP, Hanke CW, Swanson NA. Dermal implants: safety of products injected for soft tissue augmentation. *J Am Acad Dermatol* 1989; **21**: 992−8.
3 Castrow FF II, Krull EA. Injectable collagen implant − update. *J Am Acad Dermatol* 1983; **9**: 889−93.
4 Cooperman LS, Mackinnon V, Bechler G, *et al.* Injectable collagen: a six-year clinical investigation. *Aesthetic Plast Surg* 1985; **9**: 145−52.
5 Stegman SJ, Chu S, Armstrong RC. Adverse reactions to bovine collagen implant: clinical and histologic features. *J Dermatol Surg Oncol* 1988; **14** (Suppl 1): 39−48.
6 Hanke CW, Higley HR, Jolivette DM, *et al.* Abscess formation and local necrosis after treatment with Zyderm or Zyplast Collagen Implant. *J Am Acad Dermatol* 1991; **25**: 319−26.
7 DeLustro F, Mackinnon V, Swanson NA. Immunology of injectable collagen in human subjects. *J Dermatol Surg Oncol* 1988; **14** (Suppl 1): 49−55.
8 Ruiz-Esparza J. Bailin M, Bailin PL. Necrobiotic granuloma formation at a collagen implant treatment site. *Cleve Clinic Quart* 1983; **50**: 163−5.
9 Barr RJ, Stegman SJ. Delayed skin test reaction to injectable collagen implant (Zyderm). The histopathologic comparative study. *J Am Acad Dermatol* 1984; **10**: 652−8.
10 Schurig V, Konz B, Ring J, Dorn M. Granulombildung an Test- und Behandlungsstellen durch intrakutan verabreichtes, injizierbares Kollagen. *Hautarzt* 1986; **37**: 42−5.
11 Kligman AM. Histologic responses to collagen implants in human volunteers: comparison of Zyderm collagen with Zyplast implant. *J Dermatol Surg Oncol* 1988; **14** (Suppl 1): 57−65.
12 DeLustro F, Fries J, Kang A, *et al.* Immunity to injectable collagen and autoimmune disease: a summary of current understanding. *J Dermatol Surg Oncol* 1988; **14** (Suppl 1): 57−65.
13 Swanson N, Stoner JG, Siegle RJ, *et al.* Treatment site reactions to Zyderm Collagen Implantation. *J Dermatol Surg Oncol* 1983; **9**: 377−80.
14 Cooperman LS, Michaeli D. The immunogenicity of injectable collagen. II. A retrospective review of seventy-two tested and treated patients. *J Am Acad Dermatol* 1984; **10**: 647−51.
15 Siegle RJ, McCoy JP, Schade W, *et al.* Intradermal implantation of bovine collagen: humoral immune responses associated with clinical reactions. *Arch Dermatol* 1984; **120**: 183−7.
16 Ellingsworth LR, DeLustro F, Brennan JE, *et al.* The human immune response to reconstituted bovine collagen. *J Immunol* 1986; **136**: 877−82.
17 McCoy JP Jr, Schade W, Siegle RJ, *et al.* Immune responses to bovine collagen implants. Significance of pretreatment serology. *J Am Acad Dermatol* 1987; **16**: 955−60.
18 Vanderveen EE, McCoy JP Jr, Schade W, *et al.* The association of HLA and immune responses to bovine collagen implants. *Arch Dermatol* 1986; **122**: 650−4.
19 Trentham DE. Adverse reactions to bovine collagen implants. Additional evidence for immune response gene control of collagen reactivity in humans. *Arch Dermatol* 1986; **122**: 643−4.

Gelatin matrix implant

This mixture of gelatin powder and ε-aminocaproic acid in saline has caused initial skin test reactions in 1.9% of patients, and treatment site reactions in 8% of skin test-negative patients [1,2]. Treatment site reactions included transient erythema, swelling and nodules; 75% resolved in less than 2 weeks, but nodules persisted for more than a month in about 20% of patients. No significant systemic side-effects were seen.

1 Ruiz-Esparza J, Bailin M, Bailin PL. Treatment of depressed cutaneous scars with gelatin matrix implant: a multicenter study. *J Am Acad Dermatol* 1987; **16**: 1155–62.
2 Clark DP, Hanke CW, Swanson NA. Dermal implants: safety of products injected for soft tissue augmentation. *J Am Acad Dermatol* 1989; **21**: 992–8.

16.11 Silicone

Injection of pure medical-grade silicone in small amounts of less than 1 ml per session seems to be associated with few side-effects; treatment site reactions include erythema, purpura, hyperpigmentation, and altered contour [1,2]. However, injection of liquid silicone in ophthalmic or meningeal vessels has caused blindness, neurological deficit or even fatality. Subcutaneous injection in transsexual men has been associated with acute pneumonitis and respiratory distress syndrome [3]. Augmentation mammoplasty with medical-grade silicone has been associated with silicone migration, erysipelas-like reactions, and lymphatic obstruction [2], as well as with acute arthritis and renal failure in a patient [4]. The reader is referred to section 3.25 (p. 121) for discussion of silicone-induced sclerodermatous and other connective tissue reactions.

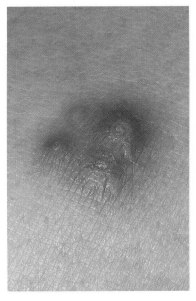

Figure 16.6 Persistent granulomatous reaction at puncture sites following a Tine test.

1 Webster RC, Fuleihan NS, Hamdan US, *et al.* Injectable silicone: report of 17 000 facial treatments since 1962. *Am J Cosmetic Surg* 1986; **3**: 41–8.
2 Clark DP, Hanke CW, Swanson NA. Dermal implants: safety of products injected for soft tissue augmentation. *J Am Acad Dermatol* 1989; **21**: 992–8.
3 Chastre J, Basset F, Viau F, *et al.* Acute pneumonitis after subcutaneous injections of silicone in transsexual men. *N Engl J Med* 1983; **308**: 764–7.
4 Uratsky NF, O'Brien JJ, Courtiss EH, *et al.* Augmentation mammoplasty associated with severe systemic illness. *Ann Plast Surg* 1979; **3**: 445–7.

16.12 Diagnostic tests for tuberculosis

Tine testing involving intradermal injection of purified protein derivative of tuberculin may result in persistent granulomatous lesions at the puncture sites (Fig. 16.6).

Chapter 17
Drugs Affecting Metabolism or Gastrointestinal Function

17.1 Hypoglycaemic drugs

Dermatological aspects of the oral hypoglycaemic drugs have been reviewed [1−3].

Biguanides

Rashes are much less frequent with metformin and phenformin than with sulphonylureas. Transient erythemas, pruritus and urticaria have been noted.

Sulphonylureas

Chlorpropamide and tolbutamide are most often prescribed, and both can give rise to toxic or allergic reactions.

Chlorpropamide

Eruptions occur in 2−3% of patients on chlorpropamide [2]. These include maculopapular rashes, photosensitivity [4], erythema annulare, erythema multiforme [5], erythema nodosum [1], lichenoid eruptions [6,7], purpura and exfoliative dermatitis [8]. Porphyria has been provoked [9]. A disulfiram-like effect, with flushing of the face, headache and palpitations after taking alcohol, occurs in up to 30% of patients [10,11]. The fact that the flush is blocked by naloxone suggests that opioids may be involved in the response.

Glibenclamide

Bullae and cholestasis have occurred together [12].

1 Beurey J, Jeandidier P, Bermont A. Les complications dermatologiques des traitements antidiabétiques. *Ann Derm Syphiligr (Paris)* 1966; **93**: 13−42.
2 Almeyda J, Baker H. Drug reactions. X. Adverse cutaneous reactions to hypoglycaemic agents. *Br J Dermatol* 1970; **82**: 634−6.
3 Harris EL. Adverse reactions to oral antidiabetic agents. *Br Med J* 1971; **3**: 29−30.
4 Hitselberger JF, Fosnaugh RP. Photosensitivity due to chlorpropamide. *JAMA* 1962; **180**: 62−3.

5 Yaffee HS. Stevens–Johnson syndrome caused by chlorpropamide: report of a case. *Arch Dermatol* 1960; **82**: 636–7.
6 Dinsdale RCW, Ormerod TP, Walker AE. Lichenoid eruption due to chlorpropamide. *Br Med J* 1968; **i**: 100.
7 Barnett JH, Barnett SM. Lichenoid drug reactions to chlorpropamide and tolazamide. *Cutis* 1984; **34**: 542–4.
8 Rothfeld EL, Goldman J, Goldberg HH, Einhorn S. Severe chlorpropamide toxicity. *JAMA* 1960; **172**: 54–6.
9 Zarowitz H, Newhouse S. Coproporphyrinuria with a cutaneous reaction induced by chlorpropamide. *N Y State J Med* 1965; **65**: 2385–7.
10 Stakosch CR, Jefferys DB, Keen H. Blockade of chlorpropamide alcohol flush by aspirin. *Lancet* 1980; **i**: 394–6.
11 Medback S, Wass JAH, Clement-Jones V, *et al*. Chlorpropamide alcohol flush and circulating met-enkephalin: a positive link. *Br Med J* 1981; **283**: 937–9.
12 Wongpaitoon V, Mills PR, Russell RI, Patrick RS. Intra-hepatic cholestasis and cutaneous bullae associated with glibenclamide therapy. *Postgrad Med J* 1981; **57**: 244–6.

17.2 Lipid lowering drugs

Acipimox

This nicotinic acid analogue causes less prostaglandin-mediated flushing and itching than nicotinic acid [1].

Clofibrate

Erythema multiforme and a variety of other erythematous rashes have been described [2].

Gemfibrozil

This lipid lowering drug has been associated with exacerbation of psoriasis [3].

1 Anonymous. Acipimox — a nicotinic acid analogue for hyperlipidaemia. *Drug Ther Bull* 1991; **29**: 57–9.
2 Murata Y, Tani M, Amano M. Erythema multiforme due to clofibrate. *J Am Acad Dermatol* 1988; **18**: 381–2.
3 Fisher DA, Elias PM, LeBoit PL. Exacerbation of psoriasis by the hypolipidemic agent, gemfibrozil. *Arch Dermatol* 1988; **124**: 854–5.

17.3 Drugs for gastrointestinal ulceration

Omeprazole

This proton pump inhibitor, indicated for gastric and duodenal ulceration and reflux oesophagitis, has been associated with diarrhoea, headache, and a variety of eruptions, including maculopapular rashes, angioedema, bullous eruption, erythema multiforme, photosensitivity, and exfoliative dermatitis [1,2].

1 Committee on Safety of Medicines. *Current Problems* 1991; **31**.
2 Langman MJS. Omeprazole. For resistant peptic ulcers and severe oesophageal reflux disease. *Br Med J* 1991; **303**: 481–2.

17.4 Laxatives

Side-effects of laxatives have been reviewed [1].

Danthron

A highly characteristic irritant erythema of the buttocks and thighs has been observed in patients who are partially incontinent. The erythema results from skin soiling by faecal matter containing a dithranol (anthralin)-like breakdown product [2].

Phenolphthalein

Fixed eruptions are well known [3,4]. Bullous erythema multiforme and a lupus-like reaction are documented.

1 Ruoff H-J. Unerwünschte Wirkungen und Wechselwirkungen von Abführmitteln. *Med Klin* 1980; **75**: 214−18.
2 Barth JH, Reshad H, Darley CR, Gibson JRA. A cutaneous complication of Dorbanex therapy. *Clin Exp Dermatol* 1984; **9**: 95−6.
3 Shelley WB, Schlappner OL, Heiss HB. Demonstration of intercellular immunofluorescence and epidermal hysteresis in bullous fixed drug eruption due to phenolphthalein. *Br J Dermatol* 1972; **6**: 118−25.
4 Wyatt E, Greaves M, Sondergaard J. Fixed drug eruption (phenolphthalein). Evidence for a blood-borne mediator. *Arch Dermatol* 1972; **106**: 671−3.

Chapter 18
Additives, Herbs, Homoeopathy and Naturopathy, and Environmental Chemicals

18.1 Food and drug additives

Dermatological complications of food and drug additives have been reviewed [1–11]; these substances have been implicated in the causation of urticaria [4–7], anaphylaxis, purpura and vasculitis [8–11]. However, a recent study suggested that common food additives are seldom if ever of significance in urticaria [11]. The necessity for double-blind placebo-controlled testing to substantiate alleged food additive allergy has been emphasized [12].

Colouring agents

Colourings in food and in medications, including some antihistamines, such as tartrazine, sunset yellow and other azo dyes, have been reported to cause urticaria [6,13,14] or vasculitis.

Flavouring agents

Aspartame

Aspartame, a synthetic dipeptide composed of aspartic acid and the methyl ester of phenylalanine used under the trade name of NutraSweet as a low-calorie artificial sweetener, has had relatively few adverse side-effects despite its widespread usage [15]. Cutaneous side-effects reported include urticaria, angioedema and other non-descript 'rashes' [16], granulomatous septal panniculitis [17], and lobular panniculitis [18]. However, in a recent study of patients with a history of aspartame sensitivity, it was not possible to identify any subject with a clearly reproducible adverse reaction [19].

Cyclamates

Cyclamates, used as sweeteners in soft drinks, have caused photosensitivity [20].

Quinine

Quinine in tonic water and other bitter drinks may cause fixed eruptions [21].

Preservatives

The food and drug preservative sodium benzoate has been associated with urticaria, angioedema, asthma, and rarely anaphylaxis [22]. Parabens used as a preservative may also cause urticaria [2,23]. Sulphites added as antioxidant preservatives may provoke urticaria, asthma, anaphylaxis and shock [24–27]. Intolerance due to meta-bisulphite as an antioxidant in a dental anaesthetic has led to angioedema; patch tests were positive [28]. Chronic urticaria was reproducibly exacerbated by the antioxidant food preservatives, butylated hydroxyanisole and butylated hydroxytoluene in two patients [12].

1 Levantine AJ, Almeyda J. Cutaneous reactions to food and drug additives. *Br J Dermatol* 1977; **91**: 359–62.
2 Simon RA. Adverse reactions to drug additives. *J Allergy Clin Immunol* 1984; **74**: 623–30.
3 Ruzicka T. Diagnostik von Nahrungsmittelallergien. *Hautarzt* 1987; **38**: 10–15.
4 Juhlin LG, Michäelsson G, Zetterström O. Urticaria and asthma induced by food-and-drug additives in patients with aspirin hypersensitivity. *J Allergy* 1972; **50**: 92–8.
5 Doeglas HMG. Reactions to aspirin and food additives in patients with chronic urticaria, including the physical urticarias. *Br J Dermatol* 1975; **93**: 135–44.
6 Supramaniam G, Warner JO. Artificial food additives intolerance in patients with angioedema and urticaria. *Lancet* 1986; **ii**: 907–9.
7 Juhlin L. Additives and chronic urticaria. *Ann Allergy* 1987; **59**: 119–23.
8 Michäelsson G, Petterson L, Juhlin L. Purpura caused by food and drug additives. *Arch Dermatol* 1974; **109**: 49–52.
9 Kubba R, Champion RI. Anaphylactoid purpura caused by tartrazine and benzoates. *Br J Dermatol* 1975; **93** Suppl 2: 61–2.
10 Eisenmann A, Ring J, von der Helm D, *et al.* Vasculitis allergica durch Nahrungsmittelallergie. *Hautarzt* 1988; **39**: 319–21.
11 Veien NK, Krogdahl A. Cutaneous vasculitis induced by food additives. *Acta Derm Venereol (Stockh)* 1991; **71**: 73–4.
12 Goodman DL, McDonnell JT, Nelson HS, *et al.* Chronic urticaria exacerbated by the antioxidant food preservatives, butylated hydroxyanisole (BHA) and butylated hydroxytoluene (BHT). *J Allergy Clin Immunol* 1990; **86**: 570–5.
13 Neuman I, Elian R, Nahum H, *et al.* The danger of 'yellow dyes' (tartrazine) to allergic subjects. *J Allergy* 1972; **50**: 92–8.
14 Miller K. Sensitivity to tartrazine. *Br Med J* 1982; **285**: 1597–8.
15 US Food and Drug Administration. Food additives permitted for direct addition to food for human consumption: aspartame. *Federal Register* 1983; **48**: 31 376–82.
16 Kulczycki A Jr. Aspartame-induced urticaria. *Ann Intern Med* 1986; **104**: 207–8.
17 Novick NL. Aspartame-induced granulomatous panniculitis. *Ann Intern Med* 1985; **102**: 206–7.
18 McCauliffe DP, Poitras K. Aspartame-induced lobular panniculitis. *J Am Acad Dermatol* 1991; **24**: 298–300.
19 Garriga MM, Berkebile C, Metcalfe DD. A combined single-blind, double-blind, placebo-controlled study to determine the reproducibility of hypersensitivity reactions to aspartame. *J Allergy Clin Immunol* 1991; **87**: 821–7.
20 Lambert SI. A new photosensitizer. The artificial sweetener cyclamate. *JAMA* 1967; **201**: 747–50.
21 Commens C. Fixed drug eruption. *Aust J Dermatol* 1983; **24**: 1–8.

22 Michils A, Vandermoten G, Duchateau J, Yernault J-C. Anaphylaxis with sodium benzoate. *Lancet* 1991; **337**: 1424−5.
23 Nagel JE, Fuscaldo JT, Fireman P. Paraben allergy. *JAMA* 1977; **237**: 1594−5.
24 Habenicht HA, Preuss L, Lovell RG. Sensitivity to ingested metabisulfites: cause of bronchospasm and urticaria. *Immunol Allergy Pract* 1983; **5**: 243−5.
25 Settipane GA. Adverse reactions to sulfites in drugs and foods. *J Am Acad Dermatol* 1984; **10**: 1077−80.
26 Twarog FJ, Leung DYM. Anaphylaxis to a component of isoetharine (sodium bisulfite). *JAMA* 1982; **248**: 2030−1.
27 Przybilla B, Ring J. Sulfit-Überempfindlichkeit. *Hautarzt* 1987; **38**: 445−8.
28 Dooms-Goosens A, Gidi de Alan A, Degreef H, Kochuyt A. Local anaesthetic intolerance due to metabisulfite. *Contact Dermatitis* 1989; **20**: 124−6.

Miscellaneous food additives

Agricultural or veterinary chemicals may leave residues in animal and plants used as human food, e.g. penicillin in milk, with resultant urticaria [1]. The exposure of a rural Turkish population to flour contaminated with hexachlorobenzene induced an outbreak of cutaneous porphyria [2]. Contaminated rapeseed cooking oil containing acetanilide resulted in the Spanish 'toxic oil syndrome'; the central feature of the illness was a toxic pneumonitis, but fixed rashes and scleroderma-like changes in survivors were seen [3−5]. Outbreaks of atypical erythema multiforme and other exanthemata in Holland were attributed to an additive in margarine [6,7]. The high arsenic content of a rural water supply in Taiwan caused arsenism [8]. Chemicals added to tobacco, e.g. menthol in cigarettes, have caused urticaria [9]. N-Nitroso compounds, which are known to be carcinogenic in animals, occur in food products and certain alcoholic drinks, but there is no direct proof as yet of a causal role in human disease [10].

1 Boonk WJ, Van Ketel WG. The role of penicillin in the pathogenesis of chronic urticaria. *Br J Dermatol* 1982; **106**: 183−90.
2 Peters HA, Gocmen A, Cripps DJ, *et al.* Epidemiology of hexachlorobenzene-induced porphyria in Turkey. *Arch Neurol* 1982; **39**: 744−9.
3 Martinez-Tello FJ, Navas-Palacios JJ, Ricoy JR, *et al.* Pathology of a new toxic syndrome caused by ingestion of adulterated oil in Spain. *Virchows Arch [Path Anat]* 1982; **397**: 261−85.
4 Leading Article. Toxic oil syndrome. *Lancet* 1983; **i**: 1257−8.
5 Rush PJ, Bell MJ, Fam AG. Toxic oil syndrome (Spanish oil disease) and chemically induced scleroderma-like conditions. *J Rheumatol* 1984; **11**: 262−4.
6 Sternberg TH, Bierman SM. Unique syndromes involving the skin induced by drugs, food additives, and environmental contaminants. *Arch Dermatol* 1963; **88**: 779−88.
7 Mali JW, Malten KE. The epidemic of polymorph toxic erythema in the Netherlands in 1960. The so-called margarine disease. *Acta Derm Venereol (Stockh)* 1966; **46**: 123−35.
8 Yeh S. Skin cancer in chronic arsenicism. *Hum Pathol* 1973; **4**: 469−85.
9 McGowan EM. Menthol urticaria. *Arch Dermatol* 1966; **94**: 62−3.
10 Tannenbaum SR. N-nitroso compounds: a perspective on human exposure. *Lancet* 1983; **i**: 628−30.

18.2 Herbal remedies, homoeopathy and naturopathy

Chinese herbal medicine

A 'tea' prepared from a decoction of herbs has been reported to be of benefit in eczema [1−3]. The decoction contains paenol (2'-hydroxy−4'-methoxyacetophenone), which is known to have platelet anti-aggregatory, analgesic, and antipyretic properties [4]. However, hepatotoxicity was described in a 9-year-old girl who consumed a Chinese herbal tea for 6 months [5] and has been reported in a further patient [6]. It has been suggested that such therapy may have immunosuppressive properties, based on the temporal association of recurrent herpes simplex with treatment in a single patient [7]. However, it has been pointed out that this association may have been simply fortuitous [8].

1 Harper JI. Chinese herbs for eczema. *Lancet* 1990; **336**: 177.
2 Atherton D, Sheehan M, Rustin MHA, *et al*. Chinese herbs for eczema. *Lancet* 1990; **336**: 1254.
3 Sheehan MP, Atherton DJ, Luo HD. Controlled trial of traditional Chinese medicinal plants in widespread non-exudative atopic eczema (Abstr). *Br J Dermatol* 1991; **125** (Suppl 38): 17.
4 Galloway JH, Marsh ID, Bittiner SB, *et al*. Chinese herbs for eczema, the active compound? *Lancet* 1991; **337**: 566.
5 Davies EG, Pollock I, Steel HM. Chinese herbs for eczema. *Lancet* 1990; **336**: 177.
6 Carlsson C. Herbs and hepatitis. *Lancet* 1990; **336**: 1068.
7 Russell Jones R. Recurrent facial herpes associated with Chinese herbal remedy. *Lancet* 1991; **338**: 55.
8 Atherton D, Sheehan MP, Rustin M. Traditional Chinese plants for eczema. *Lancet* 1991; **338**: 510.

Homoeopathic drugs

So-called natural products and homoeopathic preparations may not be as benign as imagined. Cases of erythroderma, confluent urticaria, and anaphylaxis have been reported following homoeopathic medication [1].

1 Aberer W, Strohal R. Homoeopathic preparations — severe adverse effects, unproven benefits. *Dermatologica* 1991; **182**: 253.

Naturopathy

Bizarre and unpredictable cutaneous reactions may follow topical application or ingestion of naturally occurring substances. As an example, we have seen a curious gyrate erythematous eruption in a patient following local application of onion rings as a home remedy for arthralgia (Fig. 18.1). Substantial amounts of psoralen may be absorbed from vegetables; a patient who consumed a large quantity of celery root (*Apium graveolens*) 1 hour before a visit to a suntan parlour developed a severe generalized phototoxic reaction [1].

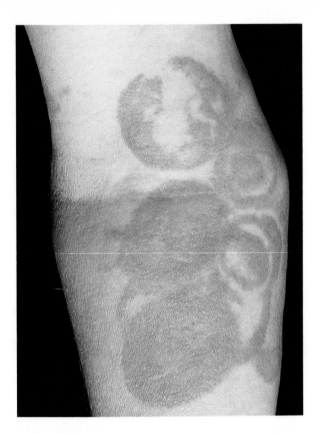

Figure 18.1 Unusual localized gyrate toxic erythema following application of onion rings for arthralgia of the elbow.

Phototoxicity has been reported from herbal remedies for vitiligo containing powdered seeds of *Psoralea corylifolia*, which contains psoralen, isopsoralen and psoralidin [2].

1 Ljunggren B. Severe phototoxic burn following celery ingestion. *Arch Dermatol* 1990; **126**: 1334–6.
2 Maurice PDL, Cream JJ. The dangers of herbalism. *Br Med J* 1989; **299**: 1204.

Miscellaneous over-the-counter preparations

Canthaxanthin, a synthetic non-provitamin A carotenoid deposited in epidermis and subcutaneous fat, caused fatal aplastic anaemia when ingested to promote tanning [1].

1 Bluhm R, Branch R, Johnston P, Stein R. Aplastic anemia associated with canthaxanthin ingested for 'tanning' purposes. *JAMA* 1990; **264**: 1141–2.

18.3 Industrial and other exposure to chemicals

The reader is referred to section 3.25 (p. 121), for discussion of sclerodermatous reactions to environmental agents. A form of fluoride toxicity occurred due to industrial poisoning in the Italian town of Chizzolo, resulting in pinkish-brown round or oval macules seen in hundreds of the local population [1]. Similar small outbreaks have occurred in North America [2]. Exfoliative dermatitis has been recorded with trichloroethylene [3]. Occupational exposure to trichloroethylene has also caused Stevens—Johnson syndrome [4].

Patients exposed to dioxin after an industrial accident at Seveso, Italy, developed early irritative lesions, comprising erythema and oedema of exposed areas, vesicobullous and necrotic lesions of the palms and fingertips, and papulonodular lesions; later lesions were those of chloracne [5]. Contamination of rice-bran cooking oil with polychlorinated biphenyls in Taiwan resulted in chloracne, and congenital abnormalities in offspring [6].

Pruritus, urticaria, and discoid and diffuse eczema may occur following the use of brominated disinfectant compounds such as 1-bromo-3-chlor-5,5-dimethyl hydantoin (Di-halo, Aquabrome) in public swimming pools [7]. Accidental occupational exposure to high concentrations of methyl bromide during a fumigation procedure resulted in erythema with multiple vesicles and large bullae, with predilection for moist flexures and pressure areas [8]. Idiopathic thrombocytopenic purpura has been associated with industrial exposure to wood preservatives [9], turpentine [10], and to insecticides such as chlordane and heptachlor [11].

1 Waldbott GC, Cecilioni VA. 'Chizzolo' maculae. *Cutis* 1970; **6**: 331—4.
2 Tabuenca JM. Toxic-allergic syndrome caused by ingestion of rapeseed oil denatured with aniline. *Lancet* 1981; **ii**: 567—8.
3 Nakayama H, Kobayashi M, Takahashi M, *et al*. Generalized eruption with severe liver dysfunction associated with occupational exposure to trichloroethylene. *Contact Dermatitis* 1988; **19**: 48—51.
4 Phoon WH, Chan MOY, Rahan VS, *et al*. Stevens—Johnson syndrome associated with occupational exposure to trichloroethylene. *Contact Dermatitis* 1984; **10**: 270—6.
5 Caputo R, Monti M, Ermacora E, *et al*. Cutaneous manifestations of tetrachlorodibenzo-*p*-dioxin in children and adolescents. *J Am Acad Dermatol* 1988; **19**: 812—19.
6 Gladen BC, Taylor JS, Wu Y-C, *et al*. Dermatological findings in children exposed transplacentally to heat-degraded polychlorinated biphenyls in Taiwan. *Br J Dermatol* 1990; **122**: 799—808.
7 Rycroft RJG, Penny PT. Dermatoses associated with brominated swimming pools. *Br Med J* 1983; **28**: 462.
8 Hezemans-Boer M, Toonstra J, Meulenbelt J, *et al*. Skin lesions due to exposure to methyl bromide. *Arch Dermatol* 1988; **124**: 917—21.
9 Hay A, Singer CRJ. Wood preservatives, solvents, and thrombocytopenic purpura. *Lancet* 1991; **338**: 766.
10 Wahlberg P, Nyman D. Turpentine and thrombocytopenic purpura. *Lancet* 1969; **ii**: 215—16.
11 Epstein SS, Ozonoff D. Leukemias and blood dyscrasias following exposure to chloradone and heptachlor. *Carcinogenesis Mutagenesis Teratogenesis* 1987; **7**: 527—40.

Chapter 19
Local and Systemic Effects of Topical Applications

Allergic contact dermatitis will not be discussed here. Many topical therapeutic agents may cause serious or even dangerous systemic side-effects if absorbed in sufficient quantity; such absorption may be facilitated through diseased skin, and with use of newer vehicles or occlusive polythene dressings. The risk of serious systemic effects is greatest in infancy and in the old and frail. The quantity absorbed in relation to body weight is greatest in infancy, when the surface area is relatively greater; moreover, neonatal skin is more permeable. Most dangerous or fatal reactions have occurred either because the physician was unaware of the potential hazard or because the patient has continued self-treatment without medical supervision.

Topical therapy

Anthralin (dithranol)

Topical anthralin used in the therapy of stable plaque psoriasis is well known to cause erythema, irritation and a sensation of burning in normal skin; it stains the skin and clothing [1]. Application of 10% triethanolamine following short contact dithranol treatment has been reported to inhibit the anthralin-induced inflammation without preventing the therapeutic effect [2]. Allergic contact dermatitis to anthralin is very rare. The natural and synthetic anthranols have toxic effects on liver, intestines and the central nervous system, but systemic toxicity in humans under therapeutic conditions has not been established [3].

1 Paramsothy Y, Lawrence CM. Time course and intensity of anthralin inflammation on involved and uninvolved psoriatic skin. *Br J Dermatol* 1987; **116**: 517−19.
2 Ramsay B, Lawrence CM, Bruce JM, Shuster S. The effect of triethanolamine application on anthralin-induced inflammation and therapeutic effect in psoriasis. *J Am Acad Dermatol* 1990; **23**: 73−6.
3 Ippen H. Basic questions on toxicology and pharmacology of anthralin. *Br J Dermatol* 1981; **105** (Suppl 20): 72−6.

Boric acid

Poisoning has usually occurred in infants treated for napkin eruptions. Almost all cases have been caused by the use of boric ointments or lotions. However, use of borated talc proved fatal in one infant [1]. Wet boric dressings caused the death of an adult woman [2].

1 Brooke C, Boggs T. Boric-acid poisoning: report of a case and review of the literature. *Am J Dis Child* 1951; **82**: 465−72.
2 Jordan JW, Crissey JT. Boric acid poisoning: report of fatal adult case from cutaneous use. A critical evaluation of this drug in dermatologic practice. *Arch Dermatol* 1957; **75**: 720−8.

Calcipotriol

This vitamin D_3 analogue has been reported to cause transient local irritation, and facial or perioral dermatitis [1]. Topical application of calcipotriol for 5 weeks to a mean of 16% of the body surface of psoriatics did not result in detectable systemic alteration of calcium metabolism [2]. The manufacturer's data sheet (Leo Laboratories) states that increased serum calcium may occur with application in daily doses of 50−100 g of the 50 µg/g ointment. Severe symptomatic hypercalcaemia developed after application of about 200 g of the ointment over 1 week to exfoliative psoriasis covering 40% of the body surface [3]. It is recommended that treatment be confined to stable mild to moderate psoriasis, and that the recommended dose of 100 g weekly should not be exceeded.

1 Kragballe K, Gjertsen BT, De Hoop D, *et al.* Double-blind, right/left comparison of calcipotriol and betamethasone valerate in treatment of psoriasis vulgaris. *Lancet* 1991; **337**: 193−6.
2 Saurat J-H, Gumowski Sunek D, Rizzoli R. Topical calcipotriol and hypercalcaemia. *Lancet* 1991; **337**: 1287.
3 Dwyer C, Chapman RS. Calcipotriol and hypercalcaemia. *Lancet* 1991; **338**: 764−5.

Chlorhexidine gluconate (Hibitane)

Urticaria, dyspnoea and anaphylactic shock have occurred following topical application as a disinfectant [1], as have contact urticaria, photosensitive dermatitis [2] and deafness.

1 Okano M, Nomura M, Hata S, *et al.* Anaphylactic symptoms due to chlorhexidine gluconate. *Arch Dermatol* 1989; **125**: 50−2.
2 Wahlberg JE, Wennersten G. Hypersensitivity and photosensitivity to chlorhexidine. *Dermatologica* 1971; **143**: 376−9.

Dequalinium chloride

Necrotic lesions have occurred following its use in the treatment of balanitis [1].

1 Coles RB, Simpson WT, Wilkinson DS. Dequalinium: a possible complication of its use in balanitis. *Lancet* 1964; **ii**: 531.

Dimethyl sulphoxide

Topical application can cause erythema, pruritus, and urticaria, but systemic reactions are very rare; a generalized contact dermatitis-like reaction followed intravesical installation in a sensitized individual [1].

1 Nishimura M, Takano Y, Toshitani Y. Systemic contact dermatitis medicamentosa occurring after intravesical dimethyl sulfoxide treatment for interstitial cystitis. *Arch Dermatol* 1988; **124**: 182–3.

Formaldehyde

Industrial exposure is recognized to be a health hazard, and a threshold limit value of 2 p.p.m. is allowed in the UK and the US [1]. Irritant or allergic dermatitis is common in exposed workers [2]. Systemic symptoms including breathlessness, headache and drowsiness have been attributed to prolonged exposure to very low levels in the home [3].

1 Leading Article. The health hazards of formaldehyde. *Lancet* 1981; **i**: 926–7.
2 Glass WI. An outbreak of formaldehyde dermatitis. *N Z Med J* 1961; **60**: 423.
3 Harris JC, Rumack BH, Aldrich FD. Toxicology of urea formaldehyde and polyurethane foam insulation. *JAMA* 1981; **245**: 243–6.

Gamma-benzene hexachloride (lindane)

Lindane has become established as the standard therapy for scabies because of its efficacy and cosmetic acceptability. However, its potential toxicity includes neurotoxicity with convulsions, especially in children [1–7]. Most reports have occurred with overexposure or misuse, but side-effects have followed single applications, particularly when the epidermal barrier has been compromised. Whether this constitutes a significant problem in normal individuals is doubtful [6]. Nevertheless, it has been suggested that permethrin may be a safer and less toxic alternative [8].

1 Lee B, Groth P. Scabies: transcutaneous poisoning during treatment. *Arch Dermatol* 1979; **115**: 124–5.
2 Pramanik AK, Hansen RC. Transcutaneous gamma benzene hexachloride absorption and toxicity in infants and children. *Arch Dermatol* 1979; **115**: 124–5.
3 Matsuoka LY. Convulsions following application of gamma benzene hexachloride. *J Am Acad Dermatol* 1981; **5**: 98–9.
4 Rasmussen JE. The problem of lindane. *J Am Acad Dermatol* 1981; **5**: 507–16.
5 Davies JE, Dehdia HV, Morgade C, *et al*. Lindane poisonings. *Arch Dermatol* 1983; **119**: 142–4.
6 Rasmussen J. Lindane: A prudent approach. *Arch Dermatol* 1987; **123**: 1008–10.
7 Friedman SJ. Lindane neurotoxic reaction in nonbullous ichthyosiform erythroderma. *Arch Dermatol* 1987; **123**: 1056–8.
8 Schultz MW, Gomez M, Hansen RC, *et al*. Comparative study of 5% permethrin cream and 1% lindane lotion for the treatment of scabies. *Arch Dermatol* 1990; **126**: 167–70.

Hexachlorophane

This substance has potential neurotoxicity. Exposure of babies to a talc containing 6.3% of hexachlorophane due to a manufacturing error resulted in deaths with ulceration, skin lesions and a characteristic demyelinating encephalopathy [1]. A 3% emulsion has produced milder neurological changes but a 0.33% concentration in talc is apparently safe. Encephalopathy has occurred in burns patients [2].

1 Martin-Bouyer G, Lebreton R, Toga M, *et al*. Outbreak of accidental hexachlorophene poisoning in France. *Lancet* 1982; **i**: 91—5.
2 Larson DL. Studies show hexachlorophene causes burn syndrome. *J Am Hosp Assoc* 1968; **42**: 63—4.

Hydroquinone

Depigmenting creams containing 6—8% of hydroquinone, used by black South African women, have caused rebound hyperpigmentation and coarsening of the skin, with ochronotic changes in the dermis, colloid degeneration and colloid milium [1,2]. Collagen degeneration may be seen histologically [2]. Similar changes have been seen in black women in the US [3] and in a Mexican—American woman [4]. Interestingly, ochronosis does not develop in areas of vitiligo [5]. The nails may be pigmented [6].

1 Findlay GH, Morrison JGL, Simson IW. Exogenous ochronosis and pigmented colloid milium from hydroquinone bleaching creams. *Br J Dermatol* 1975; **93**: 613—22.
2 Phillips JI, Isaacson C, Carman H. Ochronosis in Black South Africans who used skin lighteners. *Am J Dermatopathol* 1986; **8**: 14—21.
3 Lawrence N, Bligard CA, Reed R, Perret WJ. Exogenous ochronosis in the United States. *J Am Acad Dermatol* 1988; **18**: 1207—11.
4 Howard KL, Furner BB. Exogenous ochronosis in a Mexican—American woman. *Cutis* 1990; **45**: 180—2.
5 Hull PR, Procter PR. The melanocyte: An essential link in hydroquinone-induced ochronosis. *J Am Acad Dermatol* 1990; **22**: 529—31.
6 Garcia RL, White JW, Willis WF. Hydroquinone nail pigmentation. *Arch Dermatol* 1978; **114**: 1402—3.

Lead lotions

The use of continued wet dressings of lead subacetate in the treatment of exfoliative dermatitis caused lead poisoning with punctate basophilia and an elevated urinary lead level [1].

1 Kennedy CC, Lynas HA. Lead poisoning by cutaneous absorption from lead dressings. *Lancet* 1949; **i**: 650—2.

Mercury

Poisoning is now fortunately rare, but was seen from continued application of large amounts of a topical application, as for psoriasis

[1,2]. Idiosyncratic poisoning after much smaller doses is also recognized [3]. Intoxication has followed the use of a mercury dusting powder [4] and poisoning of a suckling infant has followed the use of perchloride of mercury lotion for cracked nipples [5]. Fever, a generalized morbilliform rash, and oedema of the extremities have been the usual clinical features. Exfoliative dermatitis and encephalopathy have developed; permanent damage to the renal tubules is manifest as persistent albuminuria or frank nephrotic syndrome [6]. Rarely, gross symptoms, such as loose teeth [7], swollen bleeding gums and weight loss may be observed.

Application of a mercury-containing cream to the face over many years can produce slate-grey pigmentation, especially on the eyelids, nasolabial folds and neck folds (exogenous ochronosis) (Fig. 19.1) [8–10]; mercury granules lie free in the dermis or within macrophages [11]. Mercury is a moderate sensitizer and leads to contact sensitivity.

1 Inman PM, Gordon B, Trinder P. Mercury absorption and psoriasis. *Br Med J* 1956; **ii**: 1202–6.
2 Young E. Ammoniated mercury poisoning. *Br J Dermatol* 1960; **72**: 449–55.
3 Williams BH, Beach WC. Idiosyncrasy to ammoniated mercury: Treatment with 2,3-dimercapto-propanol (BAL). *JAMA* 1950; **142**: 1286–8.
4 MacGregor ME, Rayner PHW. Pink disease and primary renal tubular acidosis: a common cause. *Lancet* 1964; **ii**: 1083–5.
5 Hunt GM. Mercury poisoning in infancy. *Br Med J* 1966; **i**: 1482.
6 Silverberg DS, McCall JT, Hunt JC. Nephrotic syndrome with use of ammoniated mercury. *Arch Intern Med* 1967; **20**: 581–6.
7 Bourgeois M, Dooms-Goossens A, Knockaert D, *et al.* Mercury intoxication after topical application of a metallic mercury ointment. *Dermatologica* 1986; **172**: 48–51.
8 Lamar LM, Bliss BO. Localized pigmentation of the skin due to topical mercury. *Arch Dermatol* 1966; **93**: 450–3.
9 Prigent F, Cohen J, Civatte J. Pigmentation des paupieres probablement secondaire a l'application prolongée d'une pomade ophtalmologique contenant du mercure. *Ann Dermatol Vénéréol (Paris)* 1986; **113**: 357–8.

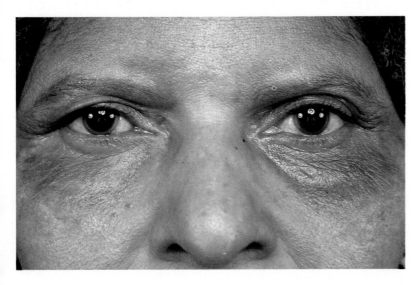

Figure 19.1 Exogenous ochronosis with peri-ocular pigmentation related to use of a mercury-containing cream. (Courtesy of St John's Institute of Dermatology, London.)

10 Aberer W. Topical mercury should be banned — dangerous, outmoded but still popular. *J Am Acad Dermatol* 1991; **24**: 150−1.
11 Burge KM, Winkelmann RK. Mercury pigmentation. An electron microscopic study. *Arch Dermatol* 1970; **102**: 51−61.

Methyl salicylate (oil of wintergreen)

Topical application of methyl salicylate and menthol as a rubifacient, with use of a heating pad, resulted in local skin necrosis and interstitial nephritis [1].

1 Heng MCY. Local necrosis and interstitial nephritis due to topical methyl salicylate and menthol. *Cutis* 1987; **39**: 442−4.

Minoxidil

Topical minoxidil, as used for male pattern alopecia, is associated with cutaneous problems in up to 10% of patients, with allergic contact dermatitis occurring in 3.7% of individuals [1].

1 Wilson C, Walkden V, Powell S, *et al*. Contact dermatitis in reaction to 2% topical minoxidil solution. *J Am Acad Dermatol* 1991; **24**: 661−2.

Neomycin

Deafness has rarely followed topical therapy, including administration of aerosol preparations containing neomycin in the treatment of extensive burns.

Phenol

Severe systemic reactions, such as abdominal pain, dizziness, haemoglobinuria, cyanosis and sometimes fatal coma have followed the application of phenol to extensive wounds. Accidental application of pure phenol to a small area of skin in an infant has proved fatal. The prolonged use of phenol as a dressing for a large ulcer may give rise to exogenous ochronosis, with darkening of the cornea and of the skin of face and hands.

Podophyllin

Excessive application may lead to severe local irritation (Fig. 19.2). There have been occasional reports of confusional states, coma, peripheral neuropathy, vomiting and even death following painting of this resin on large areas of genital warts, especially in pregnancy [1,2]. However, careful review of the reports suggests that in the majority the effects could not be attributed with certainty to podophyllin [1]. Animal experiments suggest teratogenicity; although teratogenicity is controversial in humans, the drug is best avoided in pregnancy.

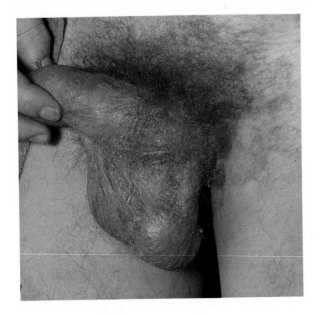

Figure 19.2 Marked irritant dermatitis following excessive self-medication with podophyllin.

1 Bargman H. Is podophyllin a safe drug to use and can it be used in pregnancy? *Arch Dermatol* 1988; **124**: 1718–20.
2 Sundharam JA, Bargman H. Is podophyllin safe for use in pregnancy? *Arch Dermatol* 1989; **125**: 1000–1.

Resorcinol

Acute resorcinol poisoning is very rare, but an ointment containing 12.5% resorcinol applied to the napkin area produced dusky cyanosis, a maculopapular eruption, haemolytic anaemia and haemoglobinuria in an infant [1]. The continued application to large leg ulcers of ointments containing resorcinol has caused myxoedema and widespread blue–grey pigmentation mimicking ochronosis [2].

1 Cunningham AA. Resorcin poisoning. *Arch Dis Child* 1956; **31**: 173–6.
2 Thomas AE, Gisburn MA. Exogenous ochronosis and myxoedema from resorcinol. *Br J Dermatol* 1961; **73**: 378–81.

Salicylic acid and salicylates

The frequent application of salicylic acid ointments to extensive lesions will produce symptoms of salicylism even in adults [1–6]. Most cases of poisoning have occurred in children with psoriasis or ichthyosis [1,2]; fatal cases have been recorded [4]. Drowsiness and delusions are followed by acidosis, coma and death from respiratory failure.

1 Young CJ. Salicylate intoxication from cutaneous absorption of salicylate acid: review of the literature and report of a case. *South Med J* 1952; **45**: 1075–7.
2 Cawley EP, Peterson NT, Wheeler CE. Salicylic acid poisoning in dermatological therapy. *JAMA* 1953; **151**: 372–4.

[357]

3 Von Weiss JF, Lever WF. Percutaneous salicylic acid intoxication in psoriasis. *Arch Dermatol* 1964; **90**: 614–19.
4 Lindsey LP. Two cases of fatal salicylate poisoning after topical application of an anti-fungal solution. *Med J Aust* 1969; **1**: 353–4.
5 Davies MG, Vella Briffa D, Greaves MW. Systemic toxicity from topically applied salicylic acid. *Br Med J* 1979; **i**: 661.
6 Anderson JAR, Ead RD. Percutaneous salicylate poisoning. *Clin Exp Dermatol* 1979; **4**: 349–51.

Silver sulphadiazine

Topical application has caused hyperpigmentation [1].

1 Dupuis LL, Shear NH, Zucker RM. Hyperpigmentation due to topical application of silver sulfadiazine cream. *J Am Acad Dermatol* 1985; **12**: 1112–14.

Topical isotretinoin

Plasma concentrations of isotretinoin and its metabolites were not measurable after topical application, and no systemic adverse reactions were reported [1].

1 Jensen BK, McGann LA, Kachevsky V, Franz TJ. The negligible systemic availability of retinoids with multiple and excessive topical application of isotretinoin 0.05% gel (Isotrex) in patients with acne vulgaris. *J Am Acad Dermatol* 1991; **24**: 425–8.

Tretinoin

Topical tretinoin, used for the management of photo-aged skin, may cause erythema, peeling, burning and itching of the skin within days [1,2]. Pink discoloration without other signs may also develop, as may inflammation in solar keratoses.

1 Weiss JS, Ellis CN, Headington JT, *et al*. Topical tretinoin improves photoaged skin: a double-blind, vehicle-controlled study. *JAMA* 1988; **259**: 527–32.
2 Weinstein GD, Nigra TP, Pochi PE, *et al*. Topical tretinoin for treatment of photodamaged skin. *Arch Dermatol* 1991; **127**: 659–65.

Vitamin E

Vitamin E in deodorants has caused contact dermatitis [1].

1 Minkin W, Cohen HJ, Frank SB. Contact dermatitis from deodorants. *Arch Dermatol* 1973; **107**: 774–5.

Warfarin

An epidemic of haemorrhagic disease with fatalities occurred due to warfarin-contaminated talcs [1]. Poisoning has also been attributed to preparation of rodent baits [2].

1 Martin-Bouyer G, Linh PD, Tuan LC, *et al.* Epidemic of haemorrhagic disease in Vietnamese infants caused by warfarin-contaminated talcs. *Lancet* 1983; i: 230–2.
2 Fristedt B, Sterner N. Warfarin intoxication from percutaneous absorption. *Arch Environ Health* 1965; **11**: 205–8.

Transdermal drug delivery systems

Transdermal delivery systems are available for clonidine, oestradiol, nitroglycerine, and scopolamine, and systems for other drugs are being developed. Erythema, irritancy, and contact sensitization are not uncommon; the occlusive element may lead to miliaria rubra [1]. Allergic skin reactions occur in up to 50% of patients with clonidine; with nitroglycerin, scopolamine, oestradiol and testosterone reactions are much less frequent [2]. Reactivation of an area of contact dermatitis may develop via oral medication rarely [2].

1 Hogan DJ, Maibach HI. Adverse dermatologic reactions to transdermal drug delivery systems. *J Am Acad Dermatol* 1990; **22**: 811–14.
2 Holdiness MR. A review of contact dermatitis associated with transdermal therapeutic systems. *Contact Dermatitis* 1989; **20**: 3–9.

Part 4
The Management of
Drug Reactions

Chapter 20
Diagnosis

20.1 General principles

Drug reactions, apart from fixed drug eruption, have non-specific clinical features, and it is often impossible to identify the offending chemical with certainty, especially when a patient with a suspected reaction is receiving many drugs simultaneously. Drug reactions may be mistaken for naturally occurring conditions, and may therefore be overlooked. By the same token, it may on occasion be very difficult to state that a given eruption is drug-induced. Experience with the type of reaction most commonly caused by particular drugs may enable the range of suspects to be narrowed, but familiar drugs may occasionally produce unfamiliar reactions, and new drugs may mimic the reactions of the familiar. The assessment of a potential adverse drug reaction always necessitates taking a careful history, and may involve a trial of drug elimination, skin tests, *in vitro* tests, and challenge by re-exposure.

A drug reaction may first become evident after the offending medication has been stopped, and depot injections may have delayed effects. Interpretation of elimination tests should be tempered by the knowledge that drug reactions may take weeks to settle. *In vivo* and *in vitro* tests are only applicable to truly allergic reactions. Skin tests, including prick and intradermal testing, and patch testing, are for the most part unreliable, even when apparently appropriate antigens are used; they may be hazardous [1]. *In vitro* tests are not widely available and are essentially research tools at the moment.

All too frequently, therefore, the diagnosis is no more than an assessment of probability. That major disagreements occurred between clinical pharmacologists asked to assess the likelihood of adverse drug reaction in two series [2,3] confirms that identification of a responsible drug is often a subjective judgement. An algorithm providing detailed criteria for ranking the probability of whether a given drug is responsible for a reaction, based on (i) previous experience, (ii) the alternative aetiologic candidates, (iii) timing of events, (iv) drug level and (v) the results of drug withdrawal and rechallenge, has been reported [4,5]. A number of other algorithms have been developed to assist in the diagnosis of which drug, if any, is the cause of a given eruption [6−9]. The difficulties inherent in the diagnosis of drug reactions have been reviewed [10,11].

1 Bruynzeel D, van Ketel W. Skin tests in the diagnosis of maculopapular drug eruptions. *Semin Dermatol* 1987; **6**: 119–24.

2 Karch FE, Smith CL, Kerzner B, *et al*. Adverse drug reactions — a matter of opinion. *Clin Pharmacol Ther* 1976; **19**: 489–92.

3 Koch-Weser J, Sellers EM, Zacest R. The ambiguity of adverse drug reactions. *Eur J Clin Pharmacol* 1977; **11**: 75–8.

4 Kramer MS, Leventhal JM, Hutchinson TA, Feinstein AR. An algorithm for the operational assessment of adverse drug reactions. I. Background, description, and instructions for use. *JAMA* 1979; **242**: 623–32.

5 Leventhal JM, Hutchinson TA, Kramer MS, Feinstein AR. An algorithm for the operational assessment of adverse drug reactions. III. Results of tests among clinicians. *JAMA* 1979; **242**: 1991–4.

6 Naranjo CA, Busto U, Sellers EM, *et al*. A method for estimating the probability of adverse drug reactions. *Clin Pharmacol Ther* 1981; **27**: 239–45.

7 Louick C, Lacouture P, Mitchell A, *et al*. A study of adverse reaction algorithms in a drug surveillance program. *Clin Pharmacol Ther* 1985; **38**: 183–7.

8 Pere J, Begaud B, Haramburu F, Albin H. Computerized comparison of six adverse drug reaction assessment procedures. *Clin Pharmacol Ther* 1986; **40**: 451–61.

9 Ghajar BM, Lanctôt KL, Shear NH, Naranjo CA. Bayesian differential diagnosis of a cutaneous reaction associated with the administration of sulfonamides. *Semin Dermatol* 1989; **8**: 213–18.

10 Ring J. Diagnostik von Arzneimittel-bedingten Unverträglichkeitsreaktionen. *Hautarzt* 1987; **38**: S16–S22.

11 Shear NH. Diagnosing cutaneous adverse reactions to drugs. *Arch Dermatol* 1990; **126**: 94–7.

20.2 Drug history

Patients should be questioned specifically about laxatives, oral contraceptives, vaccines, homoeopathic medicines, etc., as these may not be volunteered as medications, and should be asked when they last took a tablet for any reason. The history should include information on when each drug was first taken relative to the onset of the reaction, whether the same or a related drug has been administered previously, and whether there is a prior history of drug sensitivity or contact dermatitis. Allergic drug reactions do not usually develop for at least 4 days, and more commonly 7–10 days, after initial drug administration in a previously unsensitized individual. However, this time relationship cannot be relied on to differentiate between allergic and non-allergic reactions, since a previous sensitizing exposure may not have produced a clinically evident reaction.

20.3 Drug elimination

Resolution of a reaction on withdrawal of a drug is supportive incriminatory evidence but not diagnostic. Failure of a rash to subside on drug withdrawal does not necessarily exonerate it, since traces of the drug may persist for long periods, and some reactions, once initiated, continue for many days without re-exposure to the drug. The unwitting substitution of a drug which is chemically closely related may perpetuate a reaction, as when an antihistamine of phenothiazine structure is prescribed to alleviate the symptoms of a reaction caused by another phenothiazine. Elimination diets have been advocated for diagnosis of food additive intolerance leading to urticaria [1,2].

1 Rudzki E, Czubalski K, Grzywa Z. Detection of urticaria with food additives intolerance by means of diet. *Dermatologica* 1980; **161**: 57–62.
2 Metcalfe DD, Sampson HA (eds). Workshop on experimental methodology for clinical studies of adverse reactions to foods and food additives. *J Allergy Clin Immunol* 1990; **86** (Suppl): 421–42.

20.4 Skin testing

Skin testing, including prick testing and intradermal testing, may be useful in the identification of patients who present with immediate hypersensitivity reactions and are sensitive to one of a number of drugs, including penicillin and other β-lactam antibiotics, agents used in general anaesthesia, tetanus toxoid, streptokinase, chymopapain, heterologous sera, or insulin, and may thus aid in the prevention of anaphylaxis [1]. The results of skin test reactions, including intradermal testing and patch testing, were evaluated in 242 patients with delayed type (non-immediate) drug eruptions [2]. Intradermal testing was positive in 89.7% of patients, and patch tests were positive in 31.5% of cases; overall, 62% of patients had either a positive intradermal or patch test. Intradermal testing was more frequently positive in maculopapular rashes, erythema multiforme, and erythrodermic rashes than in eczematous reactions, whereas positive patch tests were comparatively frequent in erythroderma, eczematous reactions and anticonvulsant-induced reactions. It was concluded that a combination of patch testing and intradermal testing is useful in the demonstration of causative agents in delayed type drug eruptions [2]. Unfortunately, the usefulness of this approach is limited, because the significant antigenic determinants are unknown for most drugs [1]. Moreover, intradermal testing is not always safe. False negative skin testing may occur because of poor absorption through the skin, because a metabolite rather than the substance administered in the test is the sensitizing antigen, or because testing is performed either too soon after a reaction, in a refractory period, or too late, so that the patient no longer demonstrates skin test reactivity.

1 Sussman GL, Dolovich J. Prevention of anaphylaxis. *Semin Dermatol* 1989; **8**: 158–65.
2 Osawa J, Naito S, Aihara M, *et al.* Evaluation of skin test reactions in patients with non-immediate type drug eruptions. *J Dermatol (Tokyo)* 1990; **17**: 235–9.

Patch testing

Patch testing in drug eruptions may be helpful in identifying the drug responsible, especially in systemic contact-type dermatitis medicamentosa, in photosensitivity (photo-patch testing), or fixed drug reactions [1−4]. Positive patch tests have been found overall in about 15% of patients with drug eruptions [3,4] and 25% of patients with penicillin allergy [3−5]. Patients with fixed drug eruption may have positive patch tests to the causative agent [6]. In one series, local provocation in the form of patch testing at previously involved sites, but not in clinically normal skin, resulted in positive reactions in 18 of 24 patients with proven fixed drug eruptions to phenazone salicylate, a sulphonamide, doxycycline, trimethoprim, chlormezanone, a barbiturate, and carbamazepine [6]. The vehicle used as a diluent for the drug may be important in determining whether or not a reaction is seen [6]. However, most reports in the literature do not suggest that patch testing is helpful in fixed drug eruption [7]. Patch testing has supported a diagnosis of allergy, in the absence of topical sensitization, to diazepam, meprobamate and practolol [1], carbamazepine [8], tartrazine dyes [9], chloramphenicol [10], and in toxic epidermal necrolysis induced by ampicillin [11]. Antibiotics (especially penicillin, ampicillin, aminoglycosides), non-steroidal anti-inflammatory agents (pyrazolone derivatives, and occasionally aspirin), anticonvulsants (carbamazepine, hydantoin derivatives), neuroleptics (phenothiazines, barbiturates, meprobamate, benzodiazepines), β-blockers, gold salts, carbimazole, amantidine, corticosteroids, mitomycin C, heparin, and amide anaesthetics have all been associated with positive patch tests in allergic subjects [2]. However, care must be exercised, because anaphylactoid responses may occur even in response to the small amounts of drug absorbed from a patch test. Moreover, patch testing has produced exfoliative dermatitis in a sensitized patient [12]. A patch test with a solution of the drug will sometimes induce a generalized petechial reaction in patients with purpura caused by drug sensitivity, e.g. in carbromal or Sedormid purpura.

1 Felix RE, Comaish JS. The value of patch and other skin tests in drug eruptions. *Lancet* 1984; **i**: 1017−19.
2 Van Ketel WG. Immunological investigations in patients with drug-induced skin eruptions. *Arch Dermatol* 1984; **110**: 112−13.
3 Bruynzeel DP, van Ketel WG. Skin tests in the diagnosis of maculo-papular drug eruptions. *Semin Dermatol* 1987; **6**: 119−24.
4 Bruynzeel DP, van Ketel WG. Patch testing in drug eruptions. *Semin Dermatol* 1989; **8**: 196−203.
5 Bruynzeel DP, von Blomberg-van der Flier M, Scheper RJ, *et al*. Allergy for penicillin and the relevance of epicutaneous tests. *Dermatologica* 1985; **171**: 429−34.
6 Alanko K, Stubb S, Reitamo S. Topical provocation of fixed drug eruption. *Br J Dermatol* 1987; **116**: 561−7.
7 Sehgal VN, Gangwani OP. Fixed drug eruption. Current concepts. *Int J Dermatol* 1987; **26**: 67−74.
8 Houwerzijl J, de Gast GC, Nater JP. Patch test in drug eruptions. *Contact Dermatitis* 1982; **8**: 155−8.
9 Roeleveld CG, Van Ketel WG. Positive patch tests to the azo dye tartrazine. *Contact Dermatitis* 1976; **2**: 180.
10 Rudzki E, Grzywa Z, Maciejowska E. Drug reaction with positive patch tests to chloramphenicol. *Contact Dermatitis* 1976; **2**: 181.

11 Tagami H, Tatsuda K, Iwatski K, Yamada M. Delayed hypersensitivity in ampicillin-induced toxic epidermal necrolysis. *Arch Dermatol* 1983; **119**: 910–13.
12 Vaillant L, Camenen I, Lorette G. Patch testing with carbamazepine: reinduction of an exfoliative dermatitis. *Arch Dermatol* 1989; **125**: 299.

Penicillin and other β-lactam antibiotics

Potential usefulness of skin tests

For many patients with a history of an allergic reaction to penicillin or another β-lactam antibiotic, it is an easy matter to simply prescribe a drug from one of the several alternative non-cross-reacting antibiotic groups. However, sometimes the second-choice drugs used for patients suspected of penicillin allergy are clearly less effective, or less well tolerated, than the penicillins, as for example in syphilis in pregnancy [1]. The optimal therapy for these patients may then be avoided on the basis of a vague history of a possible adverse reaction to penicillin in the distant past. It is clearly important to identify those patients truly at risk of developing hypotensive episodes or fatal anaphylaxis, and skin testing could be helpful in this situation [1,2]. It has been reported that only 8–19% of patients with a history of penicillin allergy have a positive skin test reaction [3–5]. Accordingly, it has been claimed that approximately 80% of patients with a history of penicillin sensitivity do not react on comprehensive skin testing and could safely receive penicillin [2]. These figures may reflect not only a high incidence of wrongly diagnosed penicillin allergy, but also the fact that a considerable proportion of patients who have had proven allergic reactions to penicillins eventually stop producing the IgE antibody responsible.

Skin test antigens

Skin tests should be carried out using major determinant (benzylpenicilloyl polylysine, PPL) and minor determinant mixture (benzylpenicillin, benzylpenicilloate, and benzylpenilloate) antigens [6]. Procedures have been published, and the reader is referred to the original articles for details as to methodology [6,7]. Epicutaneous testing should precede intradermal testing, and positive (histamine or opiate) and negative (diluent) controls should be included. False negative results may be found after a systemic allergic reaction, as a result of a refractory period or temporary desensitization, so that skin testing should be postponed for at least 4–6 weeks [6].

Patients with a positive skin test reaction to penicillin often also have a positive reaction to other β-lactam antibiotics such as ampicillin (Fig. 20.1) and cephalosporins, e.g. cephalothin [5]. Evaluation of the skin test reactions in patients with delayed type rashes induced by penicillins and cephalosporins showed that, of those with positive oral provocation tests, 87% had positive intradermal skin test reactions [8]. These were either of Jones–Mote (cutaneous

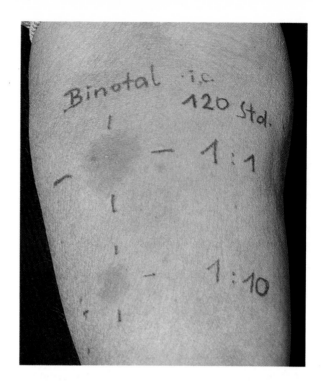

Figure 20.1 Positive intradermal tests to injection of ampicillin.

basophil hypersensitivity) type, with a peak reaction at 6–24 hours and consisting of erythema without induration, or of classical tuberculin reaction type with a peak at 48 hours. It should be appreciated that allergy to semisynthetic penicillins can occur without allergy to benzylpenicillin [9]. A case in which there was an isolated late skin test reaction at 2 hours to ampicillin only has been documented [10].

Results of skin testing

Patients treated with penicillin after a negative skin test to benzylpenicilloyl polylysine and to minor determinant mixture develop IgE-mediated reactions only very rarely, and these are almost always mild and self-limited [2]. Of patients with a history of penicillin allergy and a negative skin test, 1% develop an accelerated urticarial reaction, and 3% develop other mild reactions. Penicillin anaphylaxis has not been reported in skin test negative patients [2]. Thus, when adequately performed, negative skin tests indicate that the risk of a life-threatening reaction is almost negligible, and that any β-lactam antibiotic may be safely given. By contrast, the risk of an acute allergic reaction, including respiratory obstruction or hypotension, with a positive history and positive skin test is 50–70%; the risk in a patient with a negative history but a positive skin test is about 10% [2,6,11].

Intradermal testing is in general safe with few reactions, and does not appear to result in sensitization [3,6]. There is, however, a risk, albeit very small, of fatality from skin testing [12]. A more major problem with skin testing is that use of the major determinant, penicilloyl polylysine, alone misses about 10–25% of all positive subjects, and that even addition of benzylpenicillin G as the sole minor determinant antigen misses 5–10% of positive subjects [5,13,14]. This is significant because patients with reactivity to minor antigenic determinants are thought to be at a higher risk for anaphylaxis [6,15]. Moreover, minor determinant antigen mixture is not available commercially; mixtures of minor determinants are unstable [16]. Comprehensive skin testing is therefore only practicable in specialized centres. In addition, it has been recorded that skin tests can give both false positive and false negative reactions [17,18]. Thus it has been argued that a positive or negative result in an individual patient cannot be used to predict outcome. One group has suggested that equivocal skin test results are an indication for further testing by oral challenge [6].

Further difficulties are that skin tests have no predictive value in non-IgE-mediated reactions such as serum sickness, haemolytic anaemia, drug fever, interstitial nephritis, contact dermatitis, maculopapular exanthems, or exfoliative dermatitis; accelerated or late IgE-mediated reactions may occur despite a negative pretreatment skin test [2,6]. Skin testing is contraindicated where there is a history of exfoliative dermatitis or Stevens–Johnson syndrome. In routine practice, therefore, skin testing is held to be of limited value for penicillin allergy [19].

1 Wendel GD, Stark BJ, Jamison RB, *et al*. Penicillin allergy and desensitization in serious infections during pregnancy. *N Engl J Med* 1985; **312**: 1229–32.

2 Weiss ME, Adkinson NF. Immediate hypersensitivity reactions to penicillin and related antibiotics. *Clin Allergy* 1988; **18**: 515–40.

3 Mendelson LM, Ressler C, Rosen JP, Selcow JE. Routine elective penicillin allergy testing in children and adolescents: study of sensitization. *J Allergy Clin Immunol* 1984; **73**: 76–81.

4 Solley GO, Gleich GJ, VanDellen RG. Penicillin allergy: clinical experience with a battery of skin-test reagents. *J Allergy Clin Immunol* 1982; **69**: 238–44.

5 Sullivan TJ, Wedner HJ, Shatz GS, *et al*. Skin testing to detect penicillin allergy. *J Allergy Clin Immunol* 1981; **68**: 171–80.

6 Weber EA, Knight A. Testing for allergy to antibiotics. *Semin Dermatol* 1989; **8**: 204–12.

7 Adkinson NF Jr. Tests for immunoglobulin drug reactions. In Rose NF, Friedman H (eds) *Manual of Clinical Immunology*. American Society for Microbiology, Washington DC, 1986, pp 692–7.

8 Aihara M, Ikezawa Z. Evaluation of the skin test reactions in patients with delayed type rash induced by penicillins and cephalosporins. *J Dermatol (Tokyo)* 1987; **14**: 440–8.

9 Walley T, Coleman J. Allergy to penicillin. *Br Med J* 1991; **302**: 1462–3.

10 Dolovich J, Ruhno MB, Sauder MD, *et al*. Isolated late cutaneous skin test response to ampicillin: a distinct entity. *J Allergy Clin Immunol* 1988; **82**: 672–9.

11 Green GR, Rosenblum AH, Sweet LC. Evaluation of penicillin hypersensi-

tivity: value of clinical history and skin testing with penicilloyl-polylysine and penicillin G: a cooperative prospective study of the penicillin study group of the American Academy of Allergy. *J Allergy Clin Immunol* 1977; **60**: 339–45.

12 Dogliotti M. An instance of fatal reaction to the penicillin scratch test. *Dermatologica* 1968; **136**: 489–96.

13 Gorevic PD, Levine BB. Desensitization of anaphylactic hypersensitivity specific for the penicilloate minor determinant of penicillin and carbenicillin. *J Allergy Clin Immunol* 1981; **68**: 267–72.

14 Sogn DD. Penicillin allergy. *J Allergy Clin Immunol* 1984; **74**: 589–93.

15 Adkinson NF Jr. Risk factors for drug allergy. *J Allergy Clin Immunol* 1984; **74**: 567–72.

16 Saxon A, Bell GN, Rohr AS, Adelman DC. Immediate hypersensitivity reactions to beta-lactam antibiotics. *Ann Intern Med* 1987; **107**: 204–15.

17 Ewan P. Allergy to penicillin. *Br Med J* 1991; **302**: 1462.

18 Ewan PW, Ackroyd JF. Allergic reactions to drugs. In Wright DJM (ed.) *Immunology of Sexually Transmitted Diseases*. Kluwer Academic, The Hague, 1988, pp 237–60.

19 Assem E-SK. Tests for detecting drug allergy. In Davies DM (ed.) *Textbook of Adverse Drug Reactions*, 3rd edn. Oxford University Press, Oxford, 1985, pp 634–49.

Agents used in general anaesthesia

Intradermal [1–3] or prick [4,5] testing may be helpful in identifying drugs responsible for adverse reactions during general anaesthesia. In one recent series, no patient experienced a recurrence of anaphylaxis during subsequent general anaesthesia, for which agents producing positive skin tests (thiobarbiturates, muscle relaxants or β-lactam antibiotics) were avoided, and provided a premedication regime of prednisone and diphenhydramine was given [6].

1 Fisher MMcD. Intradermal testing in the diagnosis of acute anaphylaxis during anaesthesia — results of five years experience. *Anaesth Intensive Care* 1979; **7**: 58–61.

2 Fisher MMcD. The diagnosis of acute anaphylactoid reactions to neuromuscular blocking agents: a commonly undiagnosed condition. *Anaesth Intensive Care* 1981; **9**: 235–41.

3 Galletly DC, Treuren BC. Anaphylactoid reactions during anaesthesia. Seven years' experience of intradermal testing. *Anaesthesia* 1985; **40**: 329–33.

4 Leynadier F, Sansarricq M, Didier JM, Dry J. Prick tests in the diagnosis of anaphylaxis to general anaesthetics. *Br J Anaesth* 1987; **59**: 683–9.

5 Moneret-Vautrin DA, Laxenaire MC. Anaphylaxis to muscle relaxants: predictive tests. *Anaesthesia* 1990; **45**: 246–7.

6 Moscicki RA, Sockin SM, Corsello BF, *et al*. Anaphylaxis during induction of general anesthesia: Subsequent evaluation and management. *J Allergy Clin Immunol* 1990; **86**: 325–32.

Local anaesthetics

Avoidance of local anaesthetics on the basis of a vague or equivocal history of a prior adverse reaction may result in substantial increased pain and risk. True allergic reactions probably constitute no more than 1% of all adverse reactions to these drugs, some but not the majority of which are due to preservatives, especially parabens. Skin testing and/or incremental challenge beginning with diluted drug is a safe and effective method for identifying a drug which a patient with a history of adverse drug reaction can tolerate [1–3]. Patients with positive patch tests to local anaesthetics and a negative history of anaphylactoid reactions rarely have positive intradermal skin tests. The risk of anaphylactic reactions with amide local anaesthetics (except butanilicaine) is therefore low in such patients [3]. Conversely, patients with anaphylactic reactions to local anaesthetics are usually patch test negative [3]. Skin testing may produce systemic adverse reactions, especially with undiluted drug. False positive reactions occur, but false negative reactions have not been reported, and most skin-tested patients who tolerate a local anaesthetic are skin test negative to the drug. The choice of a drug for use in skin testing and incremental challenge may be facilitated by current concepts of non-cross-reacting groups of local anaesthetics. Thus benzoic acid esters, both those with and without *p*-aminobenzoyl groups, do not cross-react with amide local anaesthetic agents.

1 Schatz M. Skin testing and incremental challenge in the evaluation of adverse reactions of local anesthetics. *J Allergy Clin Immunol* 1984; **74**: 606–16.
2 Fisher MMcD, Graham R. Adverse responses to local anaesthetics. *Anaesth Intensive Care* 1984; **12**: 325–7.
3 Ruzicka T, Gerstmeier M, Przybilla B, Ring J. Allergy to local anesthetics: Comparison of patch test with prick and intradermal test results. *J Am Acad Dermatol* 1987; **16**: 1202–8.

Analgesics and non-steroidal anti-inflammatory agents

Prick tests were positive only in 13% of 117 patients with a history suggestive of anaphylactoid reactions to a variety of mild analgesics including non-steroidal anti-inflammatory drugs [1].

1 Przybilla B, Ring J, Harle R, Galosi A. Hauttestung mit Schmerzmittelinhaltsstoffen bei Patienten mit anaphylaktoiden Unverträglichkeitsreaktionen auf 'leichte' Analgetika. *Hautarzt* 1985; **36**: 682–7.

Heparin

Provocation testing (Fig. 20.2) may be a useful diagnostic measure [1,2]. Low molecular weight heparin analogues may be satisfactorily substituted in some patients with this reaction [1], but are not always tolerated [2]; a panel of different low molecular weight heparin preparations should be checked by subcutaneous provocation tests before re-institution of heparin therapy.

1 Zimmermann R, Harenberg J, Weber E, *et al*. Behandlung bei heparininduzierter kutaner Reaktion mit einem niedermolekularen Heparin-Analog. *Dtsch Med Wochenschr* 1984; **109**: 1326–8.

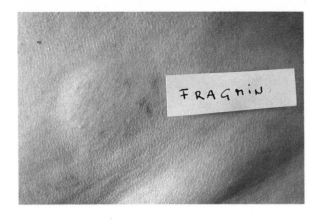

Figure 20.2 Positive intradermal test to injection of low molecular weight heparin.

2 Klein GF, Kofler H, Wol H, Fritsch PO. Eczema-like, erythematous, infiltrated plaques: A common side effect of subcutaneous heparin therapy. *J Am Acad Dermatol* 1989; **21**: 703−7.

Skin testing in urticaria

Skin tests have been advocated as useful in the investigation of chronic urticaria [1]. Patch testing with a series of penicillins was positive in 6.9% of patients, and there were positive intracutaneous tests to cilligen and/or penicillin G in 21.5% of patients. Avoidance of dietary dairy produce, which potentially might have contained penicillin, alleviated the urticaria in 50% of the penicillin allergic patients. The reported prevalence of positive intracutaneous tests to penicillin was much higher in this study than in other reported series in the literature.

1 Boonk WJ, van Ketel WG. Skin testing in chronic urticaria. *Dermatologica* 1981; **163**: 151−9.

20.5 *In vitro* tests

Tests for IgE antibody: RAST and ELISA tests

The detection of drug-specific circulating antibodies does not prove an allergy. It is important to record when a blood test is taken in relation to the evolution of a drug reaction, since the antibody response to a drug has a finite duration. For example, anti-penicillin IgE antibodies begin to disappear within 10 to 30 days. Radioallergosorbent (RAST) tests for drug-specific IgE class antibody are available for penicillin, insulin, and adrenocorticotrophic hormone. The RAST test detects specific IgE antibody to the penicilloyl determinant, and is positive in 60−90% of patients with a positive skin test to penicilloyl polylysine [1,2]; however, there is no *in vitro* test for minor determinant antigens, and therefore in practice this test is of very limited use [2,3]. Investigation of cross-reactivity of antibodies to penicillin in 123 patients with a history of penicillin allergy, using enzyme linked immunosorbent assay (ELISA) tests, detected IgE antibodies specific to amoxycillin, ampicillin, or flucloxacillin respectively in three patients [4]. These antibodies did not cross-react with other penicillin antigens, and would have been missed had testing involved only use of benzylpenicillin. Thus allergy to semisynthetic penicillins can occur without allergy to benzylpenicillin, negative tests specific for benzylpenicillin or phenoxymethylpenicillin cannot be generalized to other penicillins, and exclusive reliance on benzylpenicilloyl RAST tests to detect allergy to semisynthetic penicillins could lead to serious adverse consequences [5].

1 Wide L, Juhlin L. Detection of penicillin allergy of the immediate type by radioimmunoassay of reagins (IgE) to penicilloyl conjugates. *Clin Allergy* 1971; **1**: 171−7.
2 Weiss ME, Adkinson NF. Immediate hypersensitivity reactions to penicillin and related antibiotics. *Clin Allergy* 1988; **18**: 515−40.
3 Ewan P. Allergy to penicillin. *Br Med J* 1991; **302**: 1462.
4 Christie G, Coleman J, Newby S, *et al.* A survey of the prevalence of penicillin specific IgG, IgM and IgE antibodies detected by ELISA and defined by hapten inhibition in patients with suspected penicillin allergy and in healthy volunteers. *Br J Clin Pharmacol* 1988; **25**: 381−6.
5 Walley T, Coleman J. Allergy to penicillin. *Br Med J* 1991; **302**: 1462−3.

Miscellaneous *in vitro* tests

The histamine release test [1], the basophil degranulation test [2−4], the passive haemagglutination test [5], and the lymphocyte transformation test [6−11] are of strictly limited use. A positive basophil degranulation assay, which involves binding of drug to specific IgE on the basophil surface, has been reported with penicillin, erythromycin, sulphonamides and aspirin, but false negative results are common [3,4]. A number of drugs have been reported to induce lymphocyte proliferation, as determined by incorporation of ^{3}H-thymidine, in patients with drug eruptions, including penicillin, carbamazepine, phenytoin, frusemide, sulphamethoxazole, and hydrochlorothiazide [7,9−11]. However, in general only low levels of stimulation are observed, perhaps because the antigen responsible for the reaction is a drug metabolite rather than the parent compound, and the significance of the test is difficult to interpret. While the leucocyte and macrophage migration inhibition tests [12,13] and the lymphocyte toxicity assay [14−17] are the subject of investigation, they are essentially research tools. A patient with a fixed drug eruption to multiple drugs (codeine, tetracycline, ampicillin, dimenhydrinate, penicillin V, and co-trimoxazole), confirmed by challenge testing, showed positive macrophage migration inhibition (MIF) test results to all these, but was negative on both challenge and MIF testing to erythromycin; it was concluded that MIF testing correlated well with the results of challenge testing and could be useful in identifying causative agents [18].

1 Perelmutter L, Eisen AH. Studies on histamine release from leukocytes of penicillin-sensitive individuals. *Int Arch Allergy* 1970; **38**: 104−12.

2 Shelley WB. Indirect basophil degranulation test for allergy to penicillin and other drugs. *JAMA* 1963; **184**: 171–8.

3 Sastre Dominguez J, Sastre Castillo A. Human basophil degranulation test in drug allergy. *Allergol Immunopathol* 1986; **14**: 221–8.

4 Harrabi S, Loiseau P, Dehenry J. A technic for human basophil degranulations. *Allerg Immunol (Paris)* 1987; **19**: 287–9.

5 Thiel JA, Mitchell S, Parker CW. The specificity of hemagglutination reactions in human and experimental penicillin hypersensitivity. *J Allergy* 1964; **35**: 399–424.

6 Rocklin RE, David JR. Detection *in vitro* of cellular hypersensitivity to drugs. *J Allergy Clin Immunol* 1971; **48**: 276–82.

7 Gimenez-Camarasa JM, Garcia-Calderon P, de Moragas JM. Lymphocyte transformation test in fixed drug eruption. *N Engl J Med* 1975; **292**: 819–21.

8 Dobozy A, Hunyadi J, Kenderessy AS, Simon N. Lymphocyte transformation test in detection of drug hypersensitivity. *Clin Exp Dermatol* 1981; **6**: 367–72.

9 Sarkany I. Role of lymphocyte transformation in drug allergy. *Int J Dermatol* 1981; **8**: 544–5.

10 Roujeau JC, Albengres E, Moritz S, *et al.* Lymphocyte transformation test in drug-induced toxic epidermal necrolysis. *Int Arch Allergy Appl Immunol* 1985; **78**: 22–4.

11 Zakrzewska JM, Ivanyi L. *In vitro* lymphocyte proliferation by carbamazepine, carbamazepine-10,11-epoxide, and oxcarbazepine in the diagnosis of drug-induced hypersensitivity. *J Allergy Clin Immunol* 1988; **82**: 1826–32.

12 David JR, al-Askari S, Lawrence HS, Thomal L. Delayed hypersensitivity *in vitro*. I. The specificity of inhibition of cell migration by antigens. *J Immunol* 1964; **93**: 264–73.

13 Halevy S, Grunwald MH, Sandbank M, *et al.* Macrophage migration inhibition factor (MIF) in drug eruption. *Arch Dermatol* 1990; **126**: 48–51.

14 Shear N, Spielberg S, Grant D, *et al.* Differences in metabolism of sulfonamides predisposing to idiosyncratic toxicity. *Ann Intern Med* 1986; **105**: 179–84.

15 Shear N, Spielberg S. Anticonvulsant hypersensitivity syndrome. *In vitro* assessment of risk. *J Clin Invest* 1989; **82**: 1826–32.

16 Rieder MJ, Uetrecht J, Shear NH, *et al.* Diagnosis of sulfonamide hypersensitivity reactions by *in vitro* 'rechallenge' with hydroxylamine metabolites. *Ann Intern Med* 1989; **110**: 286–9.

17 Shear NH. Diagnosing cutaneous adverse reactions to drugs. *Arch Dermatol* 1990; **126**: 94–7.

18 Kivity S. Fixed drug eruption to multiple drugs: clinical and laboratory investigation. *Int J Dermatol* 1991; **30**: 149–51.

20.6 Challenge tests

A drug suspected of causing a drug eruption may be reliably incriminated by the reaction in response to a test dose administered after recovery. However, fatal reactions have occurred to test doses, as for example to penicillin and quinine, and provocation tests should only be performed in exceptional circumstances [1–6]. A history of Stevens–Johnson syndrome or of toxic epidermal necrolysis constitutes an absolute contraindication to drug challenge, and test dosing in reactions of anaphylactic type, blood dyscrasia, or systemic lupus erythematosus-like reaction is seldom advisable. Challenge tests are open to misinterpretation [6], because a very small challenge dose may fail to elicit a reaction which a therapeutic dose would provoke, because of false positives, and because false negatives may occur as a result of a refractory period following a reaction [7].

Test dosing in patients with drug reactions such as fixed drug eruption, which are not potentially fatal, may be helpful [5]. Topical challenge in the form of patch testing in a previously involved site may yield a positive response in a high proportion of such cases [8]. Oral provocation tests using tartrazine, and other food additives such as sodium benzoate, have been advocated for the investigation of chronic urticaria or food intolerance [9–12]. Protocols for the analysis of adverse reactions to foods and food additives have been published [13].

1 Kauppinen K. Cutaneous reactions to drugs. With special reference to severe mucocutaneous bullous eruptions and sulphonamides. *Acta Derm Venereol (Stockh)* 1972; **52** (Suppl 68): 1–89.
2 Kauppinen K. Rational performance of drug challenge in cutaneous hypersensitivity. *Semin Dermatol* 1983; **2**: 117–230.
3 Kauppinen K, Stubb S. Drug eruptions. Causative agents and clinical types. *Acta Derm Venereol (Stockh)* 1984; **64**: 320–4.
4 Girard M. Conclusiveness of rechallenge in the interpretation of adverse drug reactions. *Br J Clin Pharmacol* 1987; **23**: 73–9.
5 Kauppinen K, Alanko K. Oral provocation: uses. *Semin Dermatol* 1989; **8**: 187–91.
6 Girard M. Oral provocation: limitations *Semin Dermatol* 1989; **8**: 192–5.
7 Stevenson DD, Simon RA, Mathison DA. Aspirin-sensitive asthma: tolerance to aspirin after positive oral aspirin challenges. *J Allergy Clin Immunol* 1980; **66**: 82–8.
8 Alanko K, Stubb S, Reitamo S. Topical provocation of fixed drug eruption. *Br J Dermatol* 1987; **116**: 561–7.
9 Warin RP, Smith RJ. Challenge test battery in chronic urticaria. *Br J Dermatol* 1976; **94**: 401–6.
10 Supramaniam G, Warner JO. Artificial food additives intolerance in patients with angioedema and urticaria. *Lancet* 1986; **ii**: 907–9.
11 Wilson N, Scott A. A double blind assessment of additive intolerance in children using a 12 day challenge period at home. *Clin Exp Allergy* 1989; **19**: 267–72.
12 Michils A, Vandermoten G, Duchateau J, Yernault J-C. Anaphylaxis with sodium benzoate. *Lancet* 1991; **337**: 1424–5.
13 Metcalfe DD, Sampson HA (eds) Workshop on experimental methodology for clinical studies of adverse reactions to foods and food additives. *J Allergy Clin Immunol* 1990; **86** (Suppl): 421–42.

Chapter 21
Treatment of Drug Eruptions

21.1 General considerations

Clearly, prevention is better than cure [1,2]. Drugs implicated in a previous reaction should be avoided; the patient should be asked about allergies, and hypersensitivity records in the notes and on prescription charts should be checked. In the case of suspected penicillin allergy, an alternative antibiotic, preferably with a non-β-lactam structure, such as erythromycin, should be substituted; use of griseofulvin should be avoided, as it has a 5–10% cross-reactivity based on non-structural mechanisms [2]. However, lack of a positive history does not eliminate the possibility of an allergic reaction, as in the case of penicillin hypersensitivity [3]. Where it is essential to readminister one of a group of drugs to a patient with a previous history of an adverse reaction to a related medication, as with radiographic contrast media and agents used in general anaesthesia, then if possible preliminary skin testing should be carried out, to enable identification of safe alternative therapy. In addition, the procedure should be covered by premedication with oral corticosteroids and antihistamines, with or without adrenaline, in order to obtund the onset of an anaphylactic reaction. In the situation where there is no acceptable alternative for an essential drug, then rapid desensitization therapy should be considered.

The approach to treatment of an established presumed drug eruption obviously depends on the severity of the reaction. For many minor conditions, withdrawal of the suspected drug, and symptomatic therapy with emollients, mild to moderately potent topical corticosteroids, and systemic antihistamines where indicated, is all that is necessary. When a patient is receiving multiple drugs, it is wise to withdraw all but the essential medications, and to consider substituting alternative non-cross-reacting drugs for the remainder. A major aim of this book is to provide information which will enable the reader to make informed judgements as to the drug or drugs most likely to be responsible for a particular reaction pattern.

A course of systemic corticosteroids may be required for severe erythema multiforme/Stevens–Johnson syndrome, lichenoid eruptions, drug-induced vasculitis or serum sickness. The management of only the most severe reactions will be discussed briefly here. The reader is referred to standard dermatology textbooks for advice on the detailed management of drug reactions which mimic idiopathic disorders [4−6].

1 Sheffer AL, Pennoyer MD. Management of adverse drug reactions. *J Allergy Clin Immunol* 1984; **74**: 580−8.
2 Fellner MJ, Ledesma GN. Current comments on cutaneous allergy. Management of antibiotic allergies. *Int J Dermatol* 1991; **30**: 184−5.
3 Weber EA, Knight A. Testing for allergy to antibiotics. *Semin Dermatol* 1989; **8**: 204−12.
4 Braun-Falco O, Plewig G, Wolff HH, Winkelmann RK. *Dermatology*. Springer-Verlag, Berlin, 1991.
5 Champion RH, Burton JL, Ebling FJG (eds) *Textbook of Dermatology*, 5th edn. Blackwell Scientific Publications, Oxford, 1991.
6 Fitzpatrick TB, Eisen AZ, Wolff K, *et al. Dermatology in General Medicine*, 4th edn. McGraw-Hill Book Company, New York, 1992.

21.2 Anaphylaxis

The management of severe acute urticaria and anaphylaxis has been reviewed [1−7]. A couch, oxygen, and full resuscitation equipment including airways and that for tracheal intubation, intravenous fluids, cardiac drugs and monitors should be readily available in cases of a previous history of a severe reaction; emergency drugs should be drawn up in advance [4]. The drug dosage detailed below relates to therapy of adults.

In the case of an immediate anaphylactic reaction, administration of the causative agent should be stopped, if possible, and the patient made to lie flat. An intramuscular injection of 0.5−1 ml of a 1 in 1000 solution of adrenaline should be given at the site of administration of the causative agent. The airway should be checked and oxygen given. Chlorpheniramine maleate, 10−20 mg, diluted in up to 5 ml water for injections, should be given slowly intravenously over 1 minute. This may be followed by 4 mg orally every 6 hours. Alternatively, 25−50 mg of hydroxyzine, or of diphenhydramine, may be given intramuscularly or orally every 6 hours. A combination of H_1 and H_2 histamine antagonists has been recommended as preferable in prevention and treatment of anaphylaxis and anaphylactoid reactions by some authors [3]. Intravenous cimetidine (300 mg 6-hourly) has been advocated in the treatment of anaphylaxis refractory to conventional therapy [8,9].

An intravenous infusion with 0.9% sodium chloride or 5% glucose should be set up. Blood pressure and pulse should be monitored. Intravenous hydrocortisone 250 mg should be injected immediately; the sodium phosphate form is preferable to the sodium succinate form for emergency use as it is already in solution form. This may be followed by 100 mg every 6 hours intravenously, or oral prednisolone 40 mg daily for 3 days.

Where bronchospasm develops, intravenous aminophylline 250 mg over 5 minutes should be administered, followed by infusion of 250 mg in 500 ml 0.9% saline over 6 hours. An alternative approach is to give nebulized terbutaline, salbutamol, or metaproterenol (0.3 ml of a 5% solution of the latter in 2.5 ml of saline). Endotracheal intubation may be necessary if laryngeal or glottic oedema with increasing stridor persists. In the case of hypotension, intravenous plasma or plasma expander should be given, with central venous pressure monitoring as necessary, since up to 25% plasma volume may leak into the extravascular compartment. Glucagon (1 mg in 1 litre of aqueous dextrose solution at a rate of 5−15 ml/minute) may be useful for refractory hypotension in patients taking β-blockers. Myocardial depression with associated pulmonary oedema may develop as a rare complication of anaphylaxis [10,11]; rapid colloid fluid replacement, cardiac inotropic drugs such as dobutamine [5−20 μg/kg/minute), dopamine (2−20 μg/kg/minute), or amrinone, with or without intra-aortic balloon pump therapy, in the intensive care unit are indicated [11].

1 Sheffer AL, Pennoyer MD. Management of adverse drug reactions. *J Allergy Clin Immunol* 1984; **74**: 580−8.
2 Sussman GL, Dolovich J. Prevention of anaphylaxis. *Semin Dermatol* 1989; **8**: 158−65.
3 Lieberman P. The use of antihistamines in the prevention and treatment of anaphylaxis and anaphylactoid reactions. *J Allergy Clin Immunol* 1990; **86**: 684−6.
4 Brueton MJ, Lortan JE, Morgan DJR, Sutters CA. Management of anaphylaxis. *Hosp Update* 1991; **17**: 386−98.
5 Bochner BS, Lichtenstein LM. Anaphylaxis. *N Engl J Med* 1991; **324**: 1785−90.
6 Soter NA. Acute and chronic urticaria and angioedema. *J Am Acad Dermatol* 1991; **25**: 146−54.
7 Soter NA. Treatment of urticaria and angioedema: low-sedating H$_1$-type antihistamines. *J Am Acad Dermatol* 1991; **24**: 1084−7.
8 Mayumi H, Kimura S, Asano M, *et al*. Intravenous cimetidine as an effective treatment for systemic anaphylaxis and acute skin reactions. *Ann Allergy* 1987; **58**: 447.
9 Yarbrough JA, Moffitt JE, Brown DA, Stafford CT. Cimetidine in the treatment of refractory anaphylaxis. *Ann Allergy* 1989; **63**: 235−8.
10 Raper RF, Fisher MMcD. Profound reversible myocardial depression after anaphylaxis. *Lancet* 1988; **i**: 386−8.
11 Otero E, Onufer JR, Reiss CK, Korenblat PE. Anaphylaxis-induced myocardial depression treated with amrinon. *Lancet* 1991; **337**: 682−3.

21.3 Exfoliative dermatitis/erythroderma

The potential complications of this serious adverse drug eruption include hypothermia, fluid and electrolyte loss, infection, cardiac failure, stress-induced gastrointestinal ulceration and haemorrhage, malabsorption, and venous thrombosis due to imposed bed rest and impaired circulation [1]. Fatalities may occur, especially in the elderly, as a result of infection or high output cardiac failure resulting from increased cutaneous blood flow, and measures to prevent these complications should be undertaken [2,3]. Digitalization and use of diuretics may be indicated. Vasodilator drugs should be avoided. Hypoalbuminaemia may require intravenous albumin replacement therapy. Disturbance of central temperature regulation is frequently present, and antipyretics may be necessary in febrile patients to reduce cardiac output [4]. Hypothermia may be missed unless a low reading thermometer is used. Patients should be maintained in an optimal environmental temperature, as they are poikilothermic and tend to follow the temperature of their surroundings [2]. Therapy with potent topical, or more usually systemic, steroids should not be delayed [4]. A starting dose of 60 mg daily is appropriate [2].

1 Irvine C. 'Skin failure' — a real entity: discussion paper. *J R Soc Med* 1991; **84**: 412–13.
2 Marks J. Erythroderma and its management. *Clin Exp Dermatol* 1982; **7**: 415–22.
3 Sage T, Faure M. Conduite a tenir devant les érythrodermies de l'adulte. *Ann Dermatol Vénéréol (Paris)* 1989; **116**: 747–52.
4 Roujeau JC, Revuz J. Intensive care in dermatology. In Champion RH, Pye RJ (eds) *Recent Advances in Dermatology*. Churchill Livingstone, Edinburgh, 1990, Vol 8, pp 85–99.

21.4 Toxic epidermal necrolysis

The management of toxic epidermal necrolysis (TEN) has been reviewed [1–6]. This potentially fatal condition requires intensive therapy [6], with careful monitoring and correction of fluid and electrolyte loss (Figs 21.1–21.3), limitation of infection, and attention to maintenance of body temperature (Fig. 21.2) and nutrition (Fig. 21.1).

Admission to a burns unit, where possible, has been advocated by some authors [7,8], although others question the necessity for this [9]. Patients may be nursed on an air-fluidized bed; care must be taken to avoid dehydration as a result of a current of warm air over denuded skin. In the case of neutropenia, reverse barrier nursing is indicated. Infection control necessitates frequent cultures of mucocutaneous erosions, blood cultures, and culture of the tips of Foley catheters and intravenous lines. Topical antiseptic preparations advocated include 0.5% silver nitrate solution applied on gauze, with 10% chlorhexidine gluconate washes [10], and saline washes followed by topical polymyxin/bacitracin ointment or 2% mupirocin [9]. Silver sulphadiazine or mafenide acetate are to be avoided, in view of suspicions that they may delay epithelialization, induce neutropenia and may exacerbate TEN [4,11]. The routine use of prophylactic broad spectrum systemic antibiotics is controversial. On the one hand it may lead to emergence of resistant strains of bacteria or promote candidal infection, but on the other hand, initiation of therapy only when there is a positive blood culture may be too late to prevent fatal septic shock [4]. None the less, several authors advocate systemic antibiotics only in the case of suspected or documented infection [8,11].

Surgical removal of necrotic epidermis is indicated. Some units do not use dressings other than paraffin gauze or hydrogel dressings [4]. Other units employ biological dressings such as porcine cu-

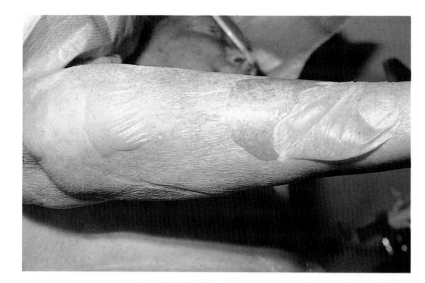

Figure 21.1 Patient with TEN with extensive fluid loss from large blisters; note nasogastric tube *in situ*.

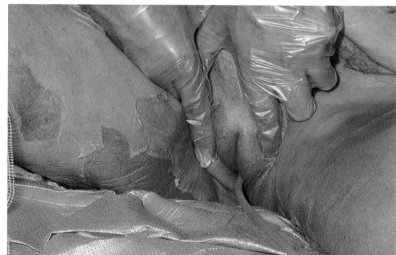

Figure 21.2 Patient with TEN; note catheter *in situ* to aid measurement of fluid balance, and aluminium foil sheeting to maintain temperature homeostasis.

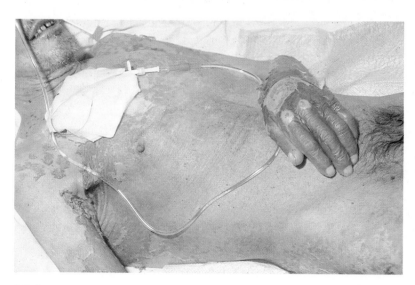

Figure 21.3 Patient recovering from TEN due to trimethoprim–sulphamethoxazole; note central line *in situ*.

taneous xenografts, cutaneous allografts, amnion or collagen-based skin substitutes [7,11]. Frequent ophthalmological assessment is necessary; antiseptic or antibiotic eye drops are required 2 hourly, and synechiae should be disrupted using a blunt instrument [6]. Monitoring of nutrition and fluid and electrolyte balance, with appropriate correction, is essential. Patients may require more than 5 litres of fluid in the first 24 hours, especially with use of an air-fluidized bed. Attention to oral hygiene enables early restoration of normal feeding. Hyperbaric oxygen has been advocated [12]. Plasmapheresis has been helpful in some [13] but not in other cases [5].

The vexed question of whether to use steroid therapy for drug-induced erythema multiforme/Stevens—Johnson syndrome and/or TEN remains controversial [2,4,11,14]. Those who favour steroid therapy do so on the basis that it may reduce inflammation and keratinocyte necrosis, although there is no definitive evidence in favour of this contention. Others suspect that high dose steroid therapy promotes or makes the signs of infection, delays healing, precipitates gastrointestinal bleeding, prolongs hospitalization, and increases mortality. Unfortunately, there have been no prospective, randomized, controlled clinical trials to resolve this issue. An un-controlled retrospective study by one group suggested that patients treated with high dose corticosteroid therapy had a higher mortality rate [1]. The mortality of TEN fell from 66% to 33% in one American burns unit simply as a result of discontinuing use of corticosteroid therapy [10]. A study from West Germany reported that TEN occurred in patients already receiving high dose glucocorticosteroid therapy, for neurosurgical complications, indicating that systemic steroids are not helpful in preventing the development of the condition [15]. The bulk of papers in the literature support the view that steroids should not be used [3,5,6,9—11]. Cyclosporin A produced improvement and stabilization within 24—48 hours in a patient with TEN secondary to phenytoin, which was previously unresponsive to prednisone and high dose methylprednisolone therapy [16].

Increasing age, widespread extent of skin lesions, neutropenia, high dose corticosteroid therapy, and raised blood urea have been reported to be associated with a poor prognosis [17,18]. Others have questioned the status of granulocytopenia as a marker for poor prognosis, and feel that reduction in the lymphocyte count is much more typical of severe TEN [19,20].

1 Garabiol B, Touraine R. Syndrome de Lyell de l'adulte: éléments de pronostic et déductions thérapeutiques. Etude de 27 cas. *Ann Méd Int (Paris)* 1976; **127**: 670—2.
2 Parsons JM. Management of toxic epidermal necrolysis. *Cutis* 1985; **36**: 305—11.
3 Ruiz-Maldonado R. Acute disseminated epidermal necrosis types 1, 2 and 3: study of sixty cases. *J Am Acad Dermatol* 1985; **13**: 623—35.
4 Revuz J, Roujeau J-C, Guillaume J-C, *et al.* Treatment of toxic epidermal necrolysis. Créteil's experience. *Arch Dermatol* 1987; **123**: 1156—8.

[381]

5 Roujeau J-C, Chosidow O, Saiag P, Guillaume J-C. Toxic epidermal necrolysis (Lyell syndrome). *J Am Acad Dermatol* 1990; **23**: 1039−58.

6 Roujeau JC, Revuz J. Intensive care in dermatology. In Champion RH, Pye RJ (eds). *Recent Advances in Dermatology*. Churchill Livingstone, Edinburgh, 1990, Vol 8, pp 85−99.

7 Pruitt BA. Burn treatment of the unburned. *JAMA* 1987; **257**: 2207−8.

8 Halebian PH, Shires GT. Burn unit treatment of acute, severe exfoliating disorders. *Annu Rev Med* 1989; **40**: 137−47.

9 Prendiville JS, Hebert AA, Greenwald MJ, *et al*. Management of Stevens−Johnson syndrome and toxic epidermal necrolysis in children. *J Pediatr* 1989; **115**: 881−7.

10 Halebian PH, Corder VJ, Madden MR, *et al*. Improved burn center survival of patients with toxic epidermal necrolysis managed without corticosteroids. *Ann Surg* 1986; **204**: 503−12.

11 Heimbach DM, Engrav JH, Marvin JA, *et al*. Toxic epidermal necrolysis. A step forward in treatment. *JAMA* 1987; **257**: 2171−5.

12 Ruocco V, Bimonte D, Luongo C, Florio M. Hyperbaric oxygen treatment of toxic epidermal necrolysis. *Cutis* 1986; **38**: 267−71.

13 Kamanabroo D, Schitz-Langraf W, Czarnetzke BM. Plasmapheresis in severe drug-induced toxic epidermal necrolysis. *Arch Dermatol* 1985; **121**: 1548−9.

14 Weston WL, Oranje AP, Rasmussen JE, *et al*. Corticosteroids for erythema multiforme? *Pediatr Dermatol* 1989; **6**: 229−50.

15 Rzany B, Schmitt H, Schöpf E. Toxic epidermal necrolysis in patients receiving glucocorticosteroids. *Acta Derm Venereol (Stockh)* 1991; **71**: 171−2.

16 Renfro L, Grant-Kels JM, Daman LA. Drug-induced toxic epidermal necrolysis treated with cyclosporin. *Int J Dermatol* 1989; **28**: 441−4.

17 Westly ED, Wechsler HL. Toxic epidermal necrolysis. Granulocytic leukopenia as a prognostic indicator. *Arch Dermatol* 1984; **120**: 721−6.

18 Revuz J, Penso D, Roujeau J-C, *et al*. Toxic epidermal necrolysis. Clinical findings and prognosis factors in 87 patients. *Arch Dermatol* 1987; **123**: 1160−5.

19 Roujeau JC, Guillaume JC, Revuz J, *et al*. Granulocytes, lymphocytes and toxic epidermal necrolysis. *Arch Dermatol* 1985; **121**: 305.

20 Bombal C, Roujeau JC, Kuentz M, *et al*. Anomalies hématologiques au cours du syndrome de Lyell: étude de 26 cas. *Ann Dermatol Vénéréol (Paris)* 1983; **110**: 113−19.

21.5 Desensitization

Avoidance of a suspected drug, and substitution of a non-cross-reacting medication, is a standard approach to the management of a drug reaction. Where the drug concerned is judged to be essential for a patient's well-being and no alternative is available, it is possible to induce a state of antigen-specific mast cell unresponsiveness in patients with type I IgE-mediated reactions. Desensitization markedly diminishes the risk of anaphylactic reactions, but not of non-IgE-mediated reactions.

Desensitization has been successfully carried out most frequently for patients with penicillin allergy, with increasing doses of penicillin being administered over 3−5 hours [1−8]. Schedules are available using either oral or parenteral methods [5−8]; it is recommended that desensitization be carried out only in an intensive care setting. β-Blocker drugs should be discontinued prior to desensitization where possible, since they may prolong and complicate treatment of anaphylactic reactions [8]. It is held to be inadvisable to premedicate with antihistamines or steroids, since these may not prevent an acute anaphylactic reaction, but may mask the early signs of such a reaction [8]. The drug is usually given orally, because many fewer preformed conjugates and drug polymers are absorbed orally, the blood levels rise gradually, and the extreme rarity of deaths following oral β-lactam drugs attests to the safety of this route [1,4−6]. Increasing doses are given, starting with a very weak concentration (e.g. 1 in 1 000 000 of the therapeutic dose) and working up to a full dose [8]. Only very occasionally is it necessary to abandon the procedure due to severe reactions [9]. There have been no severe allergic reactions recorded in patients who completed oral desensitization to penicillin; about 35% experience minor cutaneous reactions including pruritus or urticaria [4,6]. The protection afforded is usually short-lived, although tolerance can be maintained by long-term administration of low doses of oral penicillin [5]. Therefore, treatment must be initiated without delay to prevent return of sensitivity.

Desensitization has also been achieved in a patient with an allergic reaction to carbamazepine [10] and in a patient with the 'red man syndrome' related to vancomycin [11]. Patients with human immunodeficiency virus infection who have had cutaneous reactions to sulphonamides in the past have been successfully desensitized [12,13]. Mechanisms proposed to explain the development of tolerance following desensitization procedures include mediator depletion, tachyphylaxis, production of blocking antibodies, or change in the level of specific IgE antibodies [8,14].

1 Sullivan TJ, Yecies LD, Shatz GS, *et al*. Desensitization of patients allergic to penicillin using orally administered β-lactam antibiotics. *J Allergy Clin Immunol* 1982; **69**: 275−82.
2 Sullivan TJ. Antigen-specific desensitization of patients allergic to penicillin. *J Allergy Clin Immunol* 1982; **69**: 500−8.
3 Stark BJ, Gross GN, Lumry WR, Sullivan TJ. Oral desensitization of penicillin-allergic patients. *J Allergy Clin Immunol* 1984; **73**: 112.
4 Wendel GD, Stark BJ, Jamison RB, *et al*. Penicillin allergy and desensitization in serious infections during pregnancy. *N Engl J Med* 1985; **312**: 1229−32.
5 Stark BJ, Earl HS, Gross GN, *et al*. Acute and chronic desensitization of penicillin-allergic patients using oral penicillin. *J Allergy Clin Immunol* 1987; **79**: 523−32.
6 Weiss ME, Adkinson NF. Immediate hypersensitivity reactions to penicillin and related antibiotics. *Clin Allergy* 1988; **18**: 515−40.
7 Holgate ST. Penicillin allergy: how to diagnose and when to treat. *Br Med J* 1988; **296**: 1213−14.
8 Weber EA, Knight A. Testing for allergy to antibiotics. *Semin Dermatol* 1989; **8**: 204−12.
9 Earl HS, Sullivan TJ. Acute desensitization of a patient with cystic fibrosis allergic to both beta-lactam and aminoglycoside antibiotics. *J Allergy Clin Immunol* 1987; **79**: 477−83.
10 Eames P. Adverse reaction to carbamazepine managed by desensitization. *Lancet* 1989; **i**: 509−10.
11 Lin RY. Desensitization in the management of vancomycin hypersensitivity. *Arch Intern Med* 1990; **150**: 2197−8.
12 White MV, Haddad ZH, Brunner E, Sainz C. Desensitization to trimethoprim−sulfamethoxazole in patients with acquired immune deficiency syndrome and *Pneumocystis carinii* pneumonia. *Ann Allergy* 1989; **62**: 177−9.

13 Torgovnick J. Desensitization to sulfonamides in patients with HIV infection. *Am J Med* 1990; **88**: 548–9.
14 Naclerio R, Mizrahi EA, Adkinson NF Jr. Immunologic observations during desensitization and maintenance of clinical tolerance to penicillin. *J Allergy Clin Immunol* 1983; **71**: 294–301.

Index